AF412906

Pathology of Viral Hepatitis

Edited by

R D GOLDIN MD FRCPath

*Senior Lecturer at Imperial College School of
Medicine and Consultant Histopathologist at St Mary's, London, UK*

H C THOMAS PhD FRCPath FRCP

*Professor of Medicine at Imperial College School of Medicine and
Consultant Physician at St Mary's, London, UK*

The late Professor M A GERBER MD

*Formerly Professor and Chairman of the Department of Pathology,
Tulane University School of Medicine, New Orleans, USA*

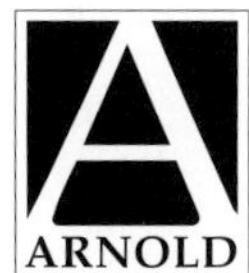

A member of the Hodder Headline Group
LONDON • SYDNEY • AUCKLAND
Co-published in the United States of America
by Oxford University Press Inc., New York

First published in Great Britain in 1998 by
Arnold, a member of the Hodder Headline Group
338 Euston Road, London NW1 3BH

http://www.arnoldpublishers.com

Co-published in the United States of America by
Oxford University Press, Inc.,
198 Madison Avenue, New York, NY10016
Oxford is a registered trademark of Oxford University Press

Whilst the advice and information in this book is believed to be true and
accurate at the date of going to press, neither the authors nor the publisher
can accept any legal responsibility or liability for any errors or omissions
that may be made. In particular (but without limiting the generality of the
preceding disclaimer) every effort has been made to check drug dosages;
however it is still possible that errors have been missed. Furthermore,
dosage schedules are constantly being revised and new side-effects
recognized. For these reasons the reader is strongly urged to consult the
drug companies' printed instructions before administering any of the drugs
recommended in this book.

British Library Cataloguing in Publication Data
A catalogue record for this book is available from the British Library

Library of Congress Cataloging-in-Publication Data
A catalog record for this book is available from the Library of Congress

ISBN 0 340 59664 3 (hb)

1 2 3 4 5 6 7 8 9 10

Publisher: Georgina Bentliff
Project Editor: Catherine Barnes
Production Editor: Liz Gooster
Production Controller: Helen Whitehorn

Typeset in 10/11pt Times by
J&L Composition Ltd, Filey, North Yorkshire
Tenon & Polert Colour Scanning Ltd
Printed in China

Dedication

This book is dedicated to the memory of Professor Mike Gerber, who contributed so much to the field of viral hepatitis.

Contents

List of Contributors

A Alberti
Professor of Internal Medicine, Department of Clinical and Experimental Medicine, University of Padova, Padova, Italy

L Chemello
Lecturer, Department of Clinical and Experimental Medicine, University of Padova, Padova, Italy

K A Fleming DPhil, MA, MB ChB, FRCPath
Dean of the Faculty of Clinical Medicine and Clinical Reader in Pathology, Nuffield Department of Pathology, John Radcliffe Hospital, Headington, Oxford, UK

G R Foster MRCP, PhD
Senior Lecturer and Honorary Consultant, The Liver Unit, St Mary's Hospital Medical School, London, UK

The late Professor M A Gerber MD
Formerly Professor and Chairman, Department of Pathology, Tulane University School of Medicine, New Orleans, USA

R D Goldin MD, FRCPath
Senior Lecturer, Imperial College School of Medicine and Consultant Histopathologist at St Mary's, London, UK

S G Hübscher MB ChB, FRCPath
Senior Lecturer in Pathology, University of Birmingham Medical School, Edgbaston, Birmingham, UK

R S Markin MD, PhD
Professor and Vice Chairman of Pathology and Associate Dean for Clinical Affairs, University of Nebraska Medical Center, Omaha, USA

P J Scheuer MD, DSc(Med), FRCPath
Professor Emeritus, Royal Free Hospital School of Medicine, London, UK

E Tabor MD
Director, Division of Transfusion Transmitted Diseases, Food and Drug Administration, Rockville, Maryland, USA

H C Thomas PhD, FRCPath, FRCP
Professor of Medicine, Imperial College School of Medicine and Consultant Physician at St Mary's, London, UK

Preface

Viral hepatitis is one of the most prevalent diseases world-wide and is the commonest cause of cirrhosis and liver cell cancer. As a rapidly evolving field, our aim has been to provide a definitive and up-to-date account of the pathology of viral hepatitis. We hope that this book will be useful to those pathologists and physicians who deal regularly with patients with viral hepatitis. While many of these work in centres where large numbers of such patients are seen, this pattern has changed somewhat in recent years. With the recognition that many patients are infected with HCV, and the growing importance of pathology in relation to natural history and treatment, this number has expanded to include pathologists and physicians who until recently have seen relatively few patients with liver disease. This book will also provide the non-specialist with a concise source of up-to-date information and the inclusion of chapters on the pathogenesis of liver damage and carcinogenesis will facilitate the entry of researchers new to the field of viral hepatitis.

Essentially the book deals with the hepatotropic viruses, an area of research which is continually progressing. This is exemplified by the discovery of HCV and the ongoing reassessment of its significance. The contribution of immunohistochemical and molecular biological techniques to the diagnosis of viral hepatitis is highlighted in Chapter 4. In immunosuppressed patients the pattern of disease caused by the hepatotropic viruses is altered and this is given special consideration in Chapter 5. Furthermore, these patients often have significant diseases caused by non-hepatotropic viruses and these are discussed in Chapter 6.

We hope that our readers find reading the book as stimulating as we found writing it and that it helps to bring more histopathologists together with their clinical and virological colleagues to focus on viral hepatitis. With the discovery of HCV, this disease is now of major importance to the developed as well as to the developing world.

R D Goldin
H C Thomas

CHAPTER 1

The hepatotropic viruses: epidemiology, natural history and virology

G R FOSTER, R D GOLDIN AND H C THOMAS

Infection with hepatotropic viruses is a major cause of morbidity and mortality worldwide. Infection may cause either an acute self-limiting hepatitis, a chronic infection or, rarely, a fulminant hepatitis. Five different hepatotropic viruses have been identified to date (Sherlock and Dooley, 1991); two viruses, hepatitis A (HAV) and E (HEV) only cause acute hepatitis, whereas hepatitis B (HBV) and C (HCV) may cause both acute and chronic infections. The final member of the hepatotropic viruses – Delta virus (HDV) – is a viroid that can only infect patients who are already infected with HBV. In addition to the well-characterised viruses, a number of new flaviviruses (GBV-A, GBV-B, GBV-C and hepatitis G; Fry *et al*, 1995; Karayiarmis and McGarvey, 1995) have recently been identified. The significance of this group is currently undergoing re-evaluation.

Hepatitis A

VIRAL STRUCTURE AND REPLICATION

HAV is extremely stable and resistant to heating and acidic conditions (Koff, 1998; Ross *et al*, 1991; Van der Poel *et al*, 1991). The structure of the HAV genome is shown in Figure 1.1 and consists of a monocistronic single strand of RNA, 7.5 kb long, that encodes four structural and seven non-structural proteins. The four structural proteins are encoded by three genes – VP1, VP3 and VP0. The latter protein is cleaved to produce VP2 and VP4 (Gauss-Muller *et al*, 1986). The non-structural proteins include a protease, a polymerase and a genome-linked protein, VPg, that binds to the viral RNA and assists in its processing (Weitz *et al*, 1986). The functions of the other proteins that can be identified by translation of the genomic sequence of HAV are, at present, poorly understood. The replication of HAV is believed to be similar to that of the picornaviruses: the genomic RNA is translated to produce a single polyprotein that is then cleaved to produce the viral enzymes and structural proteins (Palmenberg, 1987). The virally derived enzymes replicate viral RNA, but the precise details and the regulatory steps involved are largely unknown.

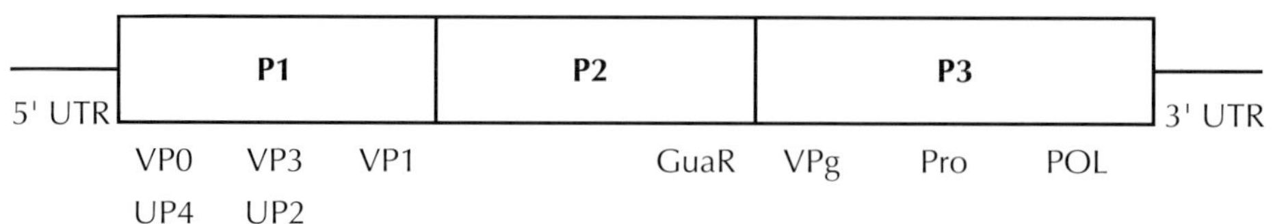

Fig 1.1   Genome structure of the hepatitis A virus. The genome consists of a 5' untranslated region (UTR), a coding region of over 7 kb and a 3' untranslated region (UTR). P1 contains the structural proteins (VP0–VP4, VP4 and VP2 being derived from the cleavage of VP0). P2 encodes a number of proteins of unknown function and includes the guanidine resistance marker (GuaR). The P3 region includes a genome-linked protein (VPg), a protease (Pro) and, probably, a virally encoded RNA polymerase (POL).

CLASSIFICATION OF HEPATITIS A

HAV has many properties typical of picornaviruses, such as morphology, biochemical characteristics and general organisation of the RNA genome (Lemon, 1992). As the predominant mode of transmission of HAV is faecal–oral, the virus was classified in the early 1980s as an enterovirus (type 72) within the *Picornaviridae* family. However, new biological and structural features of HAV have more recently been described, suggesting that it is unique among picornaviruses and thus warranting its classification within a new, separate genus. Based on the exceptional tropism for the liver of HAV, the new genus has been termed 'hepatovirus'. Distinct genotypes of HAV have been described on the basis of sequence analysis (Lemon and Robertson, 1994). A total of seven distinct genotypes has so far been defined.

CLINICAL FEATURES

Adult infection with HAV causes an acute hepatitis that is usually preceded by a prodromal syndrome of malaise and anorexia followed by jaundice with dark urine and pale stools. Clinical examination usually reveals a tender, moderately enlarged liver. The acute illness resolves within a few weeks, although many patients remain fatigued for several months (Sherlock and Dooley, 1991). Infection with HAV may be followed by a period of intrahepatic cholestasis that may last for several weeks, and a small proportion of infected individuals suffer a temporary relapse when jaundice and viraemia transiently recur during convalescence. Fulminant hepatitis is a very rare complication.

Infection with HAV in childhood is often asymptomatic and usually passes undetected. Such subclinical infections give rise to lifelong immunity. There is no unequivocal evidence that HAV ever gives rise to a chronic hepatitis.

DIAGNOSIS

Viraemia in patients with HAV infection is transient and rarely detected – by the time the patient presents to a physician, the virus is no longer present in the circulation. Faecal excretion of the virus persists, and immune electron microscopy (Humphrey *et al*, 1990) or molecular hybridisation techniques (Jansen *et al*, 1985) can be used to identify HAV directly. Such techniques are tedious and labour intensive, and are unnecessary since a specific antibody response develops early in the course of the disease. Antibodies to HAV can be detected by a variety of immunological techniques, and commercial assays are available. The most reliable assay for the diagnosis of acute HAV infection is the detection of HAV-specific IgM (Locarnini *et al*, 1979). This antibody is produced early during the icteric phase of the disease, and the absence of anti-HAV-specific IgM antibodies effectively excludes the diagnosis of HAV infection in a patient who is jaundiced. Following an acute HAV infection, IgG antibodies against the virus persist for many years – their presence in a patient with jaundice implies that the hepatitis is not due to HAV (the patient is immune), and another cause must be sought.

EPIDEMIOLOGY

HAV is excreted in faeces and is transmitted by direct patient contact or through contaminated drinking water or food. It is therefore not surprising that infection is common in Third World countries. In general, HAV infection in underdeveloped countries occurs during childhood, and most children develop a subclinical infection without overt jaundice. They subsequently develop antibodies that protect against further infection. Adults who have not been exposed are at risk if they travel to an endemic area.

Improvements in living standards are associated with a decrease in the prevalence of HAV infection. Chinese children born in the relatively affluent South Africa have a low prevalence of antibodies, whereas their parents, born in underdeveloped China, often show evidence of previous infection (Song and Kew, 1994). In developed countries, HAV is common only in travellers or specific high-risk groups, including homosexuals and intravenous drug users.

Hepatitis B

VIRAL STRUCTURE AND REPLICATION

The structure of the HBV genome is shown in Figure 1.2. The virus is a partially double-stranded DNA virus with a circular genome that is 3.2 kb long (*see* review by Ganem and Varmus, 1987; Lee, 1998). This compact genome encodes four proteins: two non-structural proteins (X and polymerase) that are involved in viral replication and two structural proteins (core and surface protein). The functions of the non-structural proteins are unclear. The protein encoded by the X gene can act as a promiscuous transactivator in tissue culture systems (Rossner, 1992) (i.e. it can activate a large number of different genes), but the significance of this is unknown. The transactivating properties of the X protein may play a role in the development of liver tumours (i.e. X may activate latent oncogenes) (Hohne *et al*, 1990). The transactivating properties of X protein have also been suggested as playing a role in the interaction of HBV and the human immunodeficiency virus as well as in the development of liver cell cancer (see Chapters 5 and 8). In infected cells, X probably acts to regulate the production of HBV-encoded proteins (Henkler and Koshy, 1996). The effects of X are concentration dependent, and, as it is difficult to measure the concentration of X in naturally infected cells, it may be some time before the physiological functions of this protein can be

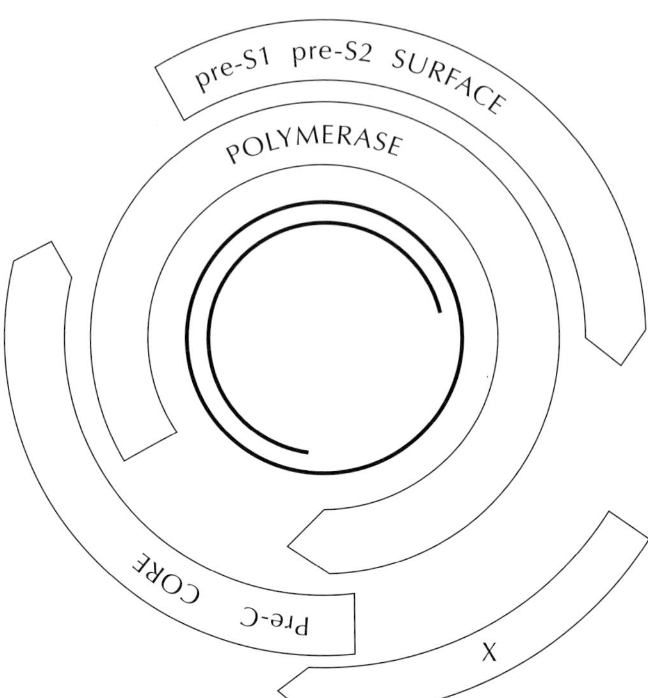

Fig 1.2   Molecular organisation of the hepatitis B virus genome. The partially double-stranded DNA encodes four open reading frames that overlap as shown.

confidently determined. The other non-structural gene (POL) encodes the viral enzymes that are necessary for HBV replication (Ganem and Varmus, 1987), but a full analysis of the structure and functions of this protein has not yet been achieved.

The structural genes of HBV are complex. The surface gene encodes three proteins that have a common carboxy terminus and an amino terminus of variable length. These three surface proteins can aggregate to form non-infectious particles that lack HBV DNA (HBsAg). Alternatively, the same proteins can form the envelope of the infectious virions that contain viral genomes as well as the other viral proteins (Dane particles). The non-infectious surface antigen particles are the majority particles released from infected cells, and their function is obscure – they may act as a decoy for virus-neutralising anti-envelope antibodies.

The core gene of HBV contains two start codons. Translation from the second codon leads to the formation of the viral nucleocapsid protein core. Translation from the first codon leads to the formation of a protein (pre-core/core) that contains a signal sequence leading to sequestration and cleavage within the endoplasmic reticulum (Standring *et al*, 1988). The cleavage product of pre-core/core is HBeAg that is released from infected cells and circulates within serum. The function of this protein is again unknown, but it may be involved in the induction of immune tolerance in fetuses since it crosses the placenta. HBeAg is not necessary for viral replication and function since mutant HBV strains exist that are unable to produce HBeAg but are able to replicate in the normal fashion.

The replication of HBV is rather unusual (Ganem and Varmus, 1987). After entry into cells, the HBV genome (partially double-stranded DNA) is converted to completely double-stranded DNA. This DNA then acts as a template for the production of an RNA molecule, pre-genomic mRNA. This mRNA is slightly longer than the template DNA from which it is derived – the mRNA is 3.5 kb long, whereas the genome is 3.2 kb in length. The overlong pre-genomic mRNA contains a terminal redundancy that is used to prime reverse transcription of the mRNA by the HBV POL protein. After reverse transcription, the first strand of the HBV DNA circularises, and the second (incomplete DNA) strand is produced. Hence, although HBV is a DNA virus, it replicates via an RNA intermediate. The reason why HBV uses this unusual replication strategy is not known, but reverse transcriptase enzymes are relatively unreliable and have a high error rate, leading to frequent mutations in the viral genome. This is not the case with enzymes that replicate DNA directly, which have a very low error rate. It is therefore possible that HBV, by replicating via an RNA intermediate, generates mutant viruses that may play a role in viral persistence.

CLINICAL FEATURES

Infection with HBV may cause an acute self-limiting hepatitis or a chronic infection. The disease that develops is dependent on the age at which infection is acquired (Sherlock and Dooley, 1991; Lee, 1998). Subjects infected in utero or at birth do not develop jaundice but become persistently infected (chronic HBV). In contrast, adult infection usually leads to an acute, self-limiting hepatitis with a prodrome of malaise and anorexia that is usually followed by jaundice and viral elimination over a period of several months. A few patients develop a very severe hepatitis (fulminant hepatitis), which is often fatal. A small proportion of infected adults (fewer than 10%) do not develop the typical acute hepatitis but have a childhood-type disease characterised by a trivial hepatitis and prolonged infection.

The clinical outcome for patients chronically infected with HBV is well characterised (Sherlock and Dooley, 1991). In many patients, the infection is asymptomatic and liver inflammation (assessed by serum transaminase measurements or liver histology) is minimal. Serological evidence of continuing infection and viraemia can be found: the patient's serum contains large amounts of HBsAg and smaller amounts of the nucleocapsid-derived antigen, HBeAg, as well as infectious virions. Other patients chronically infected with HBV develop a sub-clinical hepatitis with significant hepatic inflammation that often leads to cirrhosis. Chronically infected patients have an increased risk of developing hepatocellular carcinoma, this risk being approximately 100 times greater than for uninfected individuals (Beasley *et al*, 1981). Spontaneous viral clearance in chronic HBV infection is uncommon but is more frequent in patients with active hepatitis and rare in patients with insignificant inflammation, perhaps indicating that the inflammation in chronic HBV infection is the result of an immune response against the virus that is unable to eliminate the pathogen completely (*see* Chapter 7).

Virus eradication often proceeds in two stages. Initially, an immune response develops that destroys most virus-producing cells. The patient develops antibodies against HBeAg, and HBV DNA is often undetectable in the serum. However, at this stage, some infected cells persist, perhaps representing cells in which the HBV DNA has integrated into the host genome, and the patient continues to secrete the HBsAg. This phase of low-level infection is associated with minimal inflammatory liver disease and has a slightly increased incidence of malignant change (greater than twice the incidence when compared with the normal population). In a majority of cases, over a period of several years, the HBsAg titre declines and the patient eventually develops antibodies against this protein, the virus then being completely eliminated. In a minority of patients, after several years of minimal disease, when the patient is HBsAg-positive and anti-HBe-positive, liver disease recurs and viraemia (circulating HBV DNA) returns, despite the persistence of antibodies against HBeAg. This phase represents emergence of the HBeAg-negative virus that is unable to produce HBeAg because of a mutation at nucleotide 1896, that generates a stop codon at codon 28 of the pre-core/core reading frame from which HBeAg is translated (Carman *et al*, 1989). Overall, a majority of patients who develop chronic hepatitis spontaneously eliminate the virus, and a proportion (40%) die from either virus-induced cirrhosis or hepatocellular carcinoma.

DIAGNOSIS

The diagnosis of HBV infection is based upon immunological assays that detect viral antigens and antibodies directed against the viral proteins. Detection of the most abundant HBV-related protein, HBsAg, is relatively straightforward using commercially available immunoassays, and the presence of HBsAg in the serum indicates that the patient is suffering from an HBV infection. If the HBsAg is found in association with the nucleocapsid-derived e antigen (HBeAg), active viral replication is taking place and the patient is suffering from either acute or chronic HBV hepatitis. The distinction between an acute and a chronic infection can only be reliably determined by careful follow-up: if the hepatitis is prolonged (longer than 6 months), the infection is chronic. If, however, the hepatitis and the surface antigenaemia persist for less than 6 months, the infection can be confidently diagnosed as an acute HBV infection.

A number of supplementary tests may help to distinguish between the acute and chronic forms of HBV on a single blood sample. Acute HBV infection is usually associated with a very active hepatitis, and serum aminotransferase activity is high (>200 IU/mL). In addition, IgM antibodies directed against the core antigen of HBV (anti-HBcAg) are typically detected. In a chronic HBV infection, serum aminotransferase activity is usually lower, and although antibodies against HBcAg may be found, these are not usually of the IgM type. However, during a spontaneous or a treatment-induced seroconversion (i.e. during viral clearance), high aminotransferase activity may be found and IgM anti-HBcAb may also be detected. It may be impossible to distinguish between a chronic HBV infection that is resolving and an acute, recently acquired infection. Thus active HBV infection associated with viral replication is characterised by the presence of HBsAg and HBeAg in serum, and it may be possible to classify the infection as an acute infection if the serum contains IgM antibodies against HBcAg, although this distinction is not always possible on purely serological grounds.

As described above, chronic HBV infection may be associated with ongoing viral replication (in which case HBeAg is found in the serum), or the infection may persist in the absence of viral replication (in which case HBsAg alone is detected). Patients without active viral replication have no evidence of liver inflammation (the serum transaminase activity being normal) and, typically, the serum contains no detectable HBeAg, although it does contain antibodies directed against this protein (HBeAb). Such patients are at low risk of developing HBV-related complications and, in general, require no therapy. A small number of patients with ongoing hepatitis and antibodies against HBeAg have been identified. Such patients are typically HBsAg-positive and HBeAg-negative with antibodies against HBeAg (HBeAb). These patients are usually infected with the mutant form of HBV (Carman *et al*, 1989) that is unable to synthesise the HBeAg. The identification of such mutant viruses relies on the detection of HBV DNA in serum. This is a difficult assay that is not usually performed routinely. It is only of value in the diagnosis of patients who are HBeAg-negative with high aminotransferase activity. In such cases, the presence of HBV DNA indicates that the hepatitis is due to a mutant form of HBV; its absence suggests that the infection is due to another cause, often another virus.

EPIDEMIOLOGY

HBV is easily transmitted. It can be passed to adults through sexual intimacy as well as intravenous drug usage, and the virus is readily transmitted within families, often in utero or during vaginal delivery as well as during childhood. The natural history of HBV infection clearly favours its transmission: young children are infected early in life in conditions that result in a persistent infection that does not impair fertility and does not lead to serious complications until late in life. In early adult life, infected individuals reproduce and give birth to children who are chronically infected. Hence the virus is successfully propagated within families and the development of fatal complications does not normally occur until after the virus has been transmitted to the next generation. This ease of transmission within families explains why HBV is a common pathogen – it is estimated that over 300 million people world wide are chronically infected with HBV, and there is a very high prevalence of infection in China, Asia and Africa (Sherlock and Dooley, 1991).

Hepatitis C

VIRAL STRUCTURE AND REPLICATION

HCV is an RNA virus that has similarities to the flavi- and pestiviruses. The viral genome is over 9 kb long and encodes a number of structural and non-structural proteins (Fig. 1.3) (Choo *et al*, 1991; Bisceglie, 1998). HCV is a highly variable virus, and no two viral isolates are identical. Indeed, within an individual patient, a number of different viral isolates (quasispecies) can be detected, and the genomic sequence of these isolates changes with time (Enamoto and Sato, 1995). A number of well-conserved regions within the HCV genome (including the core gene and the untranslated 5′ region) can be identified that do not change during the course of an infection, and studies on these regions have led to the recognition that different viral strains exist (Simmonds *et al*, 1994).

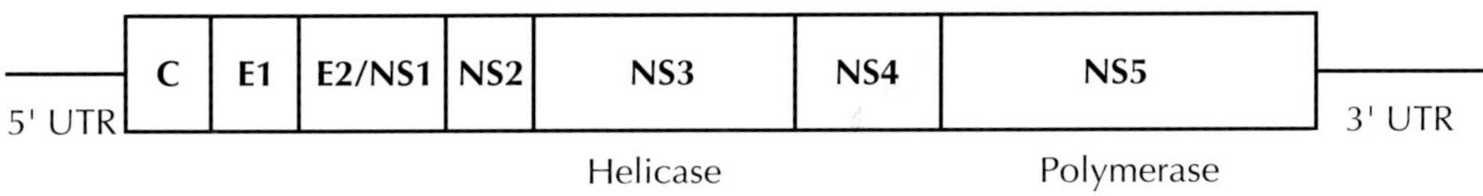

Fig 1.3   Molecular organisation of the HCV genome. The 9 kb RNA encodes a large polyprotein that is cleaved into structural proteins (core, C), envelope proteins 1 and 2 (E1 and E2) and non-structural proteins of unknown function. The non-structural protein 3 (NS3) is thought to encode a protease/helicase, and NS5 is believed to be the viral RNA polymerase. UTR, untranslated region.

At present, six major HCV subtypes have been identified and classified numerically. Within each subtype, a number of variants are found, which are classified numerically. Within each subtype, a number of variants are found, which are classified alphabetically. It is clear that there are geographical differences in the distribution of the different HCV genotypes. For example, in the UK the dominant genotypes are types 1, 2 and 3, but in the Middle East, genotype 4 predominates (Dusheiko and Simmonds, 1994). A large number of studies have examined the different HCV genotypes to see whether there are differences in the clinical outcomes of infection with different strains. There does not appear to be any great difference in the severity of the disease caused by the different genotypes (Benvegnu *et al*, 1997), although there are some data to suggest that genotype 1b causes more rapidly progressive hepatitis, and there is evidence suggesting that some genotypes may be more sensitive to IFN therapy (Simmonds, 1997). The main associations are epidemiological, genotype 1 being associated with longer disease duration and type 3 being seen mainly in young intravenous drug addicts. A relationship has been demonstrated between disease activity and the complexity of hypervariable region 1 quasispecies (Yuki *et al*, 1997).

The replication of HCV has not yet been studied in detail since no reproducible tissue culture systems exist that allow its propagation. By analogy with related viruses, it is believed that replication occurs via the formation of a polyprotein that is translated from the viral genome. This polyprotein undergoes proteolysis by virally encoded and cellular proteins to form the viral enzymes and structural proteins. These proteins then allow RNA replication and the formation of new virions.

CLINICAL FEATURES

Studies of patients who have received blood products contaminated with HCV suggest that up to 20% of infected individuals develop malaise followed by jaundice that resolves within a few weeks. These patients appear to eliminate the virus completely. However, the majority of those infected with HCV develop a chronic, persistent infection (Alter, 1992; Bisceglie, 1998). The long-term outcome for patients chronically infected with HCV is not yet clear. The majority are not obviously unwell, and liver function tests show a characteristic fluctuating pattern with periods of marked abnormality (raised serum amino transferases) interspersed with periods when the serum aminotransferases may be normal. Many of these patients probably do not develop serious sequelae.

However, a proportion of infected patients develop a hepatitis that progresses to cirrhosis and hepatocellular carcinoma. It is estimated that up to 20% of infected patients will ultimately develop cirrhosis, although this may take 20 years or more to develop, but it is still not clear which patients will progress in this way (Thursz *et al*, 1995). It is possible that there are two forms of chronic HCV: a 'benign' form that does not progress and an 'aggressive' type that does. However, it is also possible that the benign disease can accelerate into a more aggressive phase. A number of studies have tried to determine whether different HCV strains (genotypes) cause different disease types, but the data are at present conflicting: genotype 1 possibly causes more severe disease. It is currently impossible to predict an individual patient who will develop significant complications. In an important recent French study, it was shown that fibrosis increased progressively with time and that risk factors for more rapid progression included age at infection, male sex and excessive alcohol consumption. Their analysis suggested that those factors are more important than HCV genotype (Poynard *et al*, 1997). The importance of age at infection has been confirmed by other studies (Wong *et al*, 1997).

Chronic HCV infection is associated with an increased incidence of hepatocellular carcinoma in patients with cirrhosis, but it is known that this tumour develops in the absence of cirrhosis, and it is again impossible to predict which patients are at risk of malignant change (Blum, 1994).

DIAGNOSIS

The diagnosis of HCV infection is based upon detection of antibodies directed against HCV antigens. These antibodies may be detected by ELISA assays or immunoblotting procedures. Early assays relied upon the detection of antibodies directed against a single HCV antigen (C100), and after their introduction, it became clear that these assays had a high incidence of false positivity (i.e. antibodies against a single HCV antigen are not uncommon in patients who are not infected with the virus; McFarlane *et al*, 1990). This problem has been overcome by the development of assays that incorporate antigens from four different regions of the virus; if antibodies against more than two antigens are detected, it is highly likely that the patient is suffering from chronic HCV infection (Van der Poel *et al*, 1991).

In general, diagnostic tests for HCV use two assays. The first assay is an ELISA assay that includes all four antigens and detects antibodies against any of the HCV antigens included in the test. False positive assays are not uncommon, and the assay is usually followed by a confirmatory test that uses immobilised antigens on a paper strip. The antigen-containing strip is incubated with the patient's serum, and bound antibodies are detected by a chemical reaction. This assay allows the identification of antibodies binding to each of the four test antigens. If antibodies directed against more than two antigens are found, the test is positive. The final confirmation that a patient is suffering from HCV is based on direct detection of the virus. Since the virus circulates at very low levels, it can only be detected using sophisticated amplification techniques, either the polymerase chain reaction or a recently developed branched chain assay in which viral RNA is immobilised and then detected by binding to multiple, labelled oligonucleotides specific for sequences present within the viral genome (Alter *et al*, 1995). Since the vast majority of patients with antibodies to HCV antigens are actively infected with HCV, testing for viraemia is not usually required, although it may be helpful in patients with possible HCV infection who are immunosuppressed and may not be able to generate an antibody response.

EPIDEMIOLOGY

The prevalence of HCV infection varies widely. Many underdeveloped countries have a high prevalence of the disease (e.g. in Egypt, it is estimated that nearly 20% of the population are infected), but in other Third World countries, the incidence is much lower. HCV is uncommon in Europe and the USA (0.2–0.8%) but very common in Japan (0.5–2.0%). The mode of transmission of HCV is still poorly understood. It is clear that the virus can be transmitted via infected blood products, and those who use intravenous drugs have a high incidence of infection. However, the virus is relatively difficult to transmit: sexual partners of infected patients rarely become infected, and infants born to infected mothers are infrequently infected (Tibbs, 1995), although the risk of transmission appears to be increased in patients who have high levels of viraemia (e.g. patients who are immunosuppressed, for example by HIV). Since the virus is of relatively low infectivity, it is unclear why so many people are infected. One possible explanation is that the re-use of non-sterile vaccination needles may have transmitted the pathogen. HCV may therefore be a predominantly iatrogenic disease, although other possibilities, including insect vectors, have not been excluded.

Delta virus

Delta virus is a highly unusual virus that is unable to replicate or generate infectious particles in the absence of HBV (Bonino *et al*, 1986). The virus is only found in patients with HBV infection, where it increases the severity of the hepatitis. Infection with Delta virus may occur simultaneously with HBV (co-infection), or an already HBV-infected patient may acquire a second infection with Delta virus (superinfection). Co-infection with Delta virus causes a severe, sometimes fulminant, hepatitis that usually resolves completely. Co-infection can be diagnosed by the occurrence of markers of acute HBV infection (HBsAg, HBeAg and IgM antibodies directed against HBcAg) with IgM antibodies directed against the single protein produced by Delta virus – Delta antigen. Superinfection with Delta virus usually leads to chronic delta hepatitis. This chronic infection typically causes an aggressive hepatitis (Colombo *et al*, 1983) that often progresses to hepatocellular carcinoma. Chronic Delta virus infection is usually diagnosed serologically: both Delta antigen and antibodies against Delta antigen (anti-HDag) are often detected in serum using immunological assays. These assays may, however, be negative even though Delta virus is present, and the most reliable detection method is immunostaining of a liver biopsy specimen with antibodies against Delta antigen (see Chapter 4). The demonstration of Delta antigen in a liver biopsy confirms the diagnosis even when serological assays are negative. Delta virus infection is always associated with the presence of HBsAg, but the virus appears to inhibit the replication of HBV and it is not uncommon for HBeAg to be undetectable in serum.

The Delta virus consists of a single-stranded RNA genome that encodes a single protein – Delta antigen. The mature virion consists of a delta antigen/RNA core surrounded by an envelope composed of HBV-derived surface antigen. Delta virus replicates by a rolling circle-type mechanism that involves RNA-derived enzymes (ribozymes) to form new circular RNA genomes (Chen *et al*, 1986). Delta virus is rare in Western Europe and the USA, where it is usually associated with intravenous drug usage, but it is not uncommon in Mediterranean countries. The highest prevalence is in certain areas of Africa and South America. There are three major genotypes of HDV, which vary in their geographical distribution (Niro *et al*, 1997). It has been suggested that these genotypes have different pathogenicities.

Hepatitis E

HEV has recently been cloned, and its characterisation is under active investigation. The virus is a small, extremely labile particle with features that are typical of the calicivirus group (Reyes *et al*, 1990). The HEV genome is approximately 7.5 kb in length (Fig. 1.4) and contains three open reading frames (Reyes *et al*, 1990). One of these encodes a nonstructural protein that is presumed to mediate viral replication, and the other two genes are believed to encode the structural proteins of the virus. The replication strategy and structure of HEV remain to be elucidated.

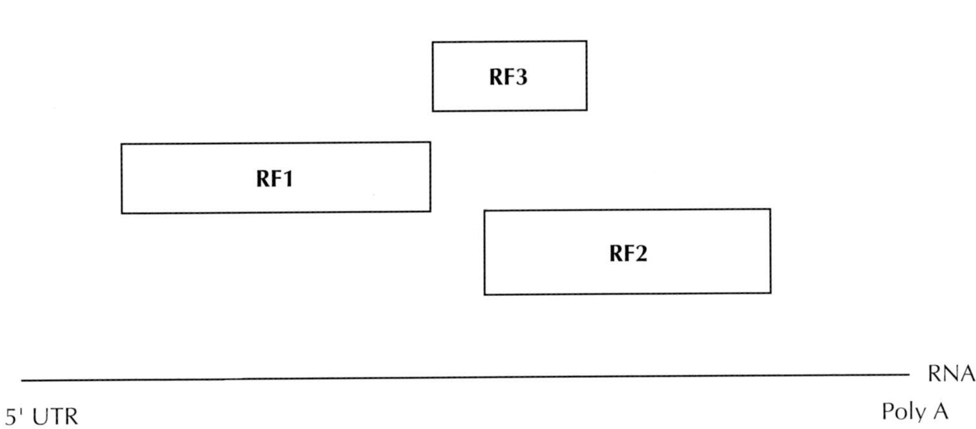

Fig 1.4 Genetic organisation of the hepatitis E virus. The virus contains a single RNA genome with an initial 5′ NCR and a poly A tail at the 3′ end. The genome encodes three open reading frames that overlap as shown. RF1 encodes non-structural proteins that probably encase a helicase and an RNA polymerase. RF2 is thought to encode structural proteins and includes immunoreactive epitopes, and RF3 encodes a protein of unknown function.

Infection with HEV follows a similar course to infection with HAV. Approximately 30% of patients develop a cholestatic jaundice, similar to that seen in HAV infections, but a recurrent form of HEV has not been described. In healthy individuals, HEV is a mild infection without significant morbidity. However, in pregnant women, a fatal, fulminant form is common, affecting up to 20% of infected patients (Reyes *et al*, 1990).

Infection with HEV appears to be common in Third World countries and occurs in epidemics as well as presenting as sporadic cases. Infection with HEV is rare in the underdeveloped world (Bradley, 1990; Bradley *et al*, 1993). Studies on the prevalence of HEV infection have been hampered by the available diagnostic tests and the poor persistence of currently detectable antibodies. At present, a number of different HEV strains have been identified (Lok and Soldevila-Pica, 1994), and it is clear that the available detection systems do not identify them all. To complicate matters still further, it is clear that antibodies against HEV may persist for only a short period of time, rendering seroprevalence studies uninformative. At present, insufficient information is available to comment on the exposure rates to HEV, but infection episodes are certainly common in the Third World and rare in Europe and USA. Patients seen in the UK, for example, have almost invariably contracted their infection elsewhere.

New hepatotropic viruses

Although the well-identified hepatotropic viruses account for the majority of cases of viral hepatitis, it is clear that other, unidentified, viruses may also cause infectious hepatitis. Thus a number of cases of post-transfusional hepatitis are not due to infection with hepatitis A, B, C or E, and it is clear that at least one other hepatotropic virus must exist. Recent advances in polymerase chain reaction technology have allowed the identification and characterisation of several novel viruses that are associated with hepatitis. The GB hepatitis viruses (Karayiarmis and McGarvey, 1995) are a group of viruses that were originally identified by transmission studies using donor serum from an infected surgeon

(GB) and tamarin monkeys. The analysis of passaged serum has led to the identification of three new viruses: GB-A, GB-B and GB-C. All of these viruses have now been passed in animal models, and it is not yet clear whether they are human or uniquely animal pathogens. Some studies in patients with hepatitis have suggested that at least one of these viruses (GB-C) is also a human pathogen (Simons *et al*, 1995).

Another research group has used serum from patients with non-A, B, C hepatitis as the starting material for polymerase chain reaction-based viral identification. This approach has identified a novel flavivirus (hepatitis G) that is associated with human hepatitis following the transfusion of contaminated blood (Fry *et al*, 1995).

GBV-C and HGV share 86% nucleotide and 96% deduced amino homology and they are considered to be different isolates of the same virus. It is a member of the *Flaviviridae* and is distantly related to HCV. The significance of this virus in the pathogenesis of viral hepatitis is currently undergoing re-evaluation (e.g. Kanda *et al*, 1997; Lopez-Alcorocho *et al*, 1997). A consensus is developing that this virus is associated with at worst only mild clinical disease (Alter *et al*, 1997a; Lemon 1997). It may be that it is a 'passenger virus' transmitted with other viruses that are associated with viral hepatitis.

In a study of acute non-A–E hepatitis, it was found that HGV was not a cause of acute disease, and although the development of chronicity is common (75%), this was not associated with chronic disease (Alter *et al*, 1997a). In another study, it was confirmed that HGV can be transmitted by transfusion. However, this virus not only was *not* associated with hepatitis, but it also had no adverse effect on concurrent HCV (Alter *et al*, 1997b). Furthermore, a detailed histological study has shown that co-infection with HGV has no impact on either disease severity or the histological features of cases of HCV (Bralet *et al*, 1997). Other, as yet unidentified, viruses capable of causing at least an acute hepatitis clearly exist (Rochling *et al*, 1997).

References

Alter, H. 1992: Chronic consequences of non-A, non-B hepatitis. In Seef, L., Lewis, R. (eds) *Current perspectives in hepatology*. New York: Plenum.

Alter, H.J., Snachez-Pescador, R., Urdea, M.S. *et al.* 1995: Evaluation of branched DNA signal amplification for the detection of hepatitis C virus RNA. *Journal of Viral Hepatitis* **2**, 121.

Alter, M., Gallagher, M., Morris, T.T. *et al.*, for the Sentinel Counties Viral Hepatitis Team. 1997a: Acute non-A–E hepatitis in the United States and the role of hepatitis G virus infection. *New England Journal of Medicine* **336**, 741–6.

Alter, H., Nakatsuji, Y., McIpolder, J. *et al.* 1997b: The incidence of transfusion-associated hepatitis G virus infection and its relation to liver disease. *New England Journal of Medicine* **336**, 747–54.

Beasley, R.P., Hwang, L.Y., Lin, C.C., Chien, C.S. 1981: Hepatocellular carcinoma and hepatitis B virus – a prospective study of 22,707 men in Taiwan. *Lancet* **ii**, 1129–33.

Benvegnu, L., Pontisso, P., Cavalletto, D., Noventa, F., Chemello, L., Alberti, A. 1997: Lack of correlation between hepatitis C virus genotypes and clinical course of hepatitis C virus-related cirrhosis. *Hepatology* **25**, 211–15.

Bisceglie, A. 1998: Hepatitis C. *Lancet* 351–5.

Blum, H.E. 1994: Does hepatitis C virus cause hepatocellular carcinoma? *Hepatology* **19**, 251–5.

Bonino, F., Heerman, K.H., Rizzetto, M., Gerlich, W.H. 1986: Hepatitis delta virus: protein composition of delta antigen and its hepatitis B virus-derived envelope. *Journal of Virology* **58**, 945–50.

Bradley, D.W. 1990: Enterically transmitted non-A, non-B hepatitis. *British Medical Bulletin* **46**, 442–61.

Bradley, D.W., Krawacyzynski, K., Purdy, M.A. 1993: Hepatitis E: epidemiology, natural history and experimental models. In Zuckerman, A.J., Thomas, H.C. (eds) *Viral hepatitis*. London: Churchill Livingstone.

Bralet, M.-P., Radot-Thoraval, F., Poulatsky, J.-M. *et al.* 1997: Histopathological impact of GB virus C infection on chronic hepatitis C. *Gastroenterology* **112**, 188–92.

Carman, W.F., Jacyna, M.R., Hadziyannis, S. *et al.* 1989: Mutation preventing formation of e antigen in patients with chronic HBV infection. *Lancet* **ii**, 588–91.

Chen, P.J., Kalpana, J., Goldberg, W. *et al.* 1986: Structure and replication of the genome of the hepatitis delta virus. *Proceedings of the National Academy of Sciences of the USA* **83**, 8774–8.

Choo, Q.L., Richman, K.H., Han, J.H. *et al.* 1991: Genetic organisation and diversity of the hepatitis C virus. *Proceedings of the National Academy of Sciences of the USA* **88**, 2451–5.

Colombo, M., Cambieri, R., Rumi, M.G. *et al.* 1983: Long term delta superinfection in hepatitis B surface antigen carriers and its relationship to the course of chronic hepatitis. *Gastroenterology* **85**, 235–9.

Dusheiko, G., Simmonds, P. 1994: Sequence variability of hepatitis C virus and its clinical relevance. *Journal of Viral Hepatitis* **1**, 3–16.

Enamoto, N., Sato, C. 1995: The significance of HCV quasispecies. *Journal of Viral Hepatitis* **1**, 267–72.

Fry, K.E., Linnen, J., Zhang-Keck, Z.-Y. *et al.* 1995: Sequence analysis of a new RNA virus (hepatitis G virus, HGV) reveals a unique virus in the Flaviviridae family. *Hepatology* **22**, 181A.

Ganem, D., Varmus, H.E. 1987: The molecular biology of the hepatitis B viruses. *Annual Review of Biochemistry* **56**, 651–93.

Gauss-Muller, V., Lottspeich, F., Deinhardt, F. 1986: Characterisation of hepatitis A virus structural proteins. *Virology* **155** 732–6.

Henkler, F., Koshy, R. 1996: Transactivating functions of the hepatitis B X protein. *Journal of Viral Hepatitis* **3**(3), 109–22.

Hohne, M., Schaefer, S., Seifer, M., Feitelson, M.A., Paul, D., Gerlich, W.H. 1990: Malignant transformation of immortalised hepatocytes after transfection with hepatitis B virus DNA. *EMBO Journal* **9**, 1137–45.

Humphrey, C.D., Cook, E.H., Bradley, D.W. 1990: Identification of enterically transmitted hepatitis virus particles by solid phase immune electron microscopy. *Journal of Virological Methods* **29**, 177–88.

Jansen, R.W., Newbold, J.E., Lemon, S.M. 1985: Combined immunoaffinity cDNA-RNA hybridisation assay for detection of hepatitis A virus in clinical specimens. *Journal of Clinical Microscopy* **221**, 984–9.

Kanda, T., Yokosuka, O., Ehata, T. *et al.* 1997: Detection of GBV-C RNA in patients with non-A–E fulminant hepatitis by reverse-transcription polymerase chain reaction. *Hepatology* **25**, 1261–5.

Karayiarmis, P., McGarvey, M.J. 1995: The GB hepatitis viruses. *Journal of Viral Hepatitis* **2**, 221–6.

Koff, R.S. 1998: Hepatitis A. *Lancet* **341**, 1643–9.

Lee, W. 1998: Hepatitis B virus infection. *New England Journal of Medicine* 1733–45.

Lemon, S.M. 1992: HAV: current concepts of the molecular virology, immunobiology and approaches to vaccine development. *Review of Medical Virology* **2**, 73–87.

Lemon, S.M. 1997: GB virus C, hepatitis G virus, or human orphan flavivirus? *Hepatology* **25**, 1285–6.

Lemon, S.M., Robertson, B.H. 1994: Taxonomic classification of hepatitis A virus. In Nishioka, K., Suzuki, H., Mishiro, S., Oda, T. (eds) *Viral hepatitis and liver disease*. New York: Springer-Verlag.

Locarnini, S.A., Coulepis, A.G., Stratton, A.M., Kaldor, J., Gust, I.D. 1979: Solid phase enzyme immunoassay for detection of hepatitis A specific immunoglobulin M. *Journal of Clinical Microscopy* **9**, 459–65.

Lok, A.S.E., Soldevila-Pica, C. 1994: Epidemiology and serologic diagnosis of hepatitis E. *Journal of Hepatology* **20**, 567–9.

Lopez-Alcorocho, J.M., Millan, A., Garcia-Trevijano, E.R. *et al.* 1997: Detection of hepatitis GB virus type C RNA in serum and liver from children with chronic viral hepatitis B and C. *Hepatology* **25**, 1258–60.

McFarlane, I.G., Smith, H.M., Johnson, P.J., Bray, G.P., Vergani, D., Williams, R. 1990: Hepatitis C virus antibodies in chronic active hepatitis: pathogenetic factor or false positive result? *Lancet* **335**, 754–7.

Niro, G.A., Smedile, A., Andriulli, A., Rizzetto, M., Gerin, J.L., Casey, J.L. 1997: The predominance of hepatitis delta virus genotype 1 among chronically infected Italian patients. *Hepatology* **25**, 728–34.

Palmenberg, A.C. 1987: Picornaviral processing: some new ideas. *Journal of Cellular Biochemistry* **33**, 191–8.

Poynard, T., Bedossa, P., Opolan, P., for the OBSVIRC, METAVIR, CLINIVIR and DOSVIRC groups. 1997: Natural history of liver fibrosis progression in patients with chronic hepatitis C. *Lancet* **249**, 825–32.

Reyes, G.R., Purdy, M.A., Kim, J.P. *et al.* 1990: Isolation of a cDNA from the virus responsible for enterically transmitted non-A, non-B hepatitis. *Science* **247**, 1335–9.

Rochling, F.A., Jones, W.F., Chau, K. *et al.* 1997: Acute sporadic non-A, non-B, non-C, non-D, non-E hepatitis. *Hepatology* **25**, 478–83.

Ross, B.C., Anderson, D.A., Gust, I.D. 1991: Hepatitis A virus and hepatitis A infection. *Advances in Virus Research* **39**, 209–53.

Rossner, M.T. 1992: Review: Hepatitis B virus X gene product: a promiscuous transcriptional activator. *Journal of Medical Virology* **36**, 101–17.

Sherlock, S., Dooley, J.S. 1991: Acute and chronic hepatitis. In *Diseases of the liver and biliary system*, 9th edn. Oxford: Blackwell Scientific.

Simmonds, P. 1997: Clinical relevance of hepatitis C virus genotypes. *Gut* **40**, 291–3.

Simmonds, P., Alberti, A., Alter, H.J. *et al.* 1994: A proposed system for the nomenclature of hepatitis C viral genotypes. *Hepatology* **19**, 1321–4.

Simons, J.N., Leary, T.P., Dawson, G.J. *et al.*, 1995: Isolation of novel virus-like sequences associated with human hepatitis. *Nature Medicine* **1**, 564–9.

Song, E., Kew, M.C. 1994: The seroepidemiology of hepatitis A infection in South African Chinese. *Journal of Viral Hepatitis* **1**, 149–53.

Standring, D.N., Ou, J., Masiarz, F.R., Rutter, W.J. 1988: A signal peptide encoded within the pre-core region of hepatitis B directs the secretion of a heterogeneous population of e antigens in *Xenopus* oocytes. *Proceedings of the National Academy of Sciences of the USA* **85**, 8405–9.

Thursz, M.R., Thomas, H.C., Hill, A.D. 1995: Host genetic factors influencing the outcome of hepatitis. *New England Journal of Medicine* **4**, 215–20.

Tibbs, C. 1995: Methods of transmission of hepatitis C. *Journal of Viral Hepatitis* **2**, 100–20.

Van der Poel, P., Cuypers, H.T.M., Reesink, H.W. *et al.* 1991: Confirmation of hepatitis C virus infection by new four-antigen recombinant immunoblot assay. *Lancet* **337**, 317–19.

Weitz, M., Baroudy, B.M., Maloy, W.L., Ticehurst, J.R., Purcell, R.H. 1986: Detection of a genome-linked protein (VPg) of hepatitis A virus and its comparison with other picornaviral VPgs. *Journal of Virology* **60**, 124–30.

Wong, V., Caronia, S., Wight, D. *et al.* 1997: Importance of age in chronic hepatitis C virus infection. *Journal of Viral Hepatitis* **4**, 255–64.

Yuki, N., Hayashi, N., Moribe, T. *et al.* 1997: Relation of disease activity during chronic hepatitis C infection to complexity of hypervariable region 1 quasispecies. *Hepatology* **25**, 439–44.

CHAPTER 2

Pathology of acute viral hepatitis

M A GERBER

Acute viral hepatitis is a diffuse necroinflammatory disease of the liver of less than 6 months' duration as a result of infection by primary hepatotropic viruses (International Group, 1971, Peters, 1975; Ishak, 1976; MacSween, 1980; Phillips and Poucell, 1981; Gerber and Thung, 1985; Thung *et al*, 1989; International Hepatology Informatics Group, 1994; Scheuer, 1994; Thung and Gerber, 1995). The differentiation between acute and chronic viral hepatitis is primarily based on the duration of the disease, using 6 months for distinction. Hepatotropic viruses infect the liver as the primary target organ and include hepatitis A, B, C, D, E and possibly G as well as probably other, yet undiscovered, hepatitis viruses. Non-hepatotropic viruses may involve the liver as part of a systemic disease. These are discussed in Chapter 6.

With some exceptions, the histological alterations produced by the different primary hepatitis viruses are similar.

Clinical features

Acute hepatitis may be asymptomatic or may present with influenza-like or gastrointestinal symptoms. The typical patient has a fairly well-defined onset with anorexia, nausea, vomiting, mild pyrexia, right upper quadrant discomfort and profound malaise. Jaundice may or may not develop. The liver is palpable and tender, and the aminotransferase activities and levels of other liver-related enzymes are elevated. Serological tests for the causative hepatitis virus or viruses are positive (*see* Chapter 1). The disease usually resolves in a few months.

Acute viral hepatitis with spotty necrosis

The classical form of acute viral hepatitis is acute hepatitis with spotty necrosis (Table 2.1). The fully developed stage is characterised by panlobular disarray, increased cellularity and pleomorphism of the hepatocytes. This appearance is caused by a combination of changes consisting of: (1) hepatocellular degeneration, apoptosis and necrosis; (2) hepatocellular regeneration; and (3) sinusoidal cell activation and inflammation (Fig. 2.1) (International Group, 1971, 1977; Peters, 1975; Ishak, 1976; MacSween, 1980; Phillips

Table 2.1 Pathology of acute viral hepatitis

Hepatocellular degeneration, necrosis and apoptosis
Sinusoidal cell activation; mononuclear inflammatory cell infiltration of lobules and portal tracts
Hepatocellular regeneration: mitoses, two-cell thick plates, bi- or multinucleated hepatocytes
Low-power diagnosis: panlobular disarray, pleomorphism of hepatocytes and hypercellularity

and Poucell, 1981; Gerber and Thung, 1985; International Hepatology Informatics Group, 1994; Scheuer, 1994; Thung and Gerber, 1995). The two types of degenerative change of hepatocytes, i.e. eosinophilic degeneration with the formation of eosinophilic or apoptotic bodies, and ballooning degeneration leading to lytic necrosis, are present focally throughout the acinar parenchyma (Fig. 2.2). Regeneration is reflected in mitoses, two-cell thick plates and increased numbers of binucleate hepatocytes. The simultaneous processes of hepatocellular degeneration and regeneration produce marked variations of size, shape and staining qualities of the hepatocytes. The parenchymal changes are always accompanied by a mesenchymal reaction in that the sinusoidal lining cells, particularly Kupffer cells, become larger and more numerous. The inflammatory cell reaction, composed predominantly of macrophages and lymphocytes, is diffuse throughout the acini. The portal tracts are also infiltrated by lymphocytes and macrophages, and a few scattered plasma cells, eosinophils and neutrophils, but significant portal fibrosis or proliferation of the bile ductules is absent. The portal tracts may be expanded by the inflammatory infiltrate and spill-over of inflammatory cells into the adjacent parenchyma. It may be extremely difficult to distinguish the latter from the piecemeal necrosis ('interface hepatitis') seen in chronic hepatitis. Endophlebitis of the terminal

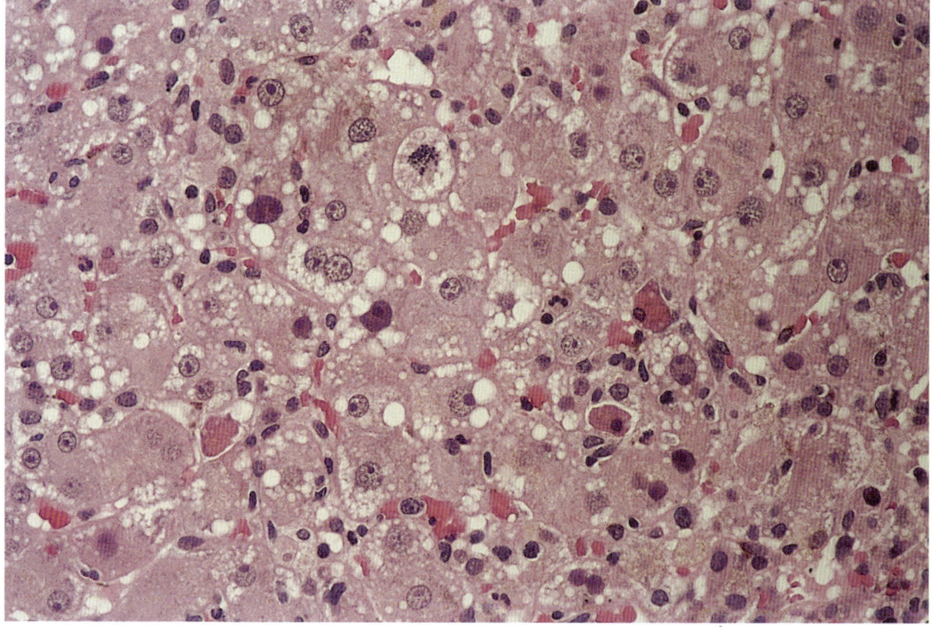

Fig 2.1 Acute viral hepatitis showing areas of focal necrosis, infiltration of sinusoids by inflammatory cells, and pleomorphism of hepatocytes (H&E, ×200).

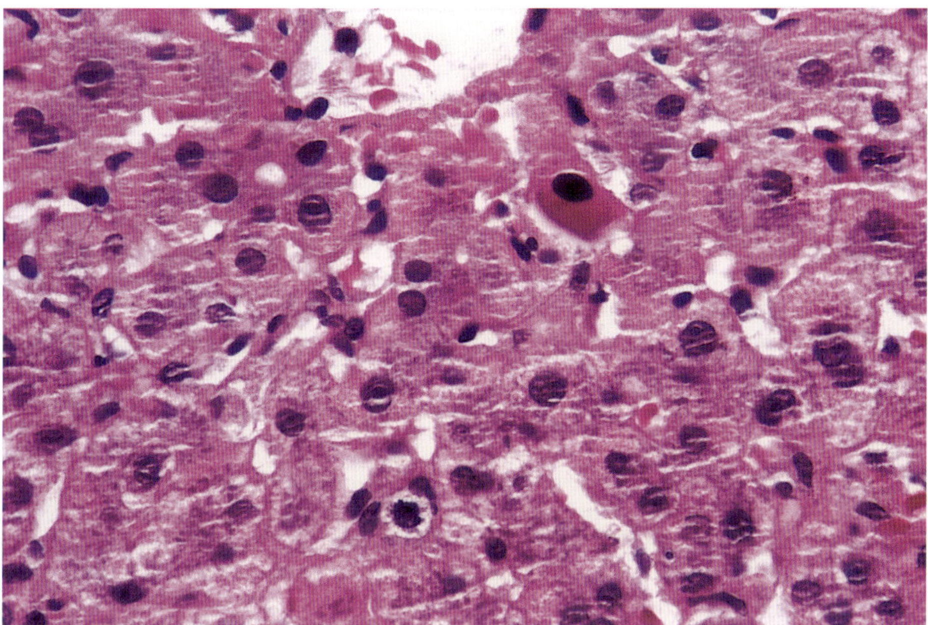

Fig 2.2 Acute viral hepatitis showing an apoptotic body and mitosis of a hepatocyte (H&E, ×400).

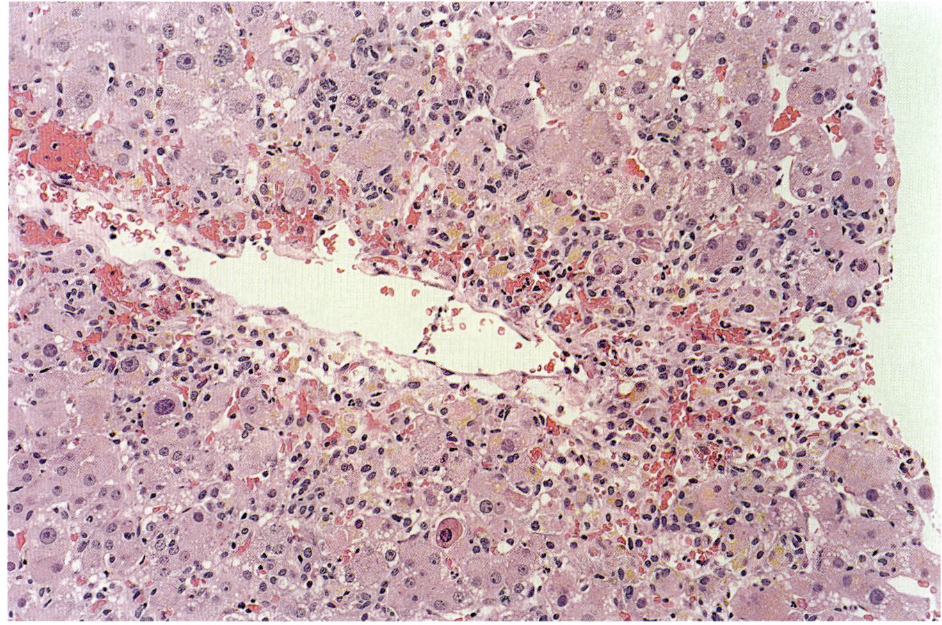

Fig 2.3 Acute viral hepatitis showing pericentral necrosis and inflammation of the central vein, so-called endophlebitis (H&E, ×400).

hepatic venules is observed (Fig. 2.3). Cholestasis, both intracellular and canalicular, is usually mild and occurs late in the course of the disease. None of the individual phenomena described above is diagnostic of acute viral hepatitis. Therefore the diagnosis is based on a combination of features described, which are best recognised under low-power magnification.

In the early stage, hepatocellular necrosis is minimal, while sinusoidal cell activation and inflammation are already present. This early lesion coincides with the first rise in aminotransferase activities. In the subsiding or late stage, hepatocellular degeneration and inflammation regress. Since the life span of DPAS-reactive macrophages is relatively long, they may persist as 'late nodules' or 'Spatknotchen' even after subsidence of the hepatitis. Small amounts of iron may also be present in these collections of macrophages.

Acute viral hepatitis with confluent necrosis

In fewer than 3% of patients with acute hepatitis, the necrosis is more extensive than spotty necrosis, leading to bridging or multilobular necrosis (Boyer and Klatskin, 1970; Ware *et al*, 1975; Bianchi, 1981; Spitz *et al*, 1981). All the other features of classic acute hepatitis are also seen. With extensive loss of the hepatocytes, the reticulin network collapses and forms passive septa or bridges between the portal tracts and central veins (Fig. 2.4). The formation of fibrous septa from active fibroplasia does not always follow. The parenchyma shows regeneration of the hepatocytes. Occasionally, more often in older persons, hepatocellular regeneration may be impaired (Peters, 1975). Although the clinical features of

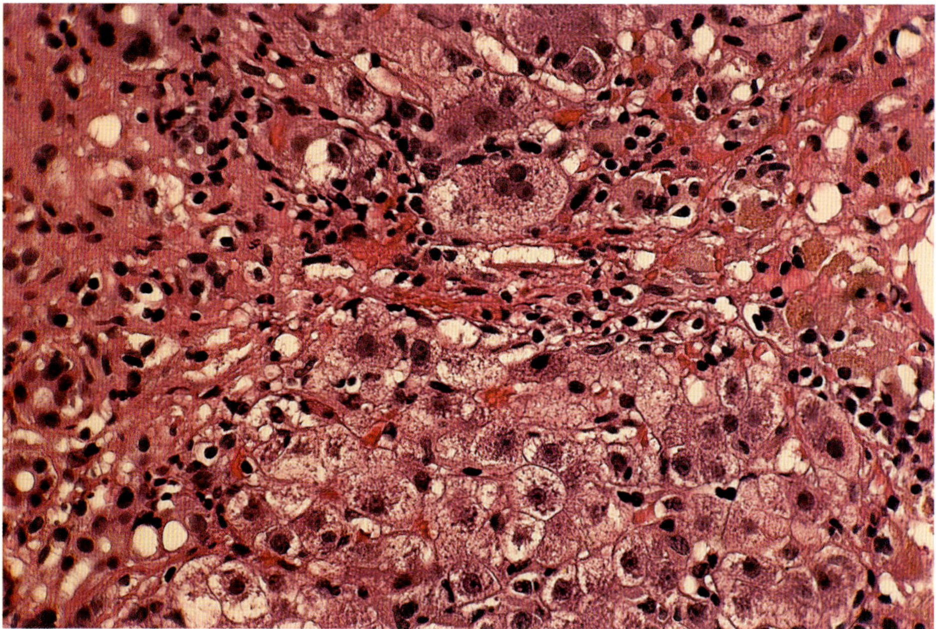

Fig 2.4 Acute viral hepatitis showing a necroinflammatory bridge between the portal tract (left) and central vein (right) (H&E, ×200).

patients with confluent necrosis are usually more severe, histopathological examination of a biopsy specimen is the only means by which bridging or multilobular necrosis can be recognised. Some cases heal, resulting in an essentially normal liver, while others progress to massive hepatic necrosis or cirrhosis (Chen and Liaw, 1988).

Acute viral hepatitis with massive necrosis

In fewer than 1% of cases with acute viral hepatitis, massive hepatic necrosis develops (Gazzard *et al*, 1975; Mathieson *et al*, 1980; Lee, 1993). In the most severe cases, patients present clinically with fulminant hepatitis and acute hepatic failure with jaundice, coagulopathy and encephalopathy. The serum aminotransferase activities, which are usually high in acute hepatitis, may decline in massive necrosis because there are few hepatocytes left to leak the enzymes. Almost all the hepatocytes are lost, resulting in collapse of the reticulin framework with approximation of the portal tracts (Fig. 2.5). This can be observed best on trichrome or reticulin stains. The sinusoids are filled with red blood cells, lymphocytes and enlarged, pigment-laden macrophages. Surviving hepatocytes, usually in a periportal location, show severe cell damage with ballooning degeneration, eosinophilic necrosis, cholestasis and enlargement with bi- or multinucleation. Steatosis is usually absent. Mononuclear inflammatory cell infiltration and endophlebitis in the lobular areas are present. The portal tracts are well preserved and show mononuclear inflammatory cell infiltration.

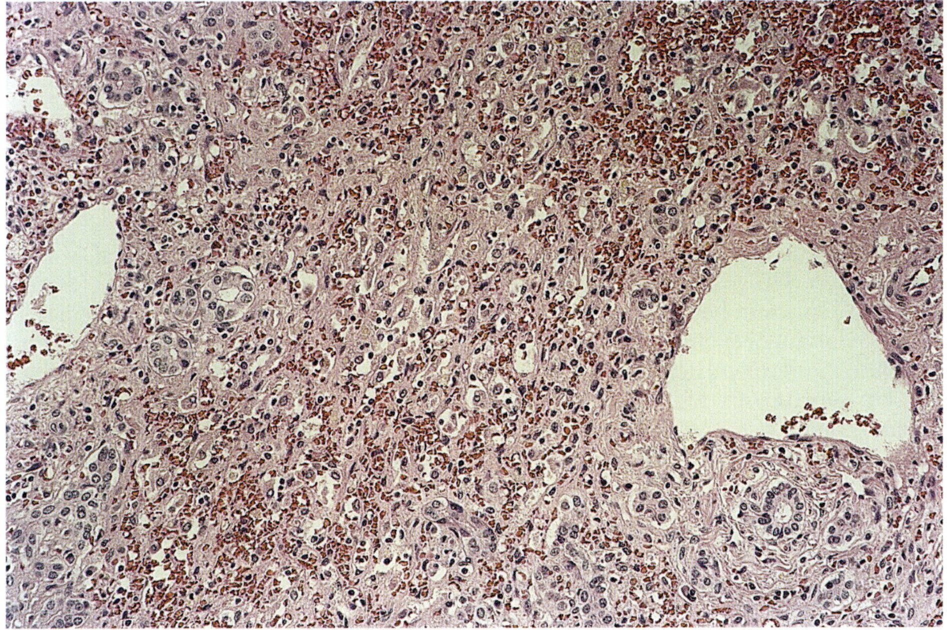

Fig 2.5   Massive hepatic necrosis showing the loss of all hepatocytes and the approximation of two portal tracts to the central vein (H&E, ×200).

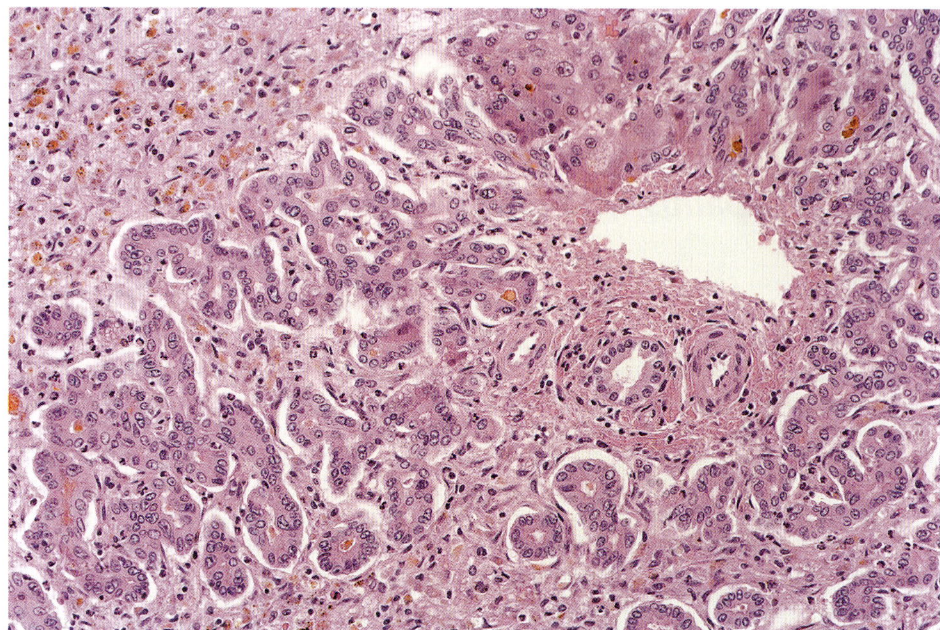

Fig 2.6   Massive hepatic necrosis showing regeneration in the form of ductular hepatocytes around the portal tract (H&E, ×200).

In patients who survive long enough, regeneration occurs, with the formation of ductular hepatocytes (Rubin *et al*, 1995; Haque *et al*, 1996) or neocholangioles in the collapsed lobules (Fig. 2.6). Sometimes regenerative nodules are formed by hepatocytes arranged in two-cell thick plates, and multinucleated hepatocytes. Survival depends largely on hepatocellular regeneration, reflected in a rise of serum alphafetoprotein level. In older patients, however, regeneration may be impaired and is associated with a poorer prognosis.

Massive hepatic necrosis may result from infection with HBV, HBV and HDV (co- or superinfection), HCV, HEV (the latter particularly in pregnant women) and, less commonly, HAV. In about half of the patients, however, the aetiology remains undetermined, even if the polymerase chain reaction for all known hepatitis viruses is used (Hytiroglou *et al*, 1995). Fulminant hepatitis D in the Amazon basin and Central Africa is characterised by hepatocytes with many small vacuoles in the cytoplasm (so-called morula cells) and granular eosinophilic necrosis, a picture that has not been observed in North America and Europe (Popper *et al*, 1983; Hadler *et al*, 1984; Buitrago *et al*, 1986); *see* Chapter 7.

Table 2.2   Extent of acute viral hepatitis

Spotty or focal necrosis
Bridging and multilobular necrosis
Massive or submassive necrosis

Transition to chronic disease

Reliable morphological criteria to suggest the transition of acute to chronic viral hepatitis have not been established, except perhaps for the presence of HBsAg-laden ground-glass hepatocytes, which may be detected during the transition of acute to chronic hepatitis B (Houthoff *et al*, 1980). However, ground-glass hepatocytes may also be seen in acute hepatitis A, D or C superimposed in a chronic HBV carrier or with reactivation of hepatitis B in an asymptomatic carrier. Other changes suggestive of a possible chronic course include bridging hepatic necrosis, extensive periportal and septal fibrosis, true piecemeal necrosis, bile ductule proliferation and heavy infiltration of the portal tracts by inflammatory cells, particularly plasma cells or lymphoid follicles (Dietrichson *et al*, 1975; Sherlock, 1976; Scheuer, 1977; Vanstapel *et al*, 1983).

Differentiation and immunopathology of acute viral hepatitis A, B, C, D and E

The parenchymal, mesenchymal and portal alterations described above represent the main features observed in acute viral hepatitis, regardless of the aetiological agent. Some features, however, are recognised as distinct and may reflect specific histological patterns of viral hepatitis A, B or C (Thung and Gerber, 1983).

In *acute viral hepatitis A*, parenchymal changes are more prominent in periportal zones than in pericentral areas, particularly in children (Tanikawa, 1979; Abe *et al*, 1982; Teixeira *et al*, 1982). Generally speaking, parenchymal alterations are less severe than in hepatitis B. The proliferation of Kupffer cells is mild, but mononuclear inflammatory cell infiltration with many plasma cells is more severe than in hepatitis B and may suggest a tendency to chronicity, which in fact is virtually absent in this disease. Microvesicular fatty change is also characteristic. Centrilobular cholestasis is frequently prominent, and the disease is more severe in adults. HAV antigen can be demonstrated in the liver for several weeks by immunohistochemical methods. The HAV antigen is expressed as fine granules in the cytoplasm of hepatocytes and Kupffer cells scattered throughout the lobules (Gerber and Thung, 1987). The virus may also be demonstrated by in situ hybridisation (*see* Chapter 4).

In *acute viral hepatitis B*, necroinflammatory lesions are often more severe in the centrilobular areas (Houthoff *et al*, 1980; Abe *et al*, 1982; McThorne *et al*, 1982). Endophlebitis is frequent. The sinusoidal cells are markedly activated, but lymphocytes predominate. They are often attached to normal or altered hepatocytes, particularly acidophilic bodies (peripolesis). These findings are consistent with the hypothesis that HBV-induced hepatocellular injury is mediated by the cytotoxic T-cells recognising virus-encoded target antigens (probably HBcAg or HBeAg) that are expressed on the hepatocellular plasma membrane during viral replication. Few or no viral components are detected by immunohistochemical methods in acute and fulminant hepatitis B, although HBcAg and HBsAg may be demonstrable during the late incubation period and in early acute hepatitis B (*see* Chapter 4).

HDV infection is always associated with HBV and may occur as co- or superinfection. HDAg can be reliably demonstrated in the nuclei and less frequently in the cytoplasm of hepatocytes (Thung *et al*, 1983; *see* Chapter 4). It is suspected that, in contrast to HBV, HDV may have a direct cytopathic effect on hepatocytes.

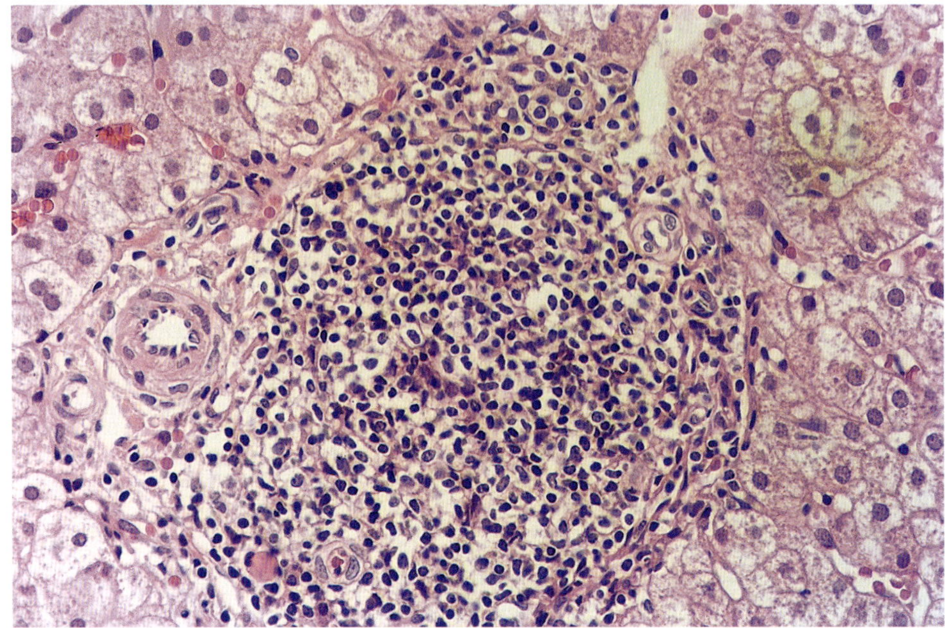

Fig 2.7 Viral hepatitis C showing a lymphoid aggregate in the portal tract (H&E, ×200).

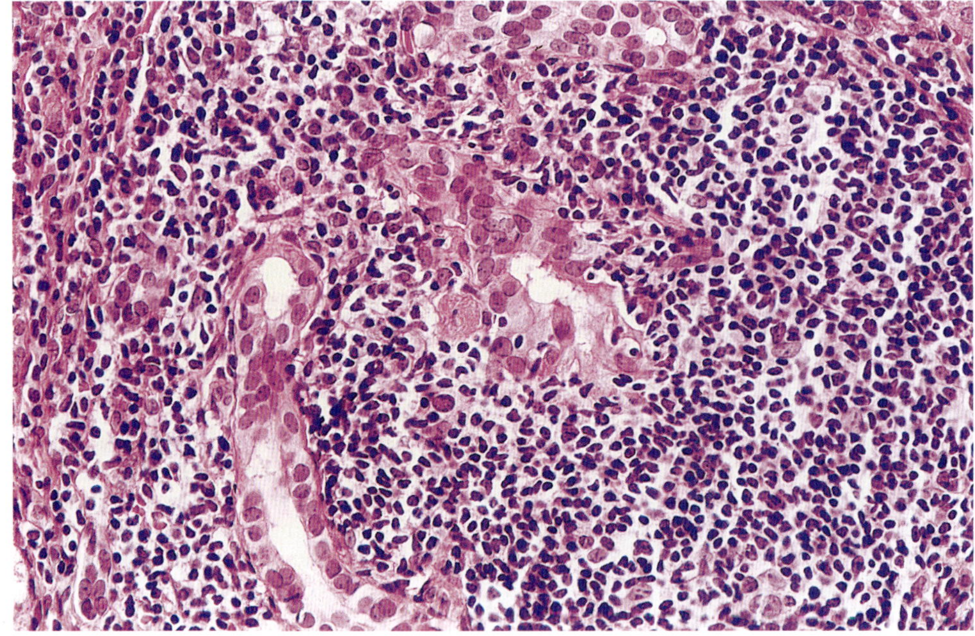

Fig 2.8 Viral hepatitis C showing disruption of the bile ducts with infiltration by lymphocytes (H&E, ×400).

In *acute viral hepatitis C*, fat accumulation in hepatocytes is often seen. Steatosis is usually mild and microvesicular, and is particularly common after exposure to blood and its products (concentrates) (Bamber *et al*, 1981a; Omata *et al*, 1981; Dienes *et al*, 1982). Bile duct alterations are frequent but are usually mild. Two types of lobular lesion are noted in acute viral hepatitis C: (1) many acidophilic bodies with only limited inflammatory reaction; and (2) conspicuous intrasinusoidal lymphocyte accumulation in the absence of clearly recognisable hepatocellular damage, similar to the changes in infectious mononucleosis and toxoplasmosis. Heavy lymphoid cell accumulation may be seen in portal triads, often forming lymphoid follicles with germinal centres (Fig. 2.7). Adjacent bile ducts are disrupted and infiltrated by lymphocytes (Fig. 2.8). Giant cell transformation may be observed in some adults with hepatitis C.

Several different ultrastructural alterations have been reported in the hepatocytes of patients or chimpanzees with hepatitis C. These include intranuclear particles, 15–29 nm in diameter, circular and tubular fused membranes in the cytoplasm, and tubular profiles in dilated cisternae of the endoplasmic reticulum (Shimizu *et al*, 1979; Thomssen *et al*, 1980; Bamber *et al*, 1981b; Desmet and DeVos, 1985). Structural and non-structural HCV antigens may be detected by immunohistochemical staining in the cytoplasm of these scattered hepatocytes, mononuclear cells and rare biliary epithelial cells (Hiramatsu *et al*, 1992; Krawczynski *et al*, 1992; Blight *et al*, 1993, 1994; Sansonno and Dammacco, 1993; Selby *et al*, 1993; Gonzalez-Peralta *et al*, 1994; Haruna *et al*, 1994; Komminoth *et al*, 1994; Tsutsumi *et al*, 1994; Ballardini *et al*, 1995; Gerber, 1995; Nouri-Aria *et al*, 1995) (*see* Chapter 4).

In *acute viral hepatitis E*, first recognised in epidemics in developing countries with a high mortality of pregnant women, but without chronic disease, cholestasis with pseudogland formation of hepatocytes is common (Bradley *et al*, 1988). Macrophages and neutrophils predominate over lymphocytes.

The original report of *acute viral hepatitis F* has not been confirmed.

The role of HGV (GBVC) in producing acute viral hepatitis is currently undergoing a re-evaluation, the most recent articles suggesting that there is no good evidence that HGV produces an acute hepatitis (Alter *et al*, 1997; Miyalowa and Moyumi, 1997).

Differential diagnosis of acute viral hepatitis

Acute viral hepatitis can usually be diagnosed on the basis of a compatible clinical history and physical examination supported by characteristic biochemical and serological tests. Liver biopsy is therefore indicated only when the aetiology of acute hepatitis is unclear or in prolonged, unresolving or relapsing hepatitis. The differential diagnosis encompasses not only hepatitis A, B, D and C, but also hepatitis caused by non-hepatotropic viruses, several bacterial infections, autoimmune processes, drugs, alcohol, acute biliary obstruction, hepatic allograft rejection and various metabolic and non-specific forms of hepatic injury (Thung *et al*, 1989).

Portal and periportal changes closely mimicking those of large bile duct obstruction may be seen in some forms, particularly in hepatitis with bridging necrosis and in cholestatic viral hepatitis. The diagnosis is usually established by observing the characteristic necroinflammatory changes in the lobules, which in acute viral hepatitis are not directly associated with cholestasis.

Drug-induced hepatitis may closely resemble acute viral hepatitis clinically, biochemically and morphologically. Certain features, however, suggest a drug-related cause; these include cytotoxic hepatocyte alterations with little inflammatory response, fatty change, granuloma formation, infiltration by eosinophils, bile duct damage and so-called induction cells (hepatocytes with increased endoplasmic reticulum).

Non-specific reactive hepatitis is particularly difficult to differentiate from the late and residual stages of acute viral hepatitis when macrophages are prominent. The necroinflammatory changes in non-specific reactive hepatitis are less pronounced.

The differentiation of acute from chronic hepatitis has been discussed above. Histologically, acute viral hepatitis with confluent necrosis, collapse, passive septa and regeneration may be mistaken for cirrhosis. However, areas of necrosis or collapse contain very few collagen and elastic fibres, in contrast to fibrous septa in chronic hepatitis and cirrhosis (Thung and Gerber, 1982).

Many viruses other than the hepatotropic viruses may affect the liver, particularly adeno- and herpes viruses (*see* Chapter 6). The extensive use of immunosuppressive treatment has increased the number of such cases. The hepatic changes consist of the activation of sinusoidal lining cells and the formation of histiocytic nodules. The focal eosinophilic necrosis of hepatocytes is a common finding and may be extensive, especially early in life and in patients with a defective immune response. Eosinophilic bodies are often seen. Nuclear or cytoplasmic viral inclusions may establish the diagnosis. Immunohistochemical studies may also be very valuable.

Damage to vessels (endothelitis) is characteristic in hepatic allograft rejection and involves the terminal hepatic venules and portal veins. Lesions of small bile ducts with vacuolation and necrosis of the epithelium are typical and more pronounced than in viral hepatitis, whereas hepatocellular damage is less severe.

Table 2.3   Differential diagnosis of acute viral hepatitis

Drug-induced hepatitis
Alcoholic hepatitis
Autoimmune hepatitis
Non-specific reactive hepatitis
Large bile duct obstruction
Chronic hepatitis
Hepatic allograft rejection

References

Abe, H., Beninger, P.R., Ikejiri, N., Setoyama, H., Sata, M., Tanikawa, K. 1982: Light microscopic findings of liver biopsy specimens from patients with hepatitis type A and comparison with type B. *Gastroenterology* **82**, 938–47.

Alter, M., Gallagher, M., Morris, T.T. *et al.* for the Sentinel Counties Viral Hepatitis Team. 1997: Acute non-A–E hepatitis in the United States and the role of hepatitis G virus infection. *New England Journal of Medicine* **336**, 741–6.

Ballardini, G., Groff, P., Giostra, F. *et al.* 1995: Hepatocellular codistribution of c100, c33, c22 and NS5 hepatitis C virus antigens detected by using immunopurified polyclonal spontaneous human antibodies. *Hepatology* **21**, 730–4.

Bamber, M., Murray, A., Lewin, J., Thomas, H.C., Sherlock, S. 1981a: Ultrastructural features in chronic non-A, non-B hepatitis: a controlled blind study. *Journal of Medical Virology* **8**, 267–75.

Bamber, M., Murray, A.K., Weller, I.V.D. *et al.* 1981b: Clinical and histologic features of a group of patients with sporadic non-A, non-B hepatitis. *Journal of Clinical Pathology* **34**, 1175–80.

Bianchi, L. 1981: Acute viral hepatitis B with bridging necrosis: a follow-up study. *Liver* **1**, 222–9.

Blight, K., Rowland, R., Hall, P.D. 1993: Immunohistochemical detection of the NS4 antigen of hepatitis C virus and its relation to histopathology. *American Journal of Pathology* **143**, 1568–73.

Blight, K., Lesniewski, R.R., LaBrooy, J.T., Gowans, E.J. 1994: Detection and distribution of hepatitis C-specific antigens in naturally infected liver. *Hepatology* **20**, 553–7.

Boyer, J.L., Klatskin, G. 1970: Pattern of necrosis of acute viral hepatitis. Prognostic value of bridging (subacute hepatic) necrosis. *New England Journal of Medicine* **283**, 1063–71.

Bradley, D.W., Krawczynski, K., Cook, E.H. Jr *et al.* 1988: Enterically transmitted non-A, non-B hepatitis: etiology of disease and laboratory studies in nonhuman primates. In Zuckerman, A.J. (ed.) *Viral hepatitis and liver disease.* New York: Alan R. Liss, 138–47.

Buitrago, B., Popper, H., Hadler, S.C., Thung, S.N., Gerber, M.A., Maynard, J.E. 1986: Specific histologic features of Santa Marta hepatitis: a severe form of hepatitis delta virus infection in Northern South America. *Hepatology* **6**, 1285–91.

Chen, T.-J., Liaw, Y.-F. 1988: The prognostic significance of bridging hepatic necrosis in chronic type B hepatitis: a histopathologic study. *Liver* **8**, 10–16.

Desmet, V.J., DeVos, R. 1985: Ultrastructural findings in non-A, non-B viral hepatitis. In Brunner, H.Y., Thaler, H. (eds.) *Hepatology: A Festschrift for Hans Popper.* New York: Raven Press, 159–75.

Dienes, H.P., Popper, H., Arnold, W., Lobeck, H. 1982: Histologic observations in human hepatitis non-A, non-B. *Hepatology* **2**, 562–71.

Dietrichson, O., Juhl, T., Christoffersen, P. *et al.* 1975: Acute viral hepatitis: factors possibly predicting chronic liver disease. *Acta Pathologica Microbiologica Scandinavica A* **83**, 183–8.

Gazzard, B.G., Portmann, B., Murray-Lyon, I.M., Williams, R. 1975: Causes of death in fulminant hepatic failure and relationship to quantitative histological assessment of parenchymal damage. *Quarterly Journal of Medicine* **44**, 615–26.

Gerber, M.A. 1995: Pathobiology of hepatitis C. *Verhandlungen der Deutschen Gesellschaft für Pathologie* **79**, 162–70.

Gerber, M.A., Thung, S.N. 1985: Viral hepatitis: pathology. In Berk, J.E. (ed.) *Bockus' Gastroenterology.* Philadelphia: WB Saunders, Volume **5**, 2825–55.

Gerber, M.A., Thung, S.N. 1987: The diagnostic value of immunohistochemical demonstration of hepatitis viral antigens in the liver. *Human Pathology* **18**, 771–4.

Gonzalez-Peralta, R.P., Fang, J.W.S., Davis, G.L. *et al.* 1994: Optimization for the detection of hepatitic C virus antigens in the liver. *Journal of Hepatology* **20**, 143–8.

Hadler, S.C., de Monzon, M., Ponzetto, A. *et al.* 1984: An epidemic of severe hepatitis due to Delta agent infection in Yucpa Indians in Venezuela. *Annals of Internal Medicine* **100**, 339–44.

Haruna, Y., Hayashi, N., Kamada, T., Hytiroglou, P., Thung, S.N., Gerber, M.A. 1994: Expression of hepatitis C virus in hepatocellular carcinoma. *Cancer* **73**, 2253–8.

Haque, S., Haruna, Y., Saito, K. *et al.* 1996: Identification of bipotential progenitor cells in human liver regeneration. *Laboratory Investigation* **75**(5), 699–705.

Hiramatsu, N., Hayashi, N., Haruna, N. *et al.* 1992: Immunohistochemical detection of hepatitis C virus-infected hepatocytes in chronic liver disease with monoclonal antibodies to core, envelope and NS3 regions of the hepatitis C virus genome. *Hepatology* **16**, 306–11.

Houthoff, H.J., Niermeijer, P., Gips, C.H., Arends, A., Hofstee, N., van Guldener, M. 1980: Hepatic morphologic findings and viral antigens in acute hepatitis B. *Virchows Archiv A: Pathologische Anatomie* **389**, 153–66.

Hytiroglou, P., Dash, S., Haruna, Y. *et al.* 1995: Detection of hepatitis B and hepatitis C viral sequences in fulminant hepatic failure of unknown etiology. *American Journal of Clinical Pathology* **104**, 588–93.

International Group 1971: Morphologic criteria in viral hepatitis. *Lancet* **i**, 333–7.

International Group 1977: Acute and chronic hepatitis revisited. *Lancet* **ii**, 914–19.

International Hepatology Informatics Group 1994: Diseases of the liver and biliary tract: standardization of nomenclature, diagnostic criteria, and progress. New York: Raven Press.

Ishak, K.G. 1976: Light microscopic morphology of viral hepatitis. *American Journal of Clinical Pathology* **65**, 787–827.

Komminoth, P., Adams, V., Roth, J. *et al.* 1994: Evaluation of methods for hepatitis C virus (HCV) detection in archival liver biopsies: comparison of immunohistochemistry, ISH, RT-PCR and in situ RT-PCR. *Pathology: Research and Practica* **190**, 1017–25.

Krawczynski, K., Beach, M.J., Bradley, D.W. *et al.* 1992: Hepatitis C virus antigen in hepatocytes: immunomorphologic detection and identification. *Gastroenterology* **103**, 622–9.

Lee, W.M. 1993: Acute liver failure. *New England Journal of Medicine* **329**, 1862–5.

MacSween, R.N.M. 1980: Pathology of viral hepatitis and its sequelae. *Clinical Gastroenterology* **9**, 23–45.

McThorne, C.H., Higgins, G.R., Ulich, T.R., Gitnick, G.L., Lewin, K.J. 1982: A histologic comparison of hepatitis B with non-A, non-B chronic active hepatitis. *Archives of Pathology and Laboratory Medicine* **106**, 433–6.

Mathieson, L.R., Skinhoj, P., Nielsen, J.O., Purcell, R.H., Wong, D., Ranek, L. 1980: Hepatitis type A, B, and non-A, non-B in fulminant hepatitis. *Gut* **21**, 72–7.

Miyakawa, Y., Mayumi, M. 1997: Hepatitis G virus – a true hepatitis virus or an accidental tourist? *New England Journal of Medicine* **336**, 795–6.

Nouri-Aria, K.T., Sallie, R., Mizokami, M., Portmann, B.C., Williams, R. 1995: Intrahepatic expression of hepatitis C virus antigens in chronic liver disease. *Journal of Pathology* **175**, 77–83.

Omata, M., Iwana, S., Masatoshi, S., Ito, Y., Okuda, K. 1981: Clinico-pathological study of acute non-A, non-B post-transfusion hepatitis: histological features of liver biopsies in acute phase. *Liver* **1**, 201–8.

Peters, R.L. 1975: Viral hepatitis: a pathologic spectrum. *American Journal of Medical Science* **270**, 17–31.

Phillips, M.J., Poucell, S. 1981: Modern aspects of the morphology of viral hepatitis. *Human Pathology* **12**, 1060–84.

Phillips, M.J., Blendis, L.M., Poucell, S. *et al.* 1991: Syncytial giant-cell hepatitis: sporadic hepatitis with distinctive pathological features, a severe clinical course, and paramyxoviral features. *New England Journal of Medicine* **324**, 455–60.

Popper, H., Thung, S.N., Gerber, M.A. *et al.* 1983: Histologic studies of severe Delta infection in Venezuelan Indians. *Hepatology* **3**, 906–12.

Rubin, E.M., Martin, A.A., Thung, S.N., Gerber, M.A. 1995: Morphometric and immunohistochemical characterization of human liver regeneration. *American Journal of Pathology* **147**(2), 397–404.

Sansonno, D., Dammacco, F. 1993: Hepatitis C virus c100 antigen in liver tissue from patients with acute and chronic infection. *Hepatology* **18**, 240–5.

Scheuer, P.J. 1977: Chronic hepatitis: a problem for the pathologist. *Histopathology* **1**, 5–19.

Scheuer, P.J. 1994: Viral hepatitis. In MacSween, R.N.M., Anthony, P.P., Scheuer, P.J. (eds) *Pathology of the liver*. Edinburgh: Churchill Livingstone, 243–67.

Selby, M.J., Choo, Q.-L., Berger, K. *et al.* 1993: Expression, identification and subcellular localization of the proteins encoded by the hepatitis C viral genome. *Journal of General Virology* **74**, 1103–13.

Sherlock, S. 1976: Predicting progression of acute type-B hepatitis to chronicity. *Lancet* **ii**, 354–6.

Shimizu, Y.K., Feinstone, S.M., Purcell, R.H. 1979: Non-A, non-B, hepatitis: ultrastructural evidence for two agents in experimentally infected chimpanzees. *Science* **205**, 197–200.

Spitz, R.D., Keren, D.F., Boitnott, J.K., Maddrey, W.C. 1981: Bridging hepatic necrosis. Etiology and prognosis. *Digestive Diseases* **23**, 1076–8.

Tanikawa, K. 1979: Acute viral hepatitis. Type A hepatitis. Its epidemiology, clinical picture and pathologic changes of the liver. *Gastroenterologica Japonica* **14**, 167–78.

Teixeira, M.R. Jr, Weller, I.V.D., Murray, A. *et al.* 1982: The pathology of hepatitis A in man. *Liver* **2**, 53–60.

Thomssen, P.R., Legler, K., Bottscher, U., Gerlich, W., Weinmann, E., Klinge, O. 1980: Experimental non-A, non-B hepatitis: four types of cytoplasmic alteration in hepatocytes in infected chimpanzees. *Virchows Archiv B (Zellpathologie)* **33**, 233–43.

Thung, S.N., Gerber, M.A. 1982: The formation of elastic fibers in livers with massive hepatic necrosis. *Archives of Pathology and Laboratory Medicine* **106**, 468–9.

Thung, S.N., Gerber, M.A. 1983: Immunohistochemical study of Delta antigen in an American metropolitan population. *Liver* **3**, 392–7.

Thung, S.N., Gerber, M.A. 1995: *Differential diagnosis in pathology: liver disorders*. New York: Igaku-Shoin Medical Publishers.

Thung, S.N., Gerber, M.A., Popper, H. 1983: Basic morphologic patterns of viral hepatitis A, B, NANB and Delta agent in animal and man. In Chisari, F.V. (ed.) *Advances in hepatitis research*. New York: Masson Publishing, 293–302.

Thung, S.N., Gerber, M.A., Popper, H. 1989: Histopathology and ultrastructural features of acute hepatitis. In Gitnick, G. (ed.) *Modern concepts of acute and chronic hepatitis*. New York, Plenum Medical, 19–34.

Tsutsumi, M., Urashima, S., Takada, A., Date, T., Tanaka, Y. 1994: Detection of antigens related to hepatitis C virus RNA encoding the NS5 region in the livers of patients with chronic type C hepatitis. *Hepatology* **19**, 265–72.

Vanstapel, M.J., Van Steenbergen, W., DeWolf-Peeters, C. *et al.* 1983: Prognostic significance of piecemeal necrosis in acute viral hepatitis. *Liver* **3**, 46–57.

Ware, A.J., Eigenbrodt, E.H., Combes, B. 1975: Prognostic significance of subacute hepatic necrosis in acute hepatitis. *Gastroenterology* **68**, 519–24.

CHAPTER 3

Pathology of chronic viral hepatitis

P J SCHEUER AND R D GOLDIN

Chronic hepatitis means prolonged inflammation of the liver; hence the term in its widest sense includes many different diseases of varied aetiology, ranging from virus-induced to metabolic and toxic disorders, and from minimal inflammatory infiltration to cirrhosis. In practice, however, the term is used in a more restricted way. Some authors include only viral, autoimmune, drug-induced and cryptogenic hepatitis (Desmet *et al*, 1994). Others add conditions that share histological characteristics with some of these, notably primary biliary cirrhosis, primary sclerosing cholangitis, the liver lesion of α_1-antitrypsin deficiency and Wilson's disease (International Working Party, 1994). Alcoholic hepatitis, although certainly inflammatory and often chronic, is not usually included. In some alcohol abusers, on the other hand, liver biopsy shows features identical to those of chronic viral hepatitis. In this chapter, chronic hepatitis will be used in its more restricted sense for the conditions listed in Table 3.1.

The question of duration must also be taken into account. Acute, self-limiting viral hepatitis runs a course of some weeks or months. Liver function tests usually return to normal well before 6 months, although they may occasionally remain abnormal for longer (*see* Chapter 2). The same is true for histological abnormalities. While it is generally not possible to establish an exact length of time after which a hepatitis in an individual patient is chronic, there is widespread agreement that chronic hepatitis should be defined as 'persistence of liver injury associated with either elevated aminotransferase levels or viral markers for greater than six months' (Leevy *et al*, 1994). This definition is helpful when, for example, different clinical trials of therapeutic regimens need to be compared. On the other hand, it has to be remembered that a hepatitis may well be destined to be chronic from its outset, and that a diagnosis of chronicity may be possible long

Table 3.1   Types and causes of chronic hepatitis

Viral hepatitis
Type B, with or without D
Type C
Other, as yet undefined, types
Autoimmune hepatitis
Drug-induced chronic hepatitis
Chronic hepatitis of unknown cause

NB. Other diseases such as primary biliary cirrhosis are included by some authors.

before the end of 6 months. The best example of this is autoimmune hepatitis; this can be definitively diagnosed serologically and is always regarded as chronic (Meeting Report, 1993). As will be seen later in this chapter, histological proof of chronicity in viral hepatitis is often difficult, especially in the first year of the disease. The importance of attempting to define and recognise the chronicity of a hepatitis is that a diagnosis of chronic hepatitis implies a potential for the development of cirrhosis.

The nomenclature of chronic hepatitis has recently undergone change. For over 25 years, the principal subdivision of chronic hepatitis has been into the histological categories of chronic persistent, chronic active (or aggressive) and chronic lobular hepatitis (Schmid, 1966; De Groote *et al*, 1968; Popper and Schaffner, 1971; International Group, 1977). Now, with increasing knowledge of the hepatitis viruses and the availability of specific therapy, emphasis has shifted from histological classification to a nomenclature dominated by aetiology and supplemented by detailed histological description (Czaja, 1993; Desmet *et al*, 1994; International Working Party, 1994; Ishak, 1994). Semiquantitative scoring of histological features is added when necessary, for example in the assessment of clinical trials (Knodell *et al*, 1981; Okuno *et al*, 1990; Ishak *et al*, 1995). The old histological categories can easily be deduced from histological descriptions if needed. The presence of piecemeal necrosis (interface hepatitis) defines chronic active hepatitis (De Groote *et al*, 1968), while substantial lobular (acinar) activity without significant portal or periportal inflammation defines chronic lobular hepatitis (Popper and Schaffner, 1971).

One important reason for this change of nomenclature is that chronic persistent and chronic active hepatitis are not separate diseases but are frequently found in a single patient at different times, as was indeed recognised by the authors of the original classification (De Groote *et al*, 1968). Another reason is the question of sampling: a liver biopsy specimen, especially if small, may not be representative of the liver as a whole. There may be different forms and degrees of severity of liver cell damage in different parts of the liver or in the same liver at different times. A further weakness of the earlier classification is its emphasis on piecemeal necrosis (interface hepatitis). This is clearly only one of several types of liver cell damage in chronic hepatitis and is not necessarily the most important. This is discussed further in the next section.

Pathological features

The essential histological features of chronic hepatitis of any cause are liver cell damage and inflammatory cell infiltration. These can be conveniently described according to their location in the hepatic acinus. In the following sections, 'acinar changes' refers to alterations throughout the acinus, while 'periportal changes' refers to changes in that part of the acinus immediately adjacent to a small (terminal) portal tract.

ACINAR CHANGES

Hepatocellular damage and death, as recorded by the histopathologist, take different forms (*see* Chapter 7). Sublethal damage is seen as liver cell swelling (also called ballooning degeneration) or as acidophilic shrinkage. These are probably the result of different processes, but it is not yet clear why different hepatocytes undergo different types of damage. Ballooned cells are enlarged and have pale-staining cytoplasm. Cells under-

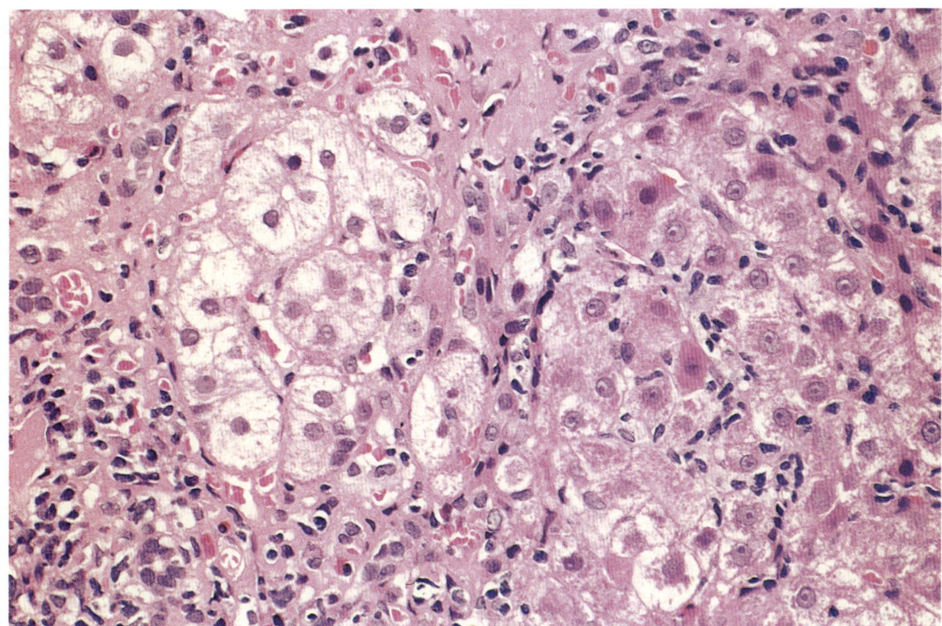

Fig 3.1   Acidophilic hepatocytes and rosette formation. Several hepatocytes (right) have intensely acidophilic cytoplasm. Gland-like clusters, rosettes, are seen to the left. The uppermost rosette has a small central lumen (H&E, ×100).

going acidophilic shrinkage (Fig. 3.1) are more eosinophilic (acidophilic) than normal and have concave outlines. They may be the precursors of apoptotic bodies, before separation of the cells from the hepatocyte plate.

The death of hepatocytes is also thought to be of two fundamentally different types: lytic necrosis and apoptosis (Alison and Sarraf, 1994). The first involves disruption of the cell membrane and its contents, while in the second, there is dehydration and fragmentation of the cell, without the triggering of a classical inflammatory response (Buja *et al*, 1993; Pileri *et al*, 1994). Apoptosis is considered to be the major form of cell death in chronic hepatitis (Powell, 1987). This is supported by the finding of Fas antigen expression on hepatocytes in chronic hepatitis B in areas of histological activity (Mochizuki *et al*, 1996) as well as in hepatitis C (Hiramatsu *et al*, 1994).

Evidence for the death of hepatocytes is usually indirect: it is assumed because hepatocytes are no longer seen in areas where they are normally present ('liver cell drop-out'). Such areas of hepatocyte loss may be small and focal, representing the loss of single cells or small groups. This is loosely called *focal necrosis* but is probably often the result of apoptosis rather than true necrosis. Larger areas result from the death of many adjacent hepatocytes and are (again loosely and perhaps incorrectly) described as *confluent necrosis* (Fig. 3.2). This may be random within the acini, zonal or in the form of bridges linking vascular structures (Fig. 3.3). The term 'bridging' was earlier used for the linking of any vascular structures (Boyer and Klatskin, 1970) but is now restricted to linking of the terminal hepatic venules (centrilobular veins in the lobular nomenclature) to the portal tracts (central–portal or C–P bridging). The distinction is important. Central–portal bridging probably represents the loss of hepatocytes from the entire zone 3 of an acinus.

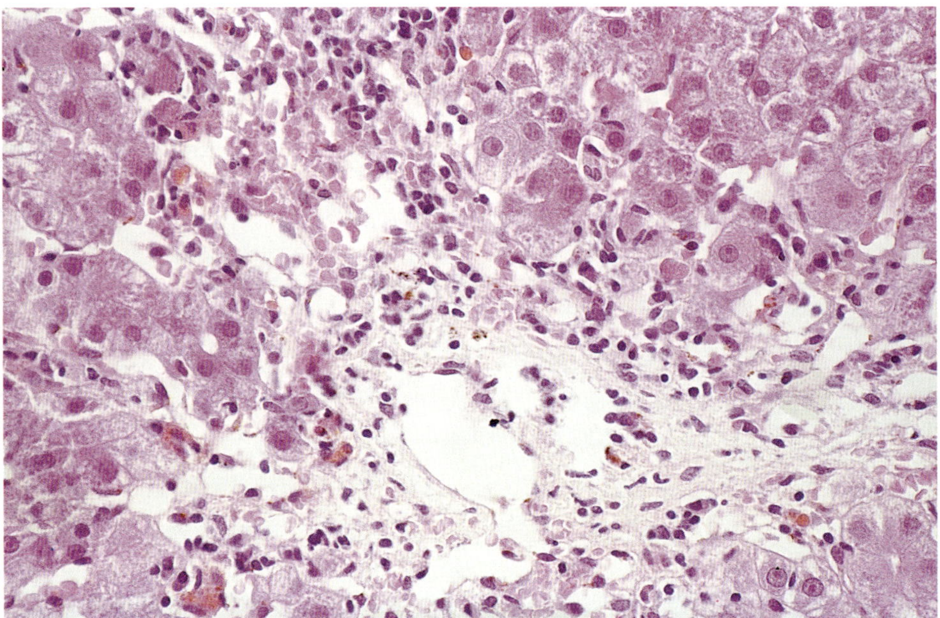

Fig 3.2 Confluent necrosis. There has been extensive loss of hepatocytes around a terminal hepatic venule (below) in this example of a chronic hepatitis with no significant portal or periportal component (H&E, ×100).

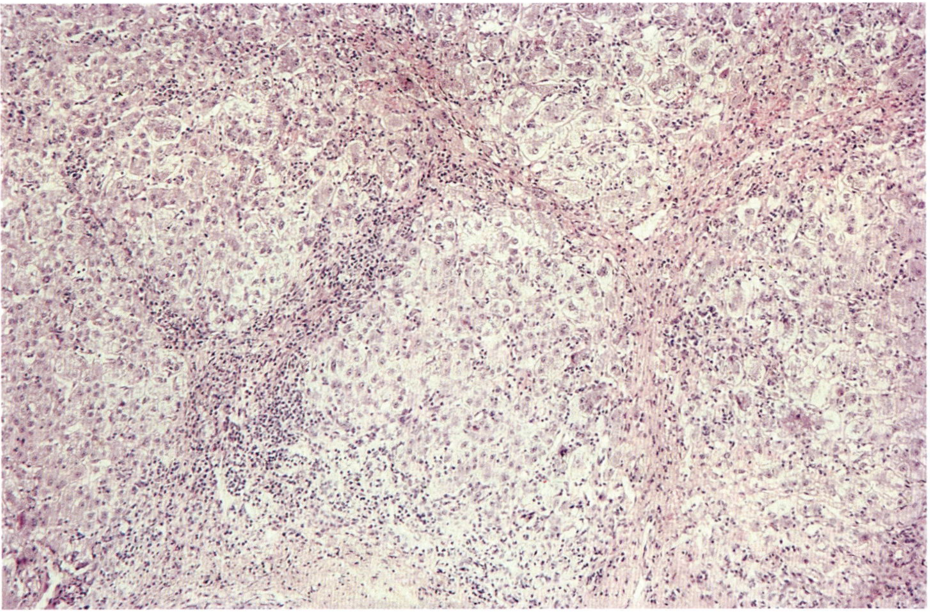

Fig 3.3 Bridging necrosis. Bridges of collapsed connective tissue and inflammatory cells link vascular structures in this example of chronic hepatitis (H&E, ×25).

Portal–portal bridging is quite different in its pathogenesis, arising as a result of widening of the portal tracts by piecemeal necrosis (*see* below). Both may be involved in the development of cirrhosis in chronic hepatitis, but their relative roles are not yet clear (Combes, 1986).

Liver-cell damage and loss results in regenerative hyperplasia of the surviving hepatocytes. This is the probable explanation for the formation of gland-like structures – hepatitic *rosettes* (*see* Fig. 3.1) in areas of severe damage near the portal tracts or, less often, elsewhere in the acini. These rosettes are bounded by compressed sinusoids and connective tissue. Some have visible central lumens homologous with normal bile canaliculi but bounded by a much larger number of hepatocytes.

Other hepatocellular alterations sometimes seen in biopsies from patients with chronic hepatitis include steatosis of the macrovesicular type. This may on occasion reflect underlying risk factors such as obesity or alcohol abuse rather than the hepatitis itself. Hepatocellular siderosis may likewise reflect other factors, notably genetic haemochromatosis. Small amounts of iron, seen mainly in Kupffer cells and endothelial cells, are relatively common in HCV infection. It has been shown that the presence of this iron is associated with more severe hepatitis (Beinker *et al*, 1996). The treatment of HCV infection with interferon (IFN) was associated with a lowering of the iron content, and the authors concluded that the fall was secondary to the decreased inflammatory activity (Boucher *et al*, 1997).

In a minority of patients with chronic hepatitis, some hepatocytes have a homogeneous eosinophilic appearance because of an abundance of closely packed mitochondria. The significance of this oncocytic change (Fig. 3.4) is uncertain (Lefkowitch *et al*, 1980;

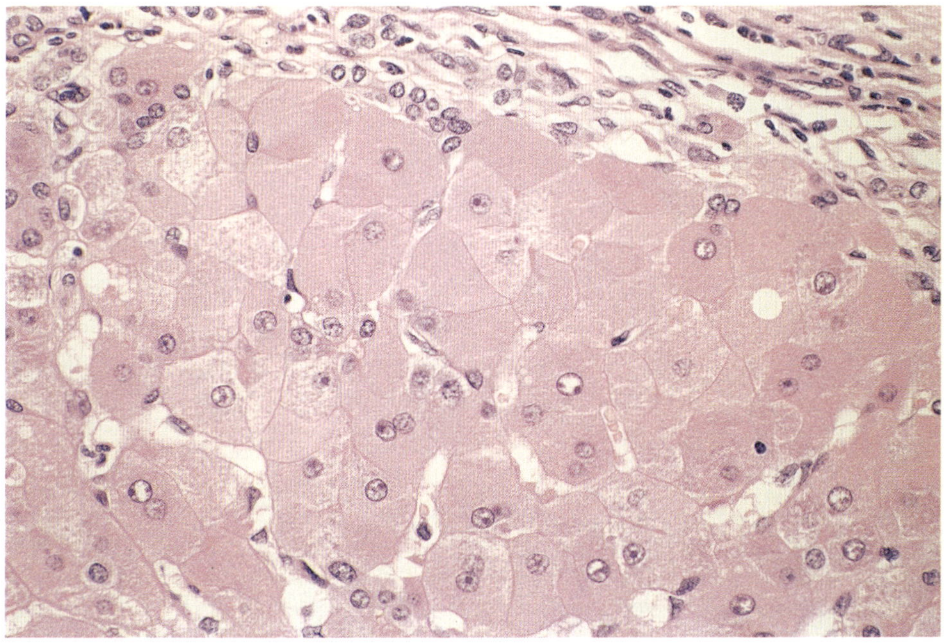

Fig 3.4   Oncocytic change. Hepatocytes in a patient with chronic hepatitis B are large and homogeneously eosinophilic because of abundant mitochondria. Compare this with the ground-glass hepatocytes in Figure 3.14 (H&E, ×100).

Gerber and Thung, 1981). Cholestasis in the form of bile thrombi in canaliculi is a relatively uncommon finding in chronic viral hepatitis and should always arouse suspicion that the hepatitis may be acute rather than chronic, or that there is a separate reason for the cholestasis (e.g. superimposed acute hepatitis, drug idiosyncrasy or biliary tract disease). Granulomas of uncertain cause are occasionally seen in chronic hepatitis, especially hepatitis C (Emile *et al*, 1993; Goldin *et al*, 1996b).

The inflammatory infiltrate that accompanies some of the above changes is predominantly composed of lymphocytes and cells of the macrophage series. As a rule, neutrophils are inconspicuous or absent from the acini except where there has been extensive necrosis. The infiltrate is thought to reflect both the mechanism of hepatocellular damage and its effects. Lymphocytes of CD8+ type are prominent, and their presence has been shown to correlate with increased expression of the adhesion molecule ICAM-1 on hepatocytes (Horiike *et al*, 1993). Various types of macrophage presumably act both as antigen-presenting cells and as scavengers following liver cell death. They may contain yellow-brown pigment of ceroid type, but this is far less prominent than in acute hepatitis. Sinusoidal endothelial cells sometimes contain eosinophilic granules (Iwamura *et al*, 1994).

PERIPORTAL CHANGES

The dominant change in this area is the process long known as piecemeal necrosis (Fig. 3.5). This was first described by Popper and his colleagues in the 1960s as a process related to immunological attack on hepatocytes (Paronetto *et al*, 1962; Popper *et al*,

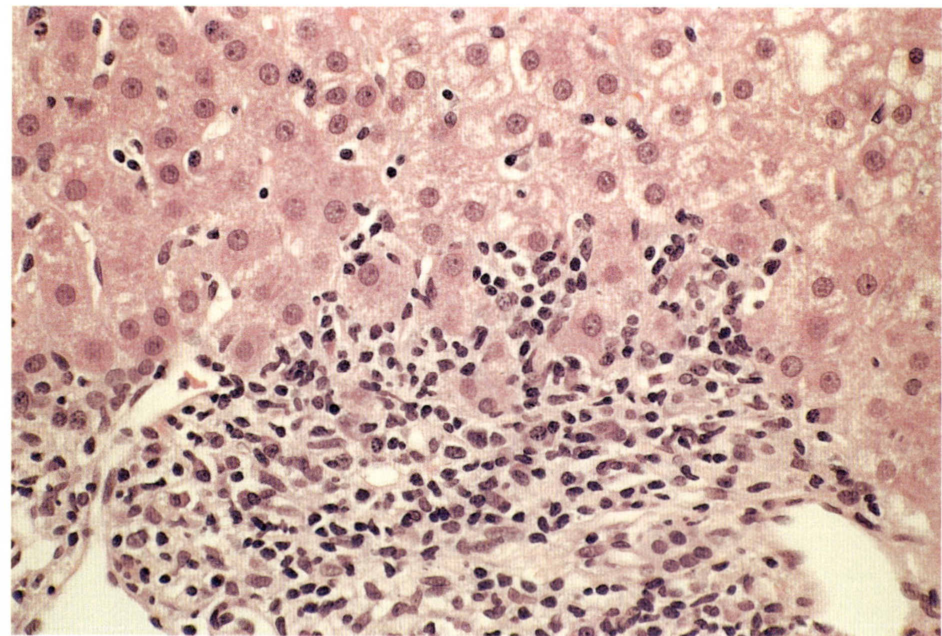

Fig 3.5   Interface hepatitis ('piecemeal necrosis'). The interface between the parenchyma and portal tract is irregular, the limiting plate has been disrupted, and the affected area is infiltrated by inflammatory cells (H&E, ×100).

1965). Later, piecemeal necrosis became the defining feature of chronic active (aggressive) hepatitis in the 1968 classification (De Groote *et al*, 1968). As already noted, the relative importance of this process and of confluent bridging necrosis has been the subject of debate (Combes, 1986). It seems likely that both contribute to the progression of the lesion, to the gradual accumulation of fibrous tissue and to the eventual development of cirrhosis in some patients.

The term 'piecemeal necrosis' was intended to convey the idea that the hepatocyte mass underwent erosion little by little, at the interface between the portal tracts or septa and the parenchyma, an erosion effected by infiltrating lymphoid cells. Later studies have suggested that the main type of liver cell damage is not necrosis but apoptosis (Powell, 1987; Mochizuki *et al*, 1996). For this reason, the term *interface hepatitis* will be used in this chapter in its place, although other authors have continued to use the term 'piecemeal necrosis'. The lesion is best recognised by irregularity of the interface and by the trapping of single and grouped hepatocytes within the inflammatory infiltrate. In assessing the severity of interface hepatitis, both the extent and the depth of the process need to be taken into account, as does the intensity of the infiltrate. The latter is, as already noted, composed mainly of lymphoid cells. These may include both small lymphocytes and plasma cells. CD4+ cells are prominent in areas of interface hepatitis (Mosnier *et al*, 1993).

A second process seen at the interface, but only in the late stages of chronic hepatitis with cirrhosis, is chronic cholestasis (so-called cholate stasis). The periportal or periseptal hepatocytes are swollen and pale-staining, and may contain bile pigment or excessive amounts of copper and copper-associated protein. In chronic biliary tract diseases such as primary biliary cirrhosis and primary sclerosing cholangitis, chronic cholestasis may appear before cirrhosis, as a result of the impaired drainage of bile (Guarascio *et al*, 1983).

PORTAL CHANGES

As in the parenchyma, the inflammatory infiltrate in the portal tracts is mainly composed of lymphocytes, plasma cells and macrophages. Smaller numbers of eosinophils and neutrophils may be seen. The infiltrate may be diffuse throughout the tract, or focal. Lymphoid follicles are common, especially but not exclusively in type C hepatitis (Fig. 3.6). They may contain germinal centres and are easily recognised by their paucity of reticulin fibres even when not obvious in haematoxylin and eosin (H&E)-stained slides (Fig. 3.7). Most portal tracts are inflamed, but the density and distribution of the infiltrate is sometimes uneven, again more in hepatitis C than in hepatitis B. In contrast to the situation in the parenchyma, the portal infiltrate is rich in B-lymphocytes and in CD4+ T-lymphocytes (van den Oord *et al*, 1990).

The small (interlobular) bile ducts often show minor alterations (Fig. 3.8) and occasionally more severe changes. The epithelium may be infiltrated by lymphocytes and show irregular distribution of the epithelial nuclei. In more severe bile duct damage, the epithelium is vacuolated and multilayered, sometimes only for part of the duct circumference. A minor degree of bile duct loss has been reported in hepatitis C (Kaji *et al*, 1994); more severe cholestatic disease is recorded but rare (Lahoti *et al*, 1994).

Ductular proliferation is usually mild or absent in the earlier stages of the disease but is found focally in areas of chronic cholestasis once cirrhosis develops. This corresponds to the ductular type of piecemeal necrosis (Portmann *et al*, 1985).

Granulomas are occasionally found, as in the acini, but are not a characteristic part of the histological picture. In intravenous drug abusers, they may be related to the inadvertent injection of talc (Min *et al*, 1974; Molos *et al*, 1987). This is seen as birefringent

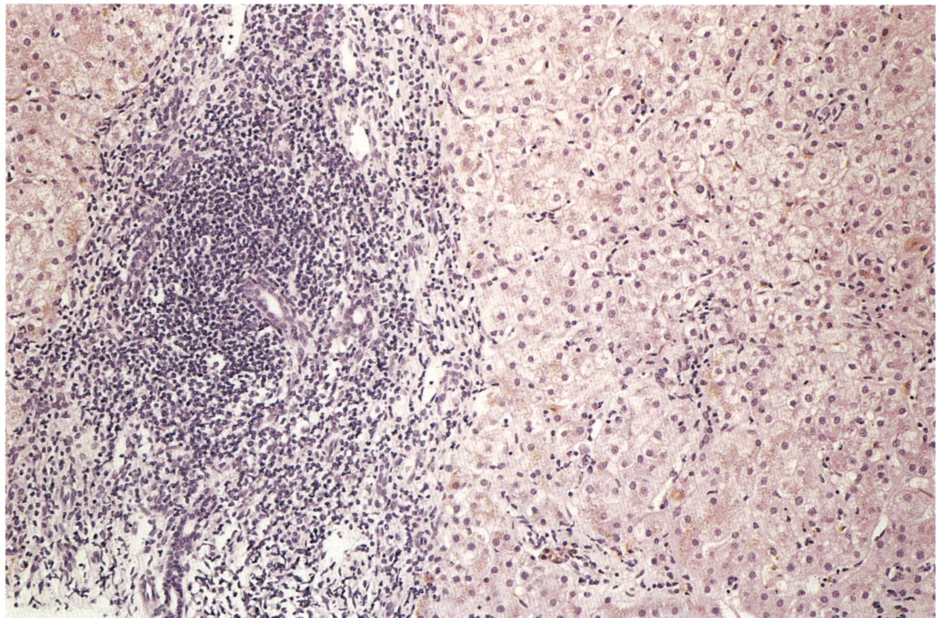

Fig 3.6   Portal inflammation with lymphoid follicle formation. The portal tract in this example of moderately severe chronic hepatitis C contains a lymphocytic follicle. Note the moderate interface hepatitis (H&E, ×40).

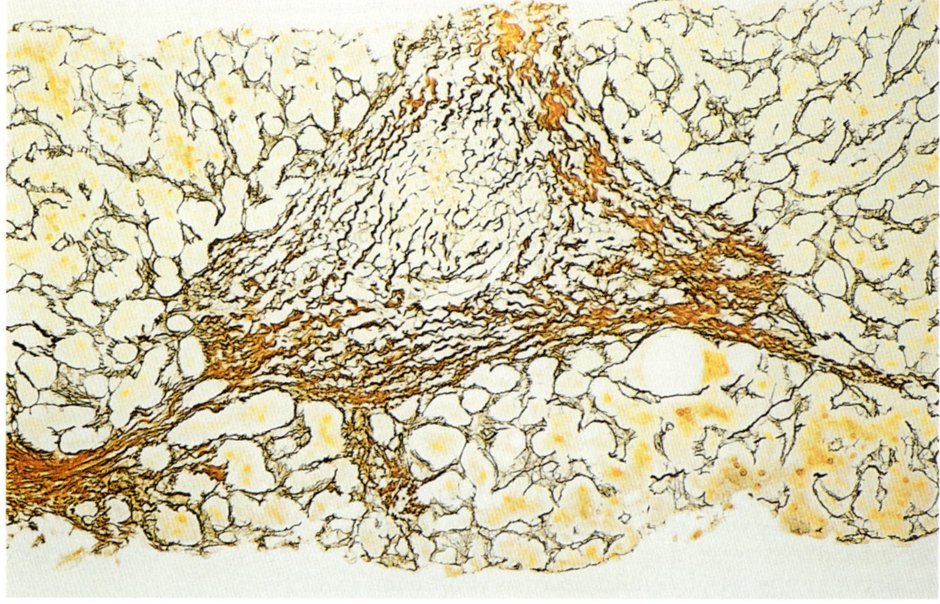

Fig 3.7   Lymphoid follicle formation. The follicle is readily seen as a pale area in this reticulin preparation (untoned reticulin, ×40).

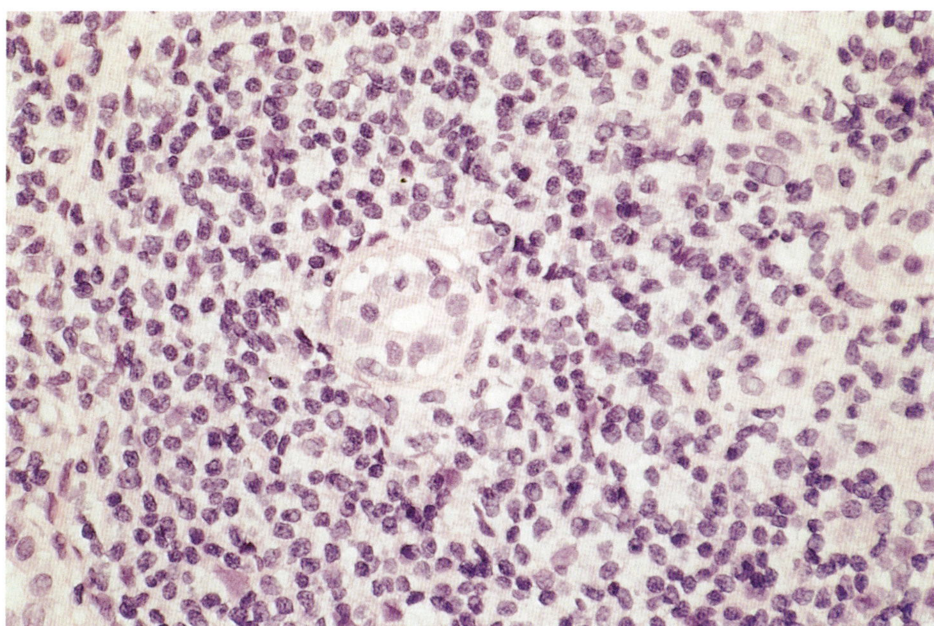

Fig 3.8 Bile duct damage in hepatitis C. A small (interlobular) bile duct at the centre of a lymphocytic infiltrate shows minor degrees of cytoplasmic vacuolation, lymphocytic infiltration and nuclear irregularity (H&E, ×100).

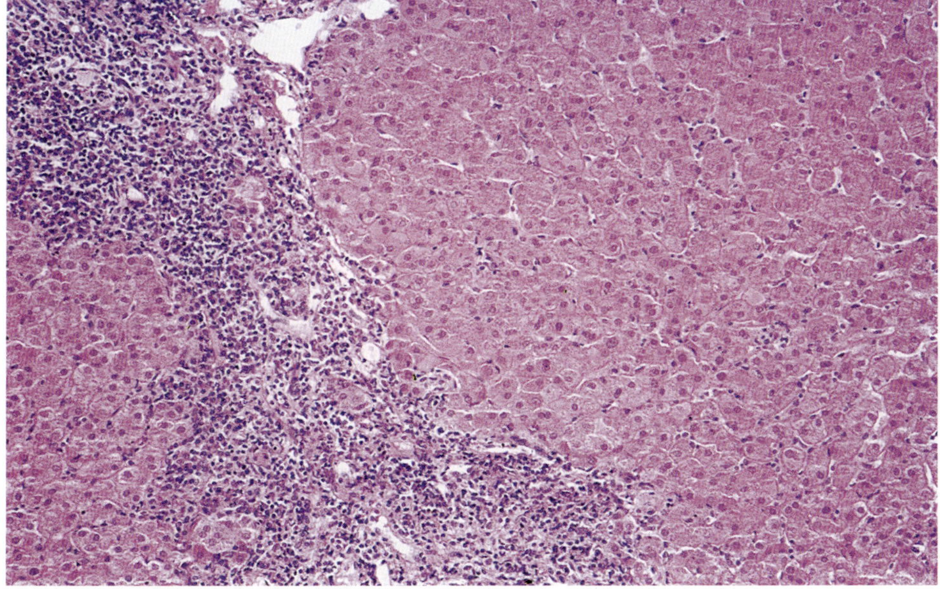

Fig 3.9 Moderately severe chronic hepatitis. The portal tract to the left is densely infiltrated by lymphocytes, and there is interface hepatitis (H&E, ×40).

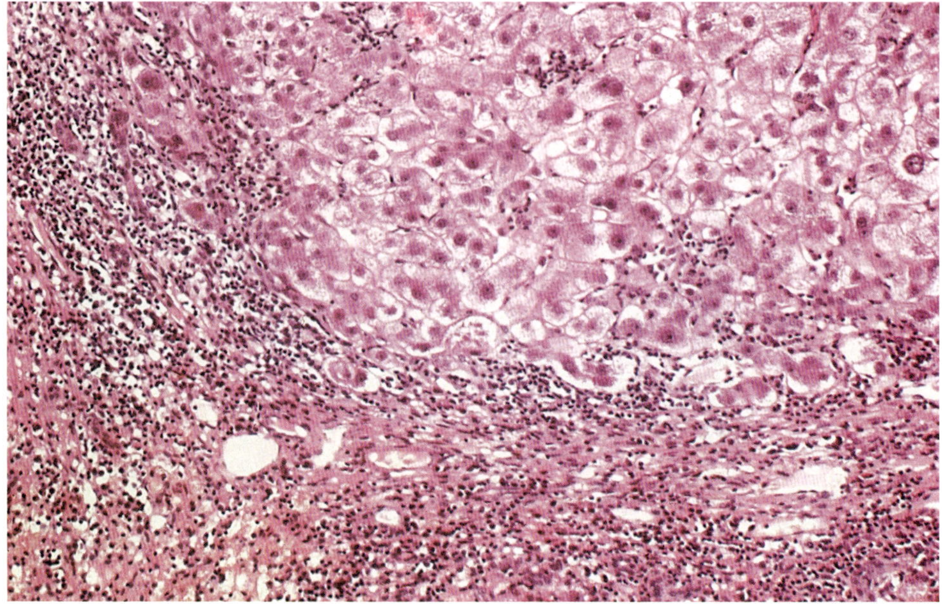

Fig 3.10   Severe chronic hepatitis with cirrhosis. Both septa and parenchyma are inflamed, and nodules have developed (H&E, ×40).

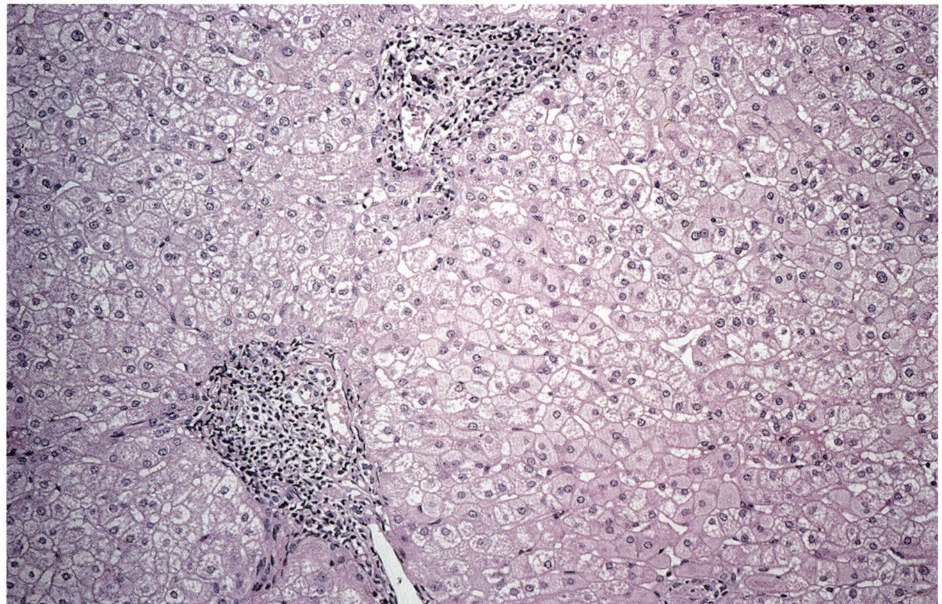

Fig 3.11   Mild chronic hepatitis. In this example, portal tracts are inflamed but the acinar architecture is intact and there is no interface hepatitis or acinar activity. This corresponds to the old category of chronic persistent hepatitis (H&E, ×40).

spicules, sometimes found also in the absence of granulomas (Allaire *et al*, 1989). As already noted, there is an association between hepatitis C and the presence of granulomas.

RELATION OF PORTAL AND PARENCHYMAL CHANGES TO NOMENCLATURE

The above changes are easily related to the old classification of chronic hepatitis. The presence of any degree of interface hepatitis corresponds to a diagnosis of chronic active hepatitis (Figs 3.9 and 3.10). The absence of any significant degree of portal or periportal inflammation, in the presence of acinar changes, corresponds to chronic lobular hepatitis (Popper and Schaffner, 1971) (*see* Fig. 3.2). Portal inflammation, with or without acinar changes but without interface hepatitis, corresponds to chronic persistent hepatitis (Fig. 3.11). As discussed earlier in this chapter, however, the old classification is no longer considered to be the most appropriate basis of nomenclature.

Biopsy diagnosis and semiquantitative assessment

The accurate diagnosis of chronic viral hepatitis requires histological information and hence liver biopsy. Without a liver biopsy, there must necessarily be uncertainty as to the diagnosis and the extent to which a chronic hepatitis has caused structural changes, including cirrhosis. It cannot be assumed that a patient with viral markers and abnormal liver function tests has a chronic hepatitis related to the virus in question. The patient may be a virus carrier with little or no liver damage due to the virus, and at the same time have an entirely different form of liver disease. For example, it is not uncommon for carriers of the hepatitis B virus to have alcohol-related liver damage. Conversely, patients may have evidence of hepatitis virus infection but normal liver function tests; the presence or absence of histological liver damage and the degree of histological activity cannot then be determined without a biopsy (Healey *et al*, 1995). In patients with known chronic viral hepatitis, biopsy helps to establish the absence or presence of cirrhosis, although this is not always easy, especially when the biopsy sample is small. The foregoing remarks indicate that liver biopsy has retained an important place in the management of the patient with chronic viral hepatitis. Indeed, the recent NIH Consensus Meeting on the management of hepatitis C concluded that liver biopsy was critical to deciding whether or not patients should be treated (National Institutes of Health Consensus Development Conference Panel Statement: Management of Hepatitis C, 1997).

The quality of the biopsy sample influences the ease of diagnosis. A Scandinavian study in which progressive lengths of biopsy tissue were uncovered indicated that, whereas in acute hepatitis the lesions were diffuse and a diagnosis could therefore be made on a small piece, classification into chronic persistent and chronic active hepatitis required a length of at least 1.5 cm (Schlichting *et al*, 1983). The recognition of cirrhosis is often very difficult in specimens taken with needles of small calibre. A liver biopsy that includes less than three portal tracts is generally considered to be too small for assessment.

Clinical trials of antiviral therapy have increasingly used histological information as part of the assessment. This has led to the elaboration of several methods for recording the severity and extent of histological changes (Knodell *et al*, 1981; Lok *et al*, 1985; Scheuer, 1991; Bedossa *et al*, 1994; Bianchi and Gudat, 1994). Some of these have been simple (Lok *et al*, 1985; Scheuer, 1991), with low inter- and intra-observer error (Goldin *et al*, 1996a). The most widely used scoring system is the Histological Activity Index (Knodell *et al*, 1981), covering different types of liver cell damage, inflammatory infiltration and structural changes and generating a wide range of scores. This has recently been updated (Ishak *et al*, 1995). Morphometric techniques have also been applied to assessing and predicting disease progression but are unlikely to be widely employed (Kage *et al*, 1997).

The histological features assessed in semiquantitative scoring systems usually include two quite separate groups of changes. The first group comprises hepatocellular damage, cell death and inflammatory infiltration. This may be conveniently described as the necroinflammatory lesion and, as already discussed, constitutes the central lesion of viral hepatitis. The second group is composed of fibrosis and architectural alterations, including cirrhosis. These are obviously related to the necroinflammatory lesion but are currently seen as secondary to it rather than part of the basic hepatitic process. Numerical assessment of the necroinflammatory process is akin to grading as used in tumour pathology, while the structural alterations provide a system of staging, that is to say a measure of the progression of the lesion (Desmet *et al*, 1994). These concepts of grading and staging, as applied to an inflammatory disease rather than to neoplasia, have been incorporated into a modification of the Histological Activity Index (Ishak *et al*, 1995) (Table 3.2). In analysing the results of grading and staging, it is of paramount importance to bear in mind that the numbers generated represent categories rather than measurements. Histological scores are increasingly being used as one of the criteria for deciding which patients with hepatitis C should be treated (National Institutes of Health Consensus Development Conference Panel Statement: Management of Hepatitis C, 1997), and their value is supported by audit of this approach (Foster *et al*, 1997).

Table 3.2 A modified Histological Activity Index (Ishak *et al*, 1995)

Grading	
A Periportal or periseptal interface hepatitis (piecemeal necrosis)	Score 0–4
B Confluent necrosis	Score 0–6
C Focal (spotty) lytic necrosis, apoptosis and focal inflammation	Score 0–4
D Portal inflammation	Score 0–4
Staging	
Architectural changes, fibrosis and cirrhosis	Score 0–6

The differential diagnosis of chronic viral hepatitis

The principal diagnoses to be considered are listed in Table 3.3. The possibility of autoimmune or drug-induced hepatitis should always be considered. While there are no entirely specific histological features of autoimmune hepatitis and a broad spectrum of

Table 3.3 Differential diagnosis of chronic viral hepatitis

Autoimmune hepatitis
Drug-induced hepatitis
Acute viral hepatitis
Primary biliary cirrhosis
Primary sclerosing cholangitis
Overlap syndromes
Chronic hepatitis of unknown cause
Non-specific reactive inflammation

changes may be seen (Dienes *et al*, 1989; Burgart *et al*, 1995), a high level of histological activity is often found in untreated patients. Plasma cells are prominent, and liver cell rosettes of hepatitic type are common. There may be lymphoid follicles, as in hepatitis C (Bach *et al*, 1992). In drug-induced chronic hepatitis, the appearances are those of chronic hepatitis in general; there is likely to be histological activity in patients who continue to receive the offending drug. When acinar activity is high, especially when there is confluent necrosis or canalicular cholestasis, the possibility arises that the hepatitis is acute rather than chronic. Extensive portal and periportal inflammation, and the presence of definite fibrosis, then support the diagnosis of chronic disease. However, it should be noted that it is very easy to mistake recent collapse for fibrosis, and an attempt should be made to assess the age of the septa by means of staining for elastic fibres; these are not normally indentifiable in the acini and only gradually accumulate over a period of several months or years (Scheuer and Maggi, 1980; Thung and Gerber, 1982). As in the case of differentiation from non-specific reactive hepatitis, clinical and serological information is important. In hepatitis A, an acute rather than chronic disease, substantial periportal inflammation and plasma cell infiltration may falsely suggest a diagnosis of chronic hepatitis (Teixeira *et al*, 1982) (*see* Chapter 2).

One of the most common problems faced by the pathologist in chronic hepatitis is its distinction from primary biliary cirrhosis and primary sclerosing cholangitis. This is because interface hepatitis is common in both these diseases (Fig. 3.12). The most helpful single differentiating criterion is ductopenia: duct loss is typical of the later stages of both the biliary diseases but is at most slight in chronic viral hepatitis. Cholestatic features in a non-cirrhotic liver also make biliary disease more likely.

In recent years, several groups of patients have been described with features of both biliary tract disease and the autoimmune type of hepatitis (Brunner and Klinge, 1987; Carrougher *et al*, 1991; Rabinovitz *et al*, 1992; Ben-Ari *et al*, 1993; Horsmans *et al*, 1994; Michieletti *et al*, 1994; Taylor *et al*, 1994; Goodman *et al*, 1995). Some patients have shown a histological picture of primary biliary cirrhosis but an antibody profile characteristic of autoimmune hepatitis. These should probably be considered as having anti-mitochondrial-negative primary biliary cirrhosis. In others, autoantibodies of the kind found in autoimmune hepatitis have been associated wtih the cholangiographic features of primary sclerosing cholangitis (Rabinovitz *et al*, 1992; Wurbs *et al*, 1995). Since interface hepatitis may be seen in such patients and is indeed occasionally severe (Berg *et al*, 1980), these conditions should be considered in the differential diagnosis of chronic viral hepatitis.

In biopsies with mild inflammatory infiltration only, or with at most a few foci of necrosis or apoptosis in the acini, non-specific reaction to nearby space-occupying lesions or to an inflammatory lesion in the portal venous drainage field should be considered. The clinical context and serological data usually clarify this issue.

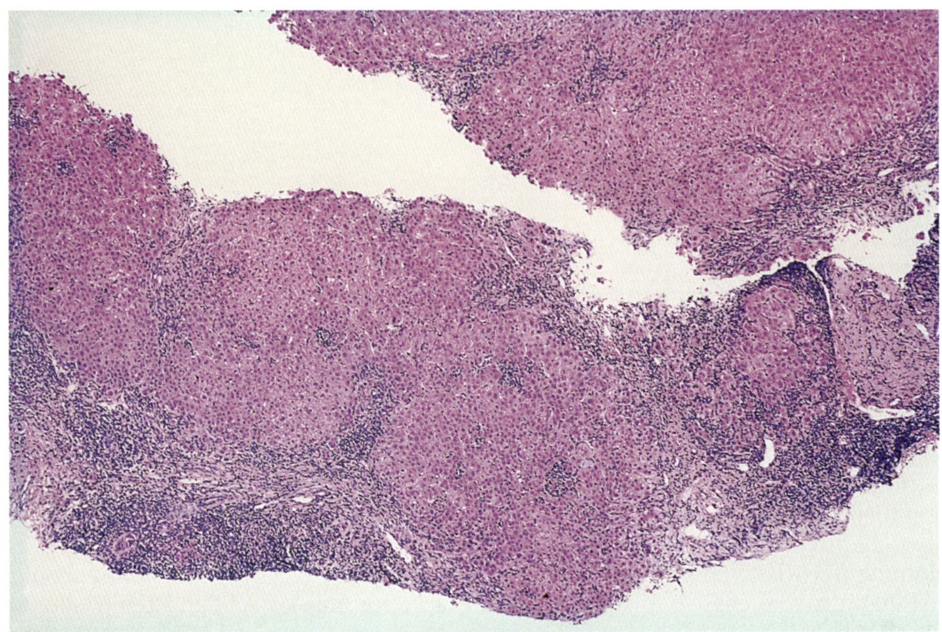

Fig 3.12   Interface hepatitis in primary biliary cirrhosis. Intense inflammatory infiltration and liver cell destruction are seen in this example (H&E, ×16).

Individual causes of chronic viral hepatitis

CHRONIC HEPATITIS B

Like all chronic hepatitis, chronic hepatitis B is characterised by the general histological features discussed above, in various proportions and degrees of severity (Fig. 3.13). There are additional characteristics typical of HBV infection. These are the presence of viral antigens in the hepatocytes and a close association between damaged hepatocytes and lymphocytes. The latter feature is not, however, specific to HBV infection. Clusters of inflammatory cells may be seen around degenerating hepatocytes. Variation in the size of hepatocyte nuclei is common, giving an appearance somewhat like large-cell dysplasia, discussed later in this chapter (Bianchi and Gudat, 1994).

Several viral antigens – the surface antigen HBsAg, the core antigen HBcAg, the e antigen HBeAg and the X antigen HBxAg (Wang *et al*, 1991) – can be demonstrated immunohistochemically (*see* Chapter 4). Of these, HBsAg and HBcAg are routinely stained for in many laboratories, while demonstration of the others generally forms part of specific research projects rather than routine diagnosis. Of the two antigens routinely stained, HBcAg is the more informative because its presence correlates well with viral replication. In particular, strong staining of cytoplasmic HBcAg is associated with active liver cell damage. Nuclear HBcAg sometimes gives the nuclei an even granular appearance ('sanded nuclei') because of the large amounts of viral protein (Bianchi and Gudat,

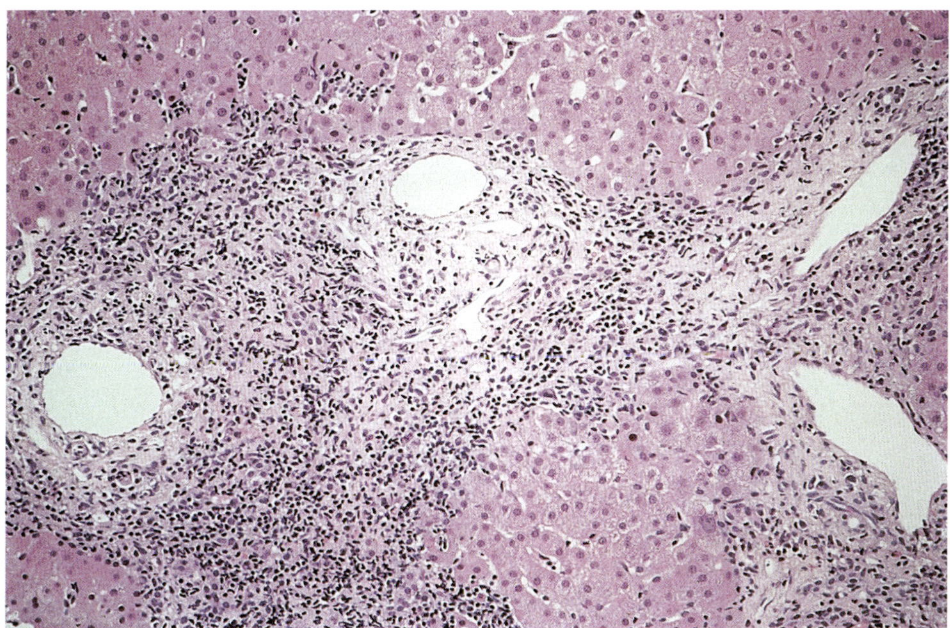

Fig 3.13 Chronic hepatitis B. Heavy inflammatory infiltration and interface hepatitis are associated with seroconversion from HBeAg positivity to the appearance of anti-HBe (H&E, ×40).

1976), but this feature has also been attributed to infection with Delta virus, HDV (*see* below). Immunohistochemical demonstration of HBV antigens in tissue sections of liver in patients with negative serum markers of replication has suggested the existence of disease caused by a 'silent' HBV mutant (Uchida *et al*, 1994a). In cases in which the precore mutant develops, HBcAg can be demonstrated immunohistochemically despite the absence of HBeAg in the serum (or in the liver).

HBsAg, the surface antigen, is usually but not always demonstrable in both the high and low viral replication phases of chronic hepatitis B. It is scanty or absent in many livers at times of intense necroinflammatory activity. It is most abundant in the characteristic *ground-glass hepatocytes*, cells with pale eosinophilic inclusions occupying much of the cytoplasm (Fig. 3.14). A pale-staining artefactual rim separates the inclusions from the remaining cytoplasm at the periphery of the cell. The inclusions consist of endoplasmic reticulum with large amounts of associated viral protein. They can be stained with orcein (Shikata *et al*, 1974), Victoria blue (Tanaka *et al*, 1981) and several other empirical stains as well as by specific antibodies. Ground-glass hepatocytes are usually found singly in the high replication phase of HBV infection, scattered randomly throughout the acini. Later in the course of the disease, when HBV replication is low, clonal clusters of HBsAg-positive cells are sometimes seen. Ground-glass cells are a feature of chronic HBV infection but not of acute hepatitis. Their presence therefore confirms chronicity (Deodhar *et al*, 1975). Differential diagnosis is from oncocytic change (Fig. 3.4), drug-induced hyperplasia of the endoplasmic reticulum, cyanamide toxicity (Vazquez *et al*, 1983; Bruguera *et al*, 1986; Vazquez, 1986), Lafora's disease and fibrinogen storage disease (Callea *et al*, 1986). The correct diagnosis is easily made with the help of staining

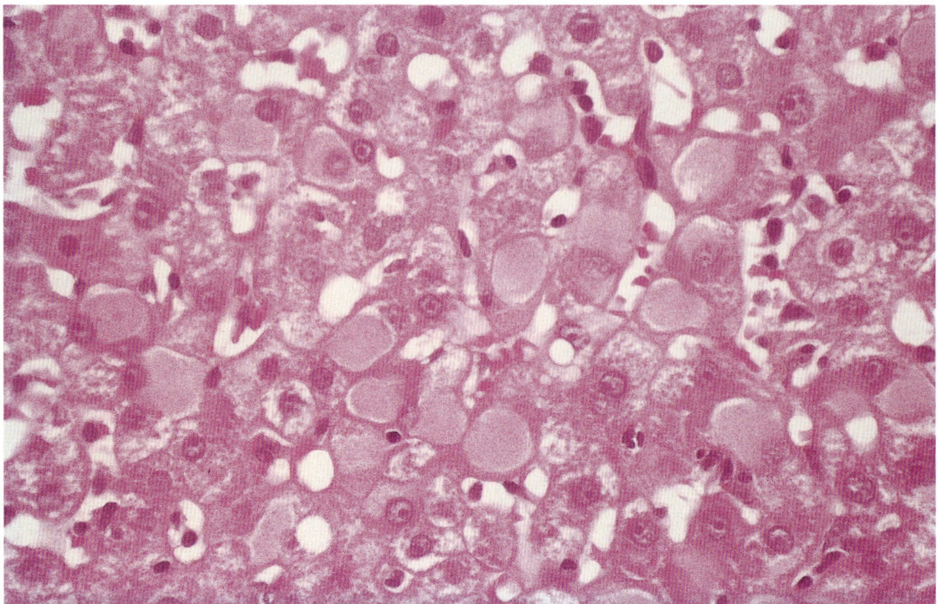

Fig 3.14   Ground-glass hepatocytes in chronic hepatitis B (H&E, ×100).

for HBsAg. Specific immunohistochemical staining also reveals HBsAg in cells without the ground-glass appearance, sometimes in a membranous or submembranous location. Hepatocyte membrane staining for HBsAg by immunofluorescence in frozen sections has been shown to correlate well with viral replication (Chu and Liaw, 1995).

Bianchi, Gudat and colleagues have used the pattern of HBsAg and HBcAg distribution to separate patients with chronic HBV infection into several groups (Gudat *et al*, 1975; Bianchi and Gudat, 1994), shown in Table 3.4. Their four reaction patterns are based on the extent to which the host is able or unable to eliminate the virus. They apply to pure infection with wild-type virus; that is to say, they are substantially modified by superinfection with the Delta virus and by the emergence of mutant strains of HBV (Bianchi and Gudat, 1994). The patterns are part of a shifting, dynamic process in any one patient, changing gradually with the evolution of the disease.

In the *elimination type*, few if any hepatocytes display viral antigens. Immunohistochemical staining reveals at most an occasional cell positive for HBsAg or HBcAg,

Table 3.4   Hepatitis B – basic reaction types of Bianchi and Gudat (Gudat *et al*, 1975; Bianchi and Gudat, 1994)

Type	HBcAg	HBsAg	Typical histology
Elimination	−	−	Acute hepatitis
Generalised HBcAg	++	+ m	Little or no acinar activity
Focal HBcAg	+	++ m	Active inflammation
HBcAg-free HBs	+/−	++ c	Minimal changes

m, predominantly membranous; c, cytoplasmic

usually at an early stage of acute hepatitis before the full immunological attack on the virus is mounted. The histology is that of acute hepatitis.

The remaining three types are characteristic of chronic HBV infection. In the *generalised HBcAg type*, seen in immunosuppressed patients and others with a defective immune response, large amounts of HBcAg are found in hepatocyte nuclei, together with HBsAg mainly in a membranous location at the periphery of the cells. The necroinflammatory lesion is mild (*see* Chapter 5). In the *focal HBcAg type*, seen in histologically active chronic disease, there is focal expression of HBcAg as well as focal or diffuse expression of HBsAg in a membranous location. Cytoplasmic HBsAg may also be seen. Histological activity is inversely related to the tissue expression of HBcAg. Finally, there is the *HBcAg-free HBs type* with mainly cytoplasmic HBsAg and little or no HBcAg or membranous HBsAg. There is no inflammation, and this pattern, representing low viral replication, is seen in carriers with low infectivity. However, HBV DNA may be integrated into the host's hepatocyte nuclei.

A different way of looking at the diversity of histological patterns in chronic HBV infection is to consider the evolution of the lesion with time. This diversity is the result of interacting viral and host factors, modified in some instances by superinfection with other viruses and the emergence of mutant forms of HBV. Chronic hepatitis B characteristically begins with a high viral replication phase, during which histological activity is often low, with or without exacerbations. This is followed after months or years by a wave of histological and biochemical activity designated as seroconversion because HBeAg in the serum is replaced by anti-HBe. At this time, both interface hepatitis and acinar activity are markedly increased. There follows a phase of low virus replication during which the patient is much less infectious, corresponding to Bianchi and Gudat's HBcAg-free HBs type. Histological activity is once again low, but the disease may undergo reactivation (Davis and Hoofnagle, 1985), often as a result of the emergence of HBeAg-negative strains. Finally, HBsAg may disappear from the serum and the only histological changes to be seen are attributable to previous liver damage and inflammation. Active disease in this phase is likely to be the result of other factors such as co-existing infection with the hepatitis C virus.

CHRONIC HEPATITIS D (DELTA INFECTION)

Co-infection or superinfection with this virus may modify the course and severity of chronic hepatitis in various ways (Craig *et al*, 1986; Govindarajan *et al*, 1986; Verme *et al*, 1986; Lin *et al*, 1989). Co-infection encourages a chronic course of both infections. Superinfection usually leads to increased severity of the histological lesion. Interface hepatitis is severe, and the development of cirrhosis is accelerated. There may be extensive acinar activity. Occasionally, superinfection by the Delta virus of a patient with chronic HBV infection leads to a fulminant clinical course. The presence of viral antigen in liver cell nuclei can easily be demonstrated immunohistochemically. The 'sanded' appearance of nuclei already noted in HBV infection has also been attributed to large numbers of Delta virus particles (Moreno *et al*, 1989). Immunohistochemical staining has a vital role to play in the diagnosis of Delta virus infection (*see* Chapter 4).

CHRONIC HEPATITIS C

Chronic hepatitis C has a number of histological characteristics that give it an easily recognisable although not completely diagnostic appearance (Table 3.5) (Bach *et al*, 1992; Gerber *et al*, 1992; Scheuer *et al*, 1992; Lefkowitch *et al*, 1993). Histological

Table 3.5   Histological characteristics of chronic hepatitis C

Acute and chronic disease may look similar
Lesion often mild, but cirrhosis is common
Lymphoid follicles
Damaged small bile ducts
Acinar activity, apoptosis
Lymphocytes in acini
Steatosis

severity correlates poorly with liver function tests (Healey *et al*, 1995). Many biopsies show mild disease, with portal inflammation but little or no interface hepatitis and a variable acinar component. The portal lesion is dominated by the presence of lymphoid follicles (*see* Fig. 3.6), ranging from a vague aggregation of the lymphocytic infiltrate to well-formed follicles with obvious germinal centres. These contain activated B-cells, around which are follicular dendritic cells and a B-cell mantle zone (Mosnier *et al*, 1993). CD4+ cells are prominent in the outer T-cell zone (Hino *et al*, 1992). The follicles are easily detected in reticulin preparations (*see* Fig. 3.7). Small bile ducts within or at one side of the infiltrate may show various degrees of abnormality, including lymphocytic infiltration, cytoplasmic vacuolation, nuclear irregularity and crowding of the epithelial cells (*see* Fig. 3.8). In the most severe cases, part of the circumference of the duct is multilayered, vacuolated and inflamed. The loss of ducts has been reported (Bach *et al*, 1992) but is rarely substantial (Kaji *et al*, 1994); this helps to distinguish chronic hepatitis C from biliary diseases such as primary biliary cirrhosis and primary sclerosing cholangitis. Lymphoid follicles and damaged bile ducts are not found in all biopsies from patients with chronic HCV infection. When present, they are also not fully diagnostic because they may be found in other diseases such as hepatitis B (Scheuer *et al*, 1992) and autoimmune hepatitis (Bach *et al*, 1992).

Within the acini, there is variable, sometimes intense, activity (Fig. 3.15). Focal acidophilic change of hepatocytes is seen, and apoptotic bodies (Councilman bodies, acidophil bodies) may be abundant. Apoptosis has also been demonstrated by means of the immunohistochemical detection of Fas antigen (Hiramatsu *et al*, 1994). Fatty change is common, and the combination of bile duct damage, lymphoid follicles and fat is highly characteristic of HCV (Lefkowitch *et al*, 1993). Clumped intracytoplasmic inclusions resembling Mallory bodies are occasionally found in periportal hepatocytes. There is focal infiltration by lymphocytes and macrophages, often around an area of liver cell loss. In some patients, sinusoids are diffusely infiltrated with lymphocytes. Granulomas of uncertain cause have been reported (Emile *et al*, 1993; Okuno *et al*, 1995; Goldin *et al*, 1996b).

Cirrhosis develops in a high proportion of patients with chronic HCV infection (Vaquer *et al*, 1994). Its characteristics are those of cirrhosis following any type of viral hepatitis, but lymphoid follicles often persist (Fig. 3.16).

A number of studies have been carried out into the possible different histological effects of the different genotypes of HCV. A recent study concluded that there were no major differences but that genotype 3a was associated with more fatty change and bile duct damage and that genotype 1b was associated with more advanced fibrosis and also increased disease duration (Mihm *et al*, 1997).

Many efforts have been made to demonstrate viral antigens in tissue sections by means of a variety of antibodies to various structural and non-structural components of the virus (Hiramatsu *et al*, 1992; Krawczynski *et al*, 1992; Yamada *et al*, 1993; Blight *et al*, 1994;

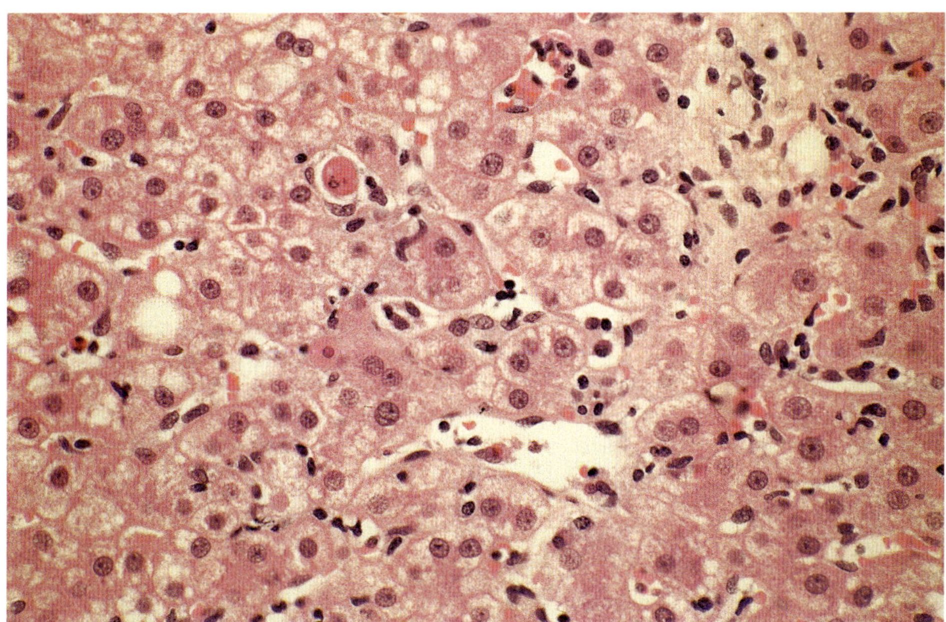

Fig 3.15 Acinar activity in chronic hepatitis C. Liver cell plates are irregular, and there is a predominantly lymphocytic infiltrate. A rounded acidophil body with nuclear remnant is seen above and to the left. There is mild steatosis (H&E, ×100).

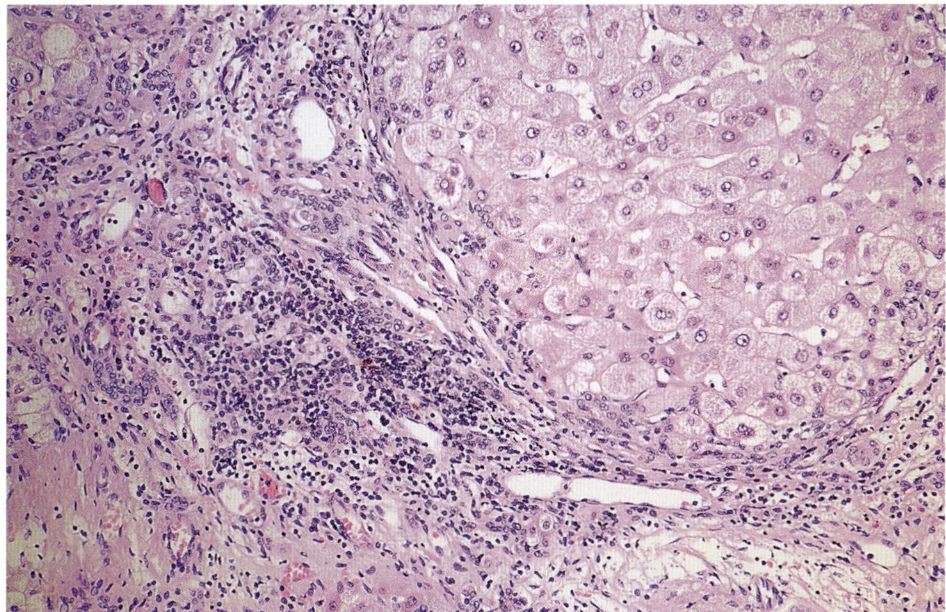

Fig 3.16 Hepatitis C with cirrhosis. The disease is still histologically active. An ill-defined lymphoid aggregate is seen (H&E, ×40).

Yap *et al*, 1994) (*see* Chapter 4). Some of these have been successful in cryostat sections and occasionally also in paraffin-embedded material (Blight *et al*, 1993; Uchida *et al*, 1994b). There have also been attempts to use in situ hybridisation to identify the virus (Haruna *et al*, 1993; Tanaka *et al*, 1993; Yamada *et al*, 1993). Neither immunohistochemical staining nor in situ hybridisation has a diagnostic role to play at the present time (Scheuer *et al*, 1997).

OTHER FORMS OF CHRONIC VIRAL HEPATITIS

The role of a flavivirus designated hepatitis G virus (HGV) or GBV-C in the causation of chronic hepatitis remains to be established. It is commonly found in the serum of patients at risk of parenteral transmission (Linnen *et al*, 1996) (*see* Chapter 1). In a detailed histological study comparing cases of HCV with or without HGV, no difference was seen in the grade or stage of the disease, the individual components of their Knodell scores or specific histological features (Bralet *et al*, 1997). However, Manolakopoulos *et al* (1998) noted more portal and periportal inflammation in patients with double infection.

Sequelae of chronic viral hepatitis

The end result of chronic viral infection depends on the extent of liver cell damage, fibrosis and regeneration, and on the persistence of viral infection. In a patient whose infection is terminated, either spontaneously or as a result of treatment, there may be little or

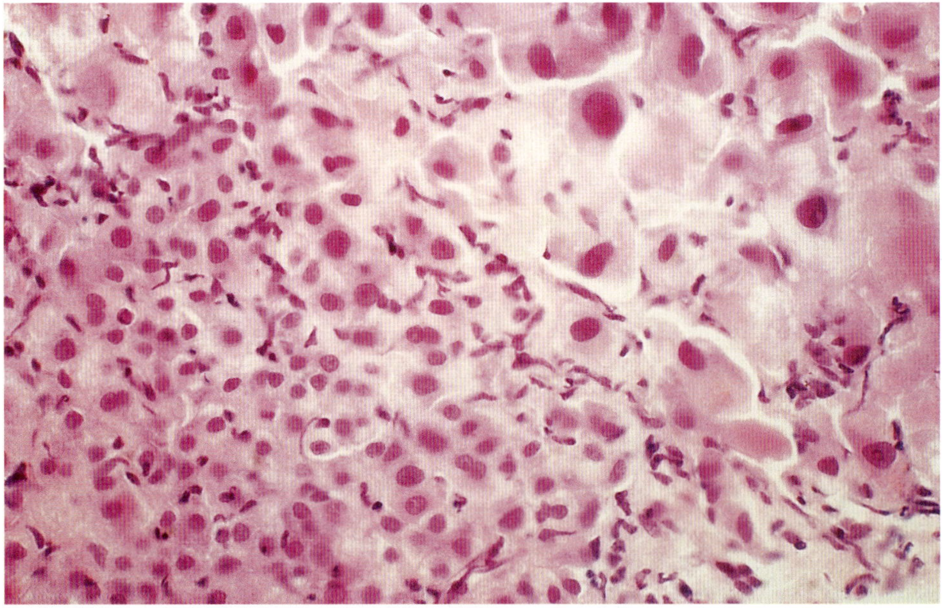

Fig 3.17 Hepatocellular dysplasia. The large-cell type is seen above and to the right; below and to the left there is small-cell dysplasia, characterised by the crowding of small hepatocytes with increased nuclear:cytoplasmic ratio (H&E, ×100).

no structural change in the liver if the disease has been mild throughout. Alternatively, episodes of necrosis, collapse, fibrosis and regeneration may have led to cirrhosis or to structural alterations short of cirrhosis. In patients with cirrhosis, and in a smaller number of patients without cirrhosis, hepatocellular carcinoma may develop (*see* Chapter 8).

Once cirrhosis has developed and also sometimes before it is established, hepatocellular dysplasia may be seen on biopsy (Fig. 3.17). The type first described (Anthony *et al*, 1973) is now known as large-cell dysplasia. In this type, the hepatocytes are enlarged, with large irregular nuclei and a normal or slightly increased nuclear:cytoplasmic ratio. There is evidence to suggest that large-cell dysplasia denotes an increased risk of the development of hepatocellular carcinoma (Borzio *et al*, 1991). It is most often seen in patients with chronic HBV infection but is by no means confined to them, and it may also be found in chronic HCV infection.

In small-cell dysplasia, the hepatocytes are smaller than normal, with an increased nuclear:cytoplasmic ratio (Crawford, 1990). This gives an appearance somewhat like that of regenerating parenchyma. Like large-cell dysplasia, small-cell dysplasia is regarded as a possible indicator of the risk of hepatocellular carcinoma. However, the exact significance and natural history of the two forms of dysplasia is not yet clear, although in many centres patients with dysplasia are more closely followed up with serial alphafetoprotein measurements and ultrasound.

References

Alison, M.R., Sarraf, C.E. 1994: Liver cell death: patterns and mechanisms. *Gut* **35**, 577–81.

Allaire, G.S., Goodman, Z.D., Ishak, K.G., Rabin, L. 1989: Talc in liver tissue of intravenous drug abusers with chronic hepatitis. A comparative study. *American Journal of Clinical Pathology* **92**, 583–8.

Anthony, P.P., Vogel, C.L., Barker, L.F. 1973: Liver cell dysplasia: a premalignant condition. *Journal of Clinical Pathology* **26**, 217–23.

Bach, N., Thung, S.N., Schaffner, F. 1992: The histological features of chronic hepatitis C and autoimmune chronic hepatitis: a comparative analysis. *Hepatology* **15**, 572–7.

Bedossa, P., Bioulac-Sage, P., Callard, P. *et al*. 1994: Intraobserver and interobserver variations in liver biopsy interpretation in patients with chronic hepatitis C. *Hepatology* **20**, 15–20.

Beinker, N.K., Voigt, M.D., Arendse, M., Smit, J., Stander, I.A., Kirsch, R.E. 1996: Threshold effect of liver iron content on hepatic inflammation and fibrosis in hepatitis B and C. *Journal of Hepatology* **25**, 633–8.

Ben-Ari, Z., Dhillon, A.P., Sherlock, S. 1993: Autoimmune cholangiopathy: part of the spectrum of autoimmune chronic active hepatitis. *Hepatology* **18**, 10–15.

Berg, P.A., Wiedmann, K.H., Sayers, T., Klopppel, G., Lindner, H. 1980: Serological classification of chronic cholestatic liver disease by the use of two different types of antimitochondrial antibodies. *Lancet* **ii**, 1329–32.

Bianchi, L., Gudat, F. 1976: Sanded nuclei in hepatitis B: eosinophilic inclusions in liver cell nuclei due to excess in hepatitis B core antigen formation. *Laboratory Investigation* **35**, 1–5.

Bianchi, L., Gudat, F. 1994: Chronic hepatitis. In MacSween, R.N.M., Anthony, P.P., Scheuer, P.J., Portmann, B., Burt, A.D. (eds) *Pathology of the liver*, 3rd edn. Edinburgh: Churchill Livingstone.

Blight, K., Rowland, R., Hall, P. de la M. *et al*. 1993: Immunohistochemical detection of the NS4 antigen of hepatitis C virus and its relation to histopathology. *American Journal of Pathology* **143**, 1568–73.

Blight, K., Lesniewski, R.R., LaBrooy, J.T., Gowans, E.J. 1994: Detection and distribution of hepatitis C-specific antigens in naturally infected liver. *Hepatology* **20** 553–7.

Borzio, M., Bruno, S., Roncalli, M. *et al.* 1991: Liver cell dysplasia and risk of hepatocellular carcinoma in cirrhosis: a preliminary report. *British Medical Journal* **302**, 1312.

Boucher, E., Bourienne, A., Adams, P., Turkin, B., Brisat, P., Deugnier, Y. 1997: Liver iron concentration and distribution in chronic hepatitis C before and after interferon treatment. *Gut* **41**, 115–20.

Boyer, J.L., Klatskin, G. 1970: Pattern of necrosis in acute viral hepatitis. Prognostic value of bridging (subacute hepatic necrosis). *New England Journal of Medicine* **283**, 1063–71.

Bralet, M.-P., Radot-Thoraud, F., Pawlotsky, J.-M. *et al.* 1997: Histopathologic impact of GB virus C infection on chronic hepatitis C. *Gastroenterology* **112**, 188–92.

Bruguera, M., Lamar, C., Bernet, M., Rodes, J. 1986: Hepatic disease associated with ground-glass inclusions in hepatocytes after cyanamide therapy. *Archives of Pathology and Laboratory Medicine* **110**, 906–10.

Brunner, G., Klinge, O. 1987: Ein der chronisch-destruierenden nicht-eitrigen Cholangitis ähnliches Krankheitsbild mit antinukleären Antikörpern (Immuncholangitis). *Deutsche Medizinische Wochenschrift* **112**, 1454–8.

Buja, L.M., Eigenbrodt, M.L., Eigenbrodt, E.H. 1993: Apoptosis and necrosis. Basic types and mechanisms of cell death. *Archives of Pathology and Laboratory Medicine* **117**, 1208–14.

Burgart, L.J., Batts, K.P., Ludwig, J., Nikias, G.A., Czaja, A.J. 1995: Recent onset autoimmune hepatitis. Biopsy findings and clinical correlations. *American Journal of Surgical Pathology* **19**, 699–708.

Callea, F., De Vos, R., Togni, R., Tardanico, R., Vanstapel, M.J., Desmet, V.J. 1986: Fibrinogen inclusions in liver cells: a new type of ground-glass hepatocyte. Immune light and electron microscopic characterization. *Histopathology* **10**, 65–73.

Carrougher, J.G., Shaffer, R.T., Canales, L.I., Goodman, Z.D. 1991: A 33-year-old woman with an autoimmune syndrome. *Seminars in Liver Disease* **11**, 256–62.

Chu, C.-M., Liaw, Y.-F. 1995: Membrane staining for hepatitis B surface antigen on hepatocytes: a sensitive and specific marker of active viral replication in hepatitis B. *Journal of Clinical Pathology* **48**, 470–3.

Combes, B. 1986: The initial morphologic lesion in chronic hepatitis, important or unimportant? *Hepatology* **6**, 518–22.

Craig, J.R., Govindarajan, S., DeCock, K.M. 1986: Delta viral hepatitis. Histopathology and course. *Pathology Annual* **21** (part 2), 1–21.

Crawford, J.M. 1990: Pathologic assessment of liver cell dysplasia and benign liver tumors: differentiation from malignant tumors. *Seminars in Diagnostic Pathology* **7**, 115–28.

Czaja, A.J. 1993: Chronic active hepatitis: the challenge for a new nomenclature. *Annals of Internal Medicine* **119**, 510–17.

Davis, G.L., Hoofnagle, J.H. 1985: Reactivation of chronic type B hepatitis presenting as acute viral hepatitis. *Annals of Internal Medicine* **102**, 762–5.

De Groote, J., Desmet, V.J., Gedigk, P. *et al.* 1968: A classification of chronic hepatitis. *Lancet* **ii**, 626–8.

Deodhar, K.P., Tapp, E., Scheuer, P.J. 1975: Orcein staining of hepatitis B antigen in paraffin sections of liver biopsies. *Journal of Clinical Pathology* **28**, 66–70.

Desmet, V.J., Gerber, M., Hoofnagle, J.H., Manns, M., Scheuer, P.J. 1994: Classification of chronic hepatitis: diagnosis, grading and staging. *Hepatology* **19**, 1513–20.

Dienes, H.P., Popper, H., Manns, M., Baumann, W., Thoenes, W., Meyer zum Büschenfelde, K.H. 1989: Histologic features in autoimmune hepatitis. *Zeitschrift für Gastroenterologie* **27**, 325–30.

Emile, J.F., Sebagh, M., Féray, C., David, F., Reynès, M. 1993: The presence of epithelioid granulomas in hepatitis C virus-related cirrhosis. *Human Pathology* **24**, 1095–7.

Foster, G.R., Goldin, R.D., Main, J., Murray-Lyon, I., Hargreaves, S., Thomas, H.C. 1997: Management of chronic hepatitis C: clinical audit of biopsy based management algorithm. *British Medical Journal* **315**, 453–8.

Gerber, M.A., Thung, S.N. 1981: Hepatitic oncocytes. Incidence, staining characteristics, and ultrastructural features. *American Journal of Clinical Pathology* **75**, 498–503.

Gerber, M.A., Krawczynski, K., Alter, M.J., Sampliner, R.E., Margolis, H.S. and Sentinel counties chronic non-A, non-B hepatitis study team 1992: Histopathology of community acquired chronic hepatitis C. *Modern Pathology* **5**, 483–6.

Goldin, R.D., Goldin, J.G., Burt, A.D. *et al.* 1996a: Intra-observer and inter-observer variation in the histopathological assessment of chronic viral hepatitis. *Journal of Hepatology* **25**, 649–54.

Goldin, R.D., Levine, T.S., Foster, G.R., Thomas, H.C. 1996b: Granulomas and hepatitis C. *Histopathology* **28**, 265–7.

Goodman, Z.D., McNally, P.R., Davis, D.R., Ishak, K.G. 1995: Autoimmune cholangitis: a variant of primary biliary cirrhosis. Clinicopathologic and serologic correlations in 200 cases. *Digestive Diseases and Sciences* **40**, 1232–42.

Govindarajan, S., De-Cock, K.M., Redeker, A.G. 1986: Natural course of delta superinfection in chronic hepatitis B virus-infected patients: histopathologic study with multiple liver biopsies. *Hepatology* **6**, 640–4.

Guarascio, P., Yentis, F., Cevikbas, U., Portmann, B., Williams, R. 1983: Value of copper-associated protein in diagnostic assessment of liver biopsy. *Journal of Clinical Pathology* **36**, 18–23.

Gudat, F., Bianchi, L., Sonnabend, W., Thiel, G., Aenishaenslin, W., Stalder, G.A. 1975: Pattern of core and surface expression in liver tissue reflects state of specific immune response in hepatitis B. *Laboratory Investigation* **32**, 1–9.

Haruna, Y., Hayashi, N., Hiramatsu, N. *et al.* 1993: Detection of hepatitis C virus RNA in liver tissues by an in situ hybridization technique. *Journal of Hepatology* **18**, 96–100.

Healey, C.J., Chapman, R.W.G., Fleming, K.A. 1995: Liver histology in hepatitis C infection: a comparison between patients with persistently normal or abnormal transaminases. *Gut* **37**, 274–8.

Hino, K., Okuda, M., Konishi, T. *et al.* 1992: Analysis of lymphoid follicles in liver of patients with chronic hepatitis C. *Liver* **12**, 387–91.

Hiramatsu, N., Hayashi, N., Haruna, Y. *et al.* 1992: Immunohistochemical detection of hepatitis C virus-infected hepatocytes in chronic liver disease with monoclonal antibodies to core, envelope and NS3 regions of the hepatitis C virus genome. *Hepatology* **16**, 306–11.

Hiramatsu, N., Hayashi, N., Katayama, K. *et al.* 1994: Immunohistochemical detection of Fas antigen in liver tissue of patients with chronic hepatitis C. *Hepatology* **19**, 1354–9.

Horiike, N., Onji,M., Kumon, I., Kanaoka, M., Michitaka, K., Ohta, Y. 1993: Intercellular adhesion molecule-1 expression on the hepatocyte membrane of patients with chronic hepatitis B and C. *Liver* **13**, 10–14.

Horsmans, Y., Piret, A., Brenard, R., Rahier, J., Geubel, A.P. 1994: Autoimmune chronic active hepatitis responsive to immunosuppressive therapy evolving into a typical primary biliary cirrhosis syndrome: a case report. *Journal of Hepatology* **21**, 194–8.

International Group 1977: Acute and chronic hepatitis revisited. *Lancet* **ii**, 914–19.

International Working Party 1994: Terminology of chronic hepatitis, hepatic allograft rejection, and nodular lesions of the liver: summary of recommendations developed by an international working party, supported by the World Congresses of Gastroenterology, Los Angeles, 1994. *American Journal of Gastroenterology* **89**, S177–S181.

Ishak, K.G. 1994: Chronic hepatitis: morphology and nomenclature. *Modern Pathology* **7**, 690–713.

Ishak, K.G., Baptista, A., Bianchi, L. *et al.* 1995: Histological grading and staging of chronic hepatitis. *Journal of Hepatology* **22**, 696–9.

Iwamura, S., Enzan, H., Saibara, T., Onishi, S., Yamamoto, Y. 1994: Appearance of sinusoidal inclusion-containing endothelial cells in liver disease. *Hepatology* **20**, 604–10.

Kage, M., Shimamatu, K., Nakashima, E., Kojiro, M., Inoue, O., Yano, M. 1997: Long-term evolution of fibrosis from chronic hepatitis to cirrhosis in patients with hepatitis C: morphometric analysis of repeated biopsies. *Hepatology* **25**, 1028–31.

Kaji, K., Nakanuma, Y., Sasaki, M. *et al.* 1994: Hepatitic bile duct injuries in chronic hepatitis C: histopathologic and immunhistochemical studies. *Modern Pathology* **7**, 937–45.

Knodell, R.G., Ishak, K.G., Black, W.C. *et al.* 1981: Formulation and application of a numerical scoring system for assessing histological activity in asymptomatic chronic active hepatitis. *Hepatology* **1**, 431–5.

Krawczynski, K., Beach, M.J., Bradley, D.W. *et al.* 1992: Hepatitis C virus antigen in hepatocytes: immunomorphologic detection and identification. *Gastroenterology* **103**, 622–9.

Lahoti, S., Murakami, C., Casey, D., Lee, W.M. 1994: Is there a cholestatic variant of hepatitis C? *Hepatology* **20**, 254A (abstract).

Leevy, C.M., Sherlock, S., Tygstrup, N., Zetterman, R. 1994: *Diseases of the liver and biliary tract. Standardization of nomenclature, diagnostic criteria, and prognosis.* New York: Raven Press.

Lefkowitch, J.H., Arborgh, B.A., Scheuer, P.J. 1980: Oxyphilic granular hepatocytes. Mitochondrion-rich liver cells in hepatic disease. *American Journal of Clinical Pathology* **74**, 432–41.

Lefkowitch, J.H., Schiff, E.R., Davis, G.L. *et al.* and the Hepatitis Interventional Therapy Group 1993: Pathological diagnosis of chronic hepatitis C: a multicenter comparative study with chronic hepatitis B. *Gastroenterology* **104**, 595–603.

Lin, H.-H., Liaw, Y.-F., Chen, T.-J., Chu, C.-M., Huang, M.-J. 1989: Natural course of patients with chronic type B hepatitis following acute hepatitis delta virus superinfection. *Liver* **9**, 129–34.

Linnen, J., Wages, J.J., Zhang-Keck, Z.-Y. *et al.* 1996: Molecular cloning and disease association of hepatitis G virus: a transfusion-transmissible agent. *Science* **271**, 505–8.

Lok, A.S.F., Lindsay, I., Scheuer, P.J., Thomas, H.C. 1985: Clinical and histological features of delta infection in chronic hepatitis B virus carriers. *Journal of Clinical Pathology* **38**, 530–3.

Manolakopoulos, S., Morris, A., Davies, S., Brown, D., Hajat, S., Dusheiko, G. 1998: Influence of GB virus C viraemia on the clinical, virological and histological features of early hepatitis C-related hepatic disease. *Journal of Hepatology* **28**, 173–8.

Meeting Report 1993: International autoimmune hepatitis group. *Hepatology* **18**, 998–1005.

Michieletti, P., Wanless, I.R., Katz, A. *et al.* 1994: Are patients with antimitochondrial antibody negative primary biliary cirrhosis a distinct syndrome of autoimmune cholangitis? *Gut* **35**, 260–5.

Mihm, S., Fayyazi, A., Hartmann, H., Ramadori, G. 1997: Analysis of histopathological manifestations of chronic hepatitis C virus infection with respect to virus genotype. *Hepatology* **25**, 735–9.

Min, K.W., Gyorkey, F., Cain, G.D. 1974: Talc granulomata in liver disease in narcotic addicts. *Archives of Pathology* **98**, 331–5.

Mochizuki, K., Hayashi, N., Hiramatsu, N. *et al.* 1996: Fas antigen expression in liver tissues of patients with chronic hepatitis B. *Journal of Hepatology* **24**, 1–7.

Molos, M.A., Litton, N., Schubert, T.T. 1987: Talc liver. *Journal of Clinical Gastroenterology* **9**, 198–203.

Moreno, A., Ramón y Cahal, S., Marazuela, M. *et al.* 1989: Sanded nuclei in delta patients. *Liver* **9**, 367–71.

Mosnier, J.-F., Degott, C., Marcellin, P., Hénin, D., Erlinger, S., Benhamou, J.-P. 1993: The intra-portal lymphoid nodule and its environment in chronic active hepatitis C: an immunohisto-chemical study. *Hepatology* **17**, 366–71.

National Institutes of Health Consensus Development Conference Panel Statement: Management of Hepatitis C. 1997: *Hepatology* **26** (Suppl 1), 25–105.

Okuno, T., Shindo, M., Arai, K., Matsumoto, M., Takeda, M. 1990: Histological improvement of chronic hepatitis B, and non-A, non-B with interferon treatment: application of a numerical scoring system for evaluating sequential morphologic changes. *Gastroenterologica Japonica* **25**, 70–7.

Okuno, T., Arai, K., Matsumoto, M., Shindo, M. 1995: Epithelioid granulomas in chronic hepatitis C: a transient pathological feature. *Journal of Gastroenterology and Hepatology* **10**, 532–7.

Paronetto, F., Rubin, E., Popper, H. 1962: Local formation of gamma-globulin in the diseased liver, and its relation to hepatic necrosis. *Laboratory Investigation* **11**, 150–8.

Pileri, S., Poggi, S., Sabattini, E. *et al.* 1994: Apoptosis as programmed cell death (PCD): *cupio dissolvi* in cell life. *Current Diagnostic Pathology* **1**, 48–55.

Popper, H., Schaffner, F. 1971: The vocabulary of chronic hepatitis. *New England Journal of Medicine* **284**, 1154–6.

Popper, H., Paronetto, F., Schaffner, F. 1965: Immune processes in the pathogenesis of liver disease. *Annals of the New York Academy of Sciences* **124**, 781–99.

Portmann, B., Popper, H., Neuberger, J., Williams, R. 1985: Sequential and diagnostic features in primary biliary cirrhosis based on serial histologic study in 209 patients. *Gastroenterology* **88**, 1777–90.

Powell, L.W. 1987: The nature of cell death in piecemeal necrosis: is order emerging from chaos? *Hepatology* **7**, 794–6.

Rabinovitz, M., Demetris, A.J., Bou-Abboud, C.F. Van Thiel, D.H. 1992: Simultaneous occurrence of primary sclerosing cholangitis and autoimmune chronic active hepatitis in a patient with ulcerative colitis. *Digestive Diseases and Sciences* **37**, 1606–11.

Scheuer, P.J. 1991: Classification of chronic viral hepatitis: a need for reassessment. *Journal of Hepatology* **13**, 372–4.

Scheuer, P.J., Maggi, G. 1980: Hepatic fibrosis and collapse: histological distinction by orcein staining. *Histopathology* **4**, 487–90.

Scheuer, P.J., Ashrafzadeh, P., Sherlock, S., Brown, D., Dusheiko, G.M. 1992: The pathology of hepatitis C. *Hepatology* **15**, 567–71.

Scheuer, P.J., Krawczynski, K., Dhillon, A.P. 1997: Histopathology and detection of hepatitis C virus in liver. *Springer Seminars in Immunopathology* **19**, 27–45.

Schlichting, P., Hølund, B., Poulsen, H. 1983: Liver biopsy in chronic aggressive hepatitis. Diagnostic reproducibility in relation to size of specimen. *Scandinavian Journal of Gastroenterology* **18**, 27–32.

Schmid, M. 1966: *Die chronische Hepatitis*. Berlin: Springer-Verlag.

Shikata, T., Uzawa, T., Yoshiwara, N., Akatsuka, T., Yamazaki, S. 1974: Staining methods of Australia antigen in paraffin section – detection of cytoplasmic inclusion bodies. *Japanese Journal of Experimental Medicine* **44**, 25–36.

Tanaka, K., Mori, W., Suwa, K. 1981: Victoria blue-nuclear fast red stain for HBs antigen detection in paraffin section. *Acta Pathologica Japonica* **31**, 93–8.

Tanaka, Y., Enomoto, N., Kojima, S. *et al.* 1993: Detection of hepatitis C virus RNA in the liver by in situ hybridization. *Liver* **13**, 203–8.

Taylor, S.L., Dean, P.J., Riely, C.A. 1994: Primary autoimmune cholangitis. An alternative to antimitochondrial antibody-negative primary biliary cirrhosis. *American Journal of Surgical Pathology* **18**, 91–9.

Teixeira, M.R. Jr, Weller, I.V.D., Murray, A. *et al.* 1982: The pathology of hepatitis A in man. *Liver* **2**, 53–60.

Thung, S.N., Gerber, M.A. 1982: The formation of elastic fibers in livers with massive hepatic necrosis. *Archives of Pathology and Laboratory Medicine* **106**, 468–9.

Uchida, T., Shimojima, S., Gotoh, K., Shikata, T., Mima, S. 1994a: Pathology of livers infected wtih 'silent' hepatitis B virus mutant. *Liver* **14**, 251–6.

Uchida, T., Shikata, T., Tanaka, E., Kiyosawa, K. 1994b: Immunoperoxidase staining of hepatitis C virus in formalin-fixed, paraffin-embedded needle liver biopsies. *Virchows Archiv* **424**, 465–9.

van den Oord, J.J., De Vos, R., Facchetti, F., Delabie, J., De Wolf-Peeters, C., Desmet, V.J. 1990: Distribution of non-lymphoid, inflammatory cells in chronic HBV infection. *Journal of Pathology* **160**, 223–30.

Vaquer, P., Canet, R., Llompart, A., Riera, J., Obrador, A., Gayá, J. 1994: Histological evolution of chronic hepatitis C. Factors related to progression. *Liver* **14**, 265–9.

Vazquez, J.J. 1986: Hepatic lesions induced by alcohol sensitizing drugs: two lesions for the price of one. *Hepatology* **6**, 748–9.

Vazquez, J.J., Guillen, F.J., Zozaya, J., Lahoz, M. 1983: Cyanamide-induced liver injury. A predictable lesion. *Liver* **3**, 225–30.

Verme, G., Amoroso, P., Lettieri, G. *et al.* 1986: A histological study of hepatitis delta virus liver disease. *Hepatology* **6**, 1303–7.

Wang, W., London, W., Lega, L., Feitelson, M. 1991: HBxAg in the liver from carrier patients with chronic hepatitis and cirrhosis. *Hepatology* **14**, 29–37.

Wurbs, D., Klein, R., Terracciano, L.-M. Berg, P.A., Bianchi, L. 1995: A 28-year-old woman with a combined hepatitic/cholestatic syndrome. *Hepatology* **22**, 1598–605.

Yamada, G., Nishimoto, H., Endou, H. *et al.* 1993: Localization of hepatitis C viral RNA and capsid protein in human liver. *Digestive Diseases and Sciences* **38**, 882–7.

Yap, S.H., Willems, M., van den Oord, J. *et al.* 1994: Detection of hepatitis C virus antigen by immuno-histochemical staining: a histological marker of hepatitis C virus infection. *Journal of Hepatology* **20**, 275–81.

CHAPTER 4

Application of immuno-histochemistry and in situ hybridisation

K A FLEMING AND R D GOLDIN

Hepatitis A virus

The diagnosis of HAV is conveniently and definitively made by the demonstration of IgM anti-HAV in the serum (see Chapter 1). Demonstration of HAV in tissue sections is therefore not of diagnostic value but has added to our understanding of the natural history of infection by this virus. Most of this work has been carried out in vitro and in animal tissue. However, having developed an in situ hybridisation technique, using radiolabelled probes, we have been able to demonstrate in tamarins (Taylor *et al*, 1992) HAV RNA in biopsies from patients with acute hepatitis (Taylor *et al*, 1994). HAV RNA was found in the cytoplasm of hepatocytes and within macrophages (confirmed by double staining), although it was not possible to demonstrate replicative intermediates. This may reflect the relatively late stage of disease at which the biopsies were taken.

Hepatitis B virus

HBV was first described as Australia antigen (Au ag) by Blumberg in 1964 and linked to liver disease in 1967. The first demonstration of Au ag in liver cells (by immunofluorescence) was published in *Nature* in 1969 (Millman *et al*, 1969). Further analysis, including the use of electron microscopy (Nowoslawski *et al*, 1970), was achieved by the mid-1970s, and 'ground-glass' cells were identified as being particularly strongly positive for Au ag in 1973 (Hadziyannis *et al*, 1973). The availability of antibodies to different parts of the virus, particularly the nucleocapsid core protein (HBcAg) and the viral envelope surface protein (HBsAg), showed that the topographic and cellular localisation of the various antigens varied with the patient's disease and immune status. This information helped to show that the hepatitis is not dependent on viral cytopathy but primarily reflects the patient's immune response (Gudat, *et al*, 1975; Ray *et al*, 1976; Huang and Neurath, 1979), particularly the T-cell response directed against immunodominant epitopes of the nucleocapsid protein (HBcAg) (see Chapter 7). Subsequently, molecular techniques for the detection of HBV DNA allowed the identification of viral replication and permitted the correlation of this with the cellular detection of viral antigens and with liver pathology (Hsu *et al*, 1987).

An additional advance in the investigation of the liver distribution of HBV antigens during this time was the development of improved immunohistological techniques, permitting both increased sensitivity and the analysis of formalin-fixed paraffin sections (Burns, 1975). The availability of monoclonal antibodies – allowing the unambiguous assessment of antigen distribution because of the monospecificity of the antibody – was a further technical advance. This latter clarified the relationship between core and 'e' antigen (HBeAg), an area in which early work had been fraught because of the cross-reactivity of polyclonal antisera (Mondelli *et al*, 1988). As a result of all these investigations, the immunodetection of HBV antigens can currently provide insight into the state of viral replication, the likelihood of active disease, and thus prognosis, and whether or not the virus is integrated.

The following sections will describe the distribution of HBsAg, HBcAg and HBeAg in acute and chronic HBV hepatitis. They will also briefly describe the significance in terms of viral replication, severity of disease and outcome. Certain other HBV antigens will only be mentioned briefly as these are not currently of major significance in either diagnosis or prognosis. It should be noted that HBV antigens have largely only been described in the hepatocyte (and Kupffer cell for HBsAg) (Hadziyannis *et al*, 1973), with no convincing demonstration in either biliary or endothelial cells. This is in contrast to the results of in situ hybridisation (*see* below).

IMMUNOLOCALISATION OF HBcAg, HBeAg AND HBsAg

Acute viral hepatitis

Little or no positivity of either HBsAg or HBcAg is found in acute HBV hepatitis (Ray *et al*, 1976; Yamada *et al*, 1978). A few scattered hepatocytes are positive for HBsAg in a cytoplasmic or plasma membrane distribution, while a few cells contain nuclear or membranous HBcAg. However, when the disease shows evidence of transition towards chronicity, there is then increased detection of both HBcAg and HBsAg. It is thought that this sparsity of positivity in acute viral hepatitis reflects the rapid elimination of infected cells in the immune-competent individual: experimental work on chimpanzees has shown HBsAg membrane positivity during the incubation period, presumably allowing the immune-mediated destruction of these cells, producing the hepatitic illness (Barker *et al*, 1973).

Chronic hepatitis

The natural history of chronic HBV infection may involve the following phases (Chu *et al*, 1985):

1. high replication, low immunity, high tolerance, little or no inflammation;
2. low replication, immune-mediated clearance, active inflammation;
3. low/no replication, inactive, integrated HBV.

There is transition between these phases. The distribution of HBV antigens differs in each of these three phases. In some cases, there may be reactivation of the disease associated with the emergence of the pre-core mutant (*see* Chapter 2).

HBcAg expression is normally found in the nucleus alone (Fig. 4.1) and reflects viral replication (phase 1). When viral replication is very high, HBcAg is also found in the hepatocyte cytoplasm (Fig. 4.2) (Burrell *et al*, 1985; Hsu *et al*, 1987). In these cases, cytoplasmic localisation increases with viral replication, with a concomitant decrease in nuclear localisation. Active inflammation (phase 2), the duration of which determines prognosis, is also associated with HBcAg expression, particularly cytoplasmic localisation (Hsu *et al*, 1987). The relative distribution of HBcAg between nucleus and cytoplasm may reflect cell proliferation (Yeh *et al*, 1993).

HBeAg expression also reflects viral replication (Hadziyannis *et al*, 1983). Like HBcAg, it can be found in both the nucleus and/or cytoplasm (Mondelli *et al*, 1988). However, unlike that of HBcAg, HBeAg expression, while associated with high viral replication, is not associated with active liver disease (Naoumov *et al*, 1990). This has been taken to support the concept that the immune response, and hence liver cell destruction, is directed against HBcAg epitopes that are not found in HBeAg (Yeh *et al*, 1993).

HBsAg is usually cytoplasmic in distribution (Fig. 4.3). However, on occasions, HBsAg is found in and beneath the plasma membranes (Fig. 4.4), and this has been shown to be associated with HBcAg expression and with high viral replication (phase 1) (Gudat *et al*, 1975; Ray *et al*, 1976; Huang and Neurath, 1979; Hsu *et al*, 1987). However, as with HBeAg this membranous distribution of HBsAg is not associated with marked inflammatory activity (Hsu *et al*, 1988), again suggesting that the immune response is primarily directed against nucleocapsid epitopes.

In carriers with high immunity and low tolerance (phase 3), there is low or absent viral replication with widespread viral integration. In these cases, there is variable cytoplasmic HBsAg expression, resulting in 'ground-glass' cells. These are sometimes very numerous, for example comprising more than 20% of all hepatocytes (Yamada *et al*, 1978). In cases in which the pre-core mutant developes, HBcAg can be detected in the liver despite the absence of HBeAg from the serum (or liver).

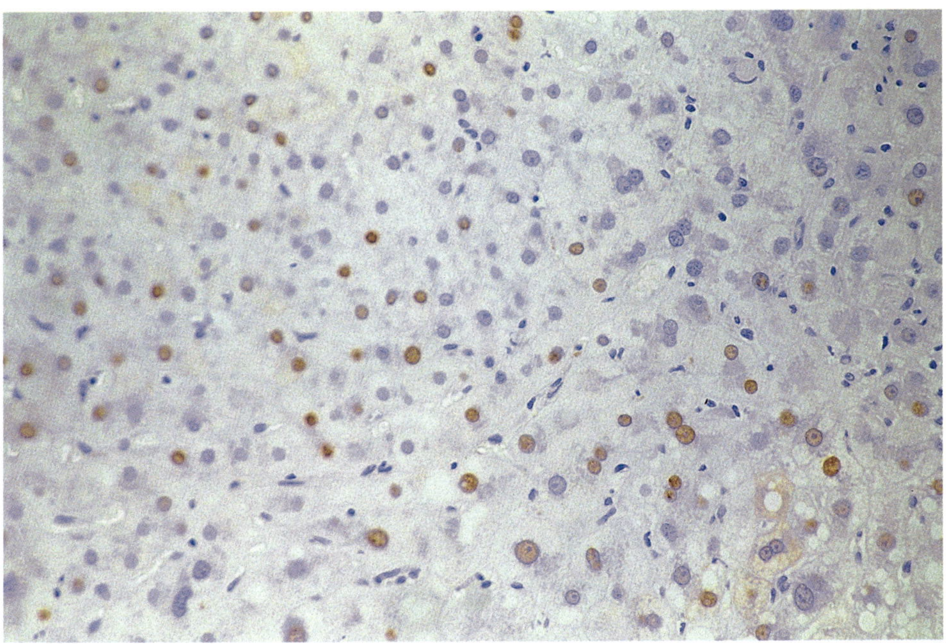

Fig 4.1   Immunohistochemical localisation of HBcAg in a clump of hepatocyte nuclei. Note the absence of inflammation (indirect immunoperoxidase with DAB).

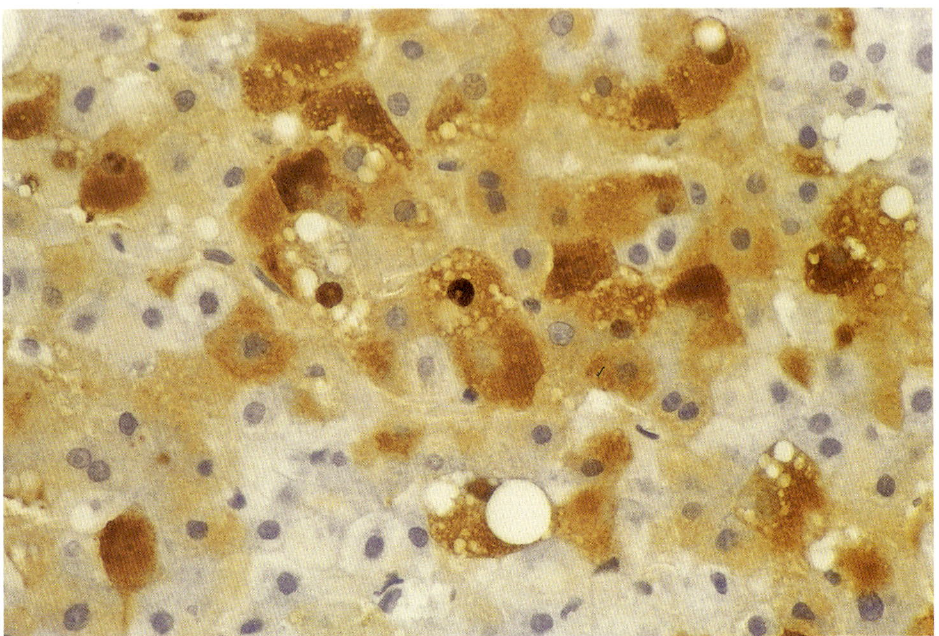

Fig 4.2 HBcAg in the cytoplasm of infected hepatocytes.

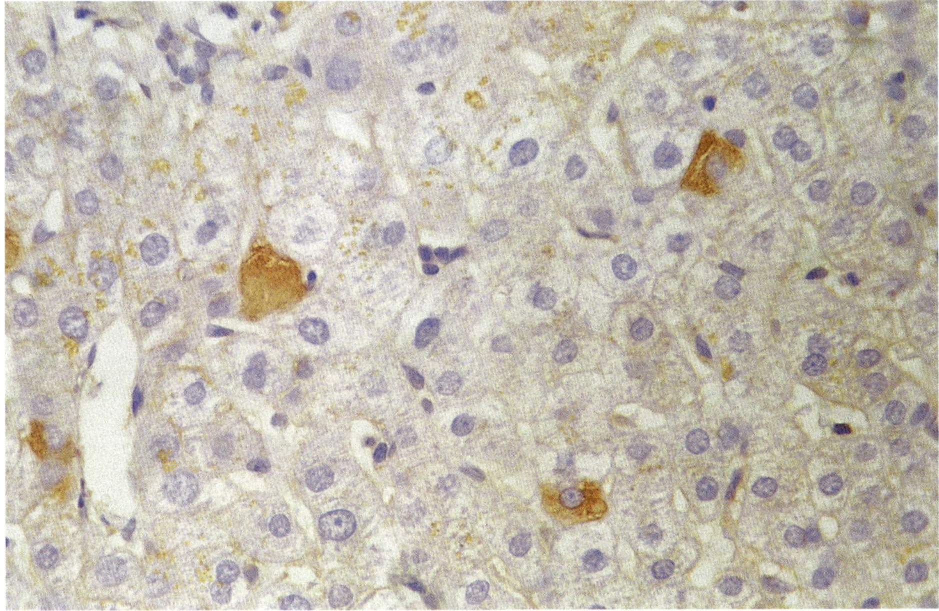

Fig 4.3 Hepatocyte cytoplasmic granular positivity for HBsAg, reflecting integrated virus. Note the absence of nuclear staining and the negativity of most cells (indirect immunoperoxidase with DAB).

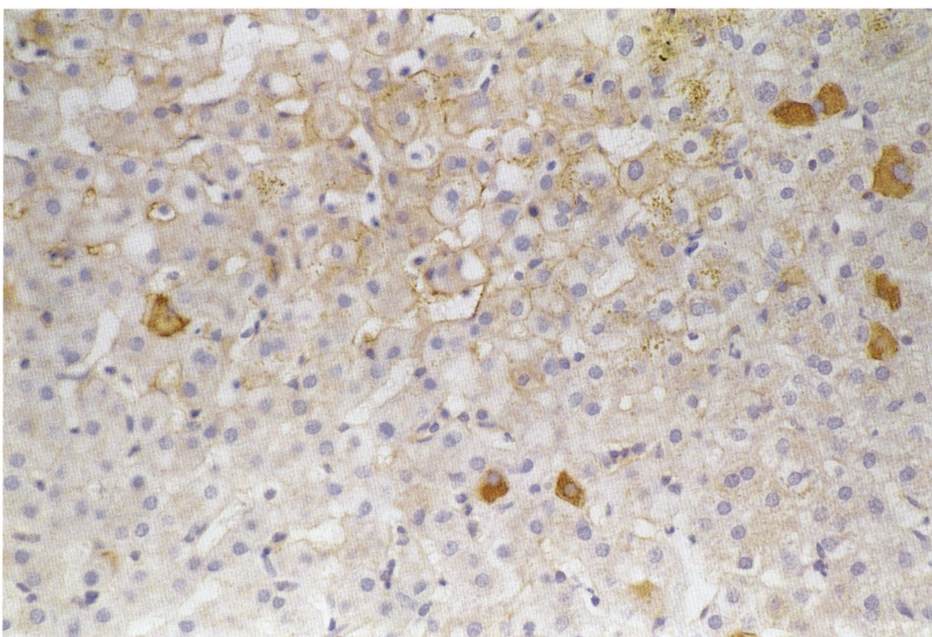

Fig 4.4 Membranous staining for HBsAg in a group of hepatocytes. The cells around the periphery of the field are negative. There is clear membranous and submembranous staining. There is no inflammation (indirect immunoperoxidase with DAB).

The mechanisms responsible for the cytoplasmic or membranous distribution of HBsAg expression are unclear. However, it has been suggested that when complete virion formation occurs, viral particles will have HBsAg in a configuration that can complex with the polyalbumin receptor. This receptor can bind to the plasma membrane of hepatocytes and thus result in a membranous distribution of HBsAg. In contrast, incomplete viral replication, with absence of Dane particle formation, produces HBsAg in the absence of the rest of the virus. This incomplete HBsAg is unable to bind the polyalbumin receptor and thus does not have a membranous localisation (Chu and Liau, 1987). This latter phase is frequently associated with integrated virus as opposed to episomal virus.

An additional feature of the integrated virus, compared with episomal virus, is the expression of HBsAg by groups of contiguous hepatocytes, often without HBcAg or HBeAg expression. It is thought that this focality reflects clonal expression of the hepatocytes containing integrated HBV (Hsu *et al*, 1988). It is frequently seen in cirrhosis, where the hepatocytes of adjacent nodules can be all completely positive or negative.

It is worth noting here that the immunohistological detection of viral antigens on the cell membrane has been suggested to be irrelevant to cell-mediated immunity (Naoumov and Eddleston, 1994). The latter is directed against viral oligopeptides (rather than whole molecules) in the HLA groove on the cell surface, which are probably inaccessible to the antibodies used in immunohistology (*see* Chapter 7). Thus immunolocalisation may not be detecting molecules actively involved in the host cell-mediated immune response. Nevertheless, in pragmatic terms, the associations between HBAg subcellular localisation and disease activity described above are valid.

There are, however, several variations on the above. In the post-transplant liver, where the patient is immunosuppressed, about 20% of patients develop an unusual form of reinfection with HBV, called fibrosing cholestatic hepatitis (Lau *et al*, 1992) (*see* Chapter 5). This is characterised by vast amounts of HBAg on the liver cells and significant liver cell damage. However, there is little or no inflammatory reaction. It has therefore been suggested that direct viral cytoplasmic damage is occurring as a result of the intracellular synthesis of large amounts of HBVAg, particularly HBsAg. An analogous situation is mice transgenic for the HBsAg (Chisari *et al*, 1987). Many of the mouse hepatocytes synthesise large amounts of HBsAg, and it has been claimed that a cytopathic effect is present, despite the complete absence of an immune response (*see* Chapter 7). There is also a tissue culture model, in which the transfection of HBV into HepG2 cells produces high HBVAg expression and results in cell death (Roingeard *et al*, 1990), again in the absence of an immune response.

OTHER HBV ANTIGENS

Recent work has examined the localisation of the three forms of the HBs protein. These three forms are named large (LHBs), middle (MHBs) and small (SHBs) HB surface protein. The large form contains both the pre-S1 and pre-S2 gene products, as well as the S gene product; the middle contains the pre-S2 and S products; while the small consists solely of the S gene product. Using monoclonal antibodies, it has been shown that, in viraemic patients, the predominant form of HBsAg in the liver cells is the small and middle HB, while in non-viraemic patients the large HB is the predominant molecule (Dienes *et al*, 1990). This latter is associated with 'ground-glass' cells. This accumulation of vast amounts of LHB is thought to reflect the presence of pre-S1 in the cell: pre-S1 has been shown to inhibit the secretion of HBsAg. Accordingly, significant amounts of LHB in cells are associated with low serum levels of HBs (Kuroki *et al*, 1989). It has been possible to detect hepatitis B X protein in cirrhotic livers (as well as liver cell cancers). It was demonstrated, in over 50% of cases, in the cytoplasm of hepatocytes (Su *et al*, 1998).

Finally, recent work has used the immunolocalisation of HBV DNA polymerase as a more specific marker for viral replication (McGarvey *et al*, 1996). Particularly, high levels of replication are seen in immunosuppressed individuals.

ELECTRON MICROSCOPY OF HBV

The ultrastructural appearance of the virus is well known, early descriptions using material from the serum of HBV patients. This showed three forms: a 42 nm diameter envelope-coated, core-containing particle, which is the intact virion (Dane particle), and 22 nm diameter tubules and spheres (Dane *et al*, 1970). It was soon recognised that the tubules and spheres represented excess surface antigen secreted by the hepatocytes, and that the central core of the Dane particle contained HBcAg, viral DNA and DNA polymerase. The 7 nm thick outer layer of the Dane particle contained the HBsAg (Almeida *et al*, 1971).

Examination of liver tissue by electron microscopy and immune electron microscopy has confirmed the subcellular localisation of the various HBV antigens shown by light microscopy. Thus HBcAg is present on spherical, virus-like, intranuclear particles and in the cytoplasm as non-particulate material (Yamada *et al*, 1978). This latter is particularly seen near ribosomes and nuclear pores. HBsAg is not seen in the nucleus but is seen in the perinuclear space and the cisternae of the endoplasmic reticulum, as tubular and spherical forms. Intact Dane particles are also localised to the endoplasmic reticulum. Accordingly, it has been proposed that the intracellular synthesis and assembly of HBV proceeds as follows. HBcAg and HBsAg are produced separately. HBcAg migrates from the ribosomes, through nuclear pores, to the nucleus, where it is assembled into a core particle, incorporating viral DNA. These particles exit into the endoplasmic reticulum and are enveloped by HBsAg, to form intact Dane particles, which are then released extracellularly (Yamada *et al*, 1978).

IN SITU HYBRIDISATION FOR HBV

The localisation of HBV DNA in liver tissue was first reported in the early 1980s (Gowans *et al*, 1981), early investigations using radiolabelled probes. More recent investigations have commonly used non-radioactive probes, primarily because of improved resolution, speed, safety and expense. The cellular localisation of HBV DNA by in situ hybridisation has largely confirmed the results of antigen detection. However, an unexpected observation has been the detection of HBV DNA in cells other than hepatocytes. Thus Blum and Haase demonstrated HBV DNA in biliary epithelial cells and in endothelial cells using ^{125}I-labelled probes (Blum *et al*, 1984). The most consistent non-hepatocyte localisation of HBV DNA has been in mononuclear cells in sinusoids. The current view is that these represent blood monocytes or lymphoid cells (Hadchuel *et al*, 1988) circulating through the liver; it is well accepted that such cells form a non-hepatic reservoir of virus and are probably the source of reinfection in transplanted livers (*see* Chapter 5). A more recent report (Mason *et al*, 1993) has claimed the detection of HBV DNA in endothelial cells, macrophages/monocytes, haemopoietic precursors, basal keratinocytes, mucosal epithelial cells, stromal fibroblasts and sustentacular and neuronal cells.

HBV DNA has been localised to both the nucleus and the cytoplasm of hepatocytes (Gowans *et al*, 1981; Naoumov *et al*, 1993) (Fig. 4.5), presumably reflecting the synthesis and transport of the virus particles. The correlation of cellular localisation of HBV DNA with viral antigens has, in general, not revealed any unexpected results. Thus cells with HBcAg and HBsAg may contain both nuclear and cytoplasmic HBV DNA (Han *et al*, 1993), with high replication (HBcAg-positivity) being associated with cytoplasmic viral DNA (Burrell *et al*, 1982).

Investigations of the relationship between the localisation of HBV DNA and inflammation have also been performed. Correlation of HBV DNA with HLA class I expression showed that HLA class I expression is *not* enhanced by the presence of HBV DNA in hepatocytes (Lau *et al*, 1993). The authors suggested that this may reflect a mechanism for the inadequate elimination of infected hepatocytes, as the HBV-containing, non-HLA expressing cells would not be the target of T-cell cytotoxicity. Another investigation examining the correlation of HBV DNA with inflammation showed that those cases with HBcAg, and with cytoplasmic HBV DNA, had chronic hepatitis, with a prominent necroinflammatory component, while those without cytoplasmic HBV DNA did not have active inflammation, suggesting that the pattern of replication may in some way influence the development of inflammatory liver damage (Naoumov *et al*, 1993).

In conclusion, the results of in situ hybridisation for HBV DNA have largely confirmed the results of other techniques. Thus, although in situ hybridisation for HBV DNA is technically relatively simple, it is of little diagnostic use at present, immunohistochemistry for HBc or HBsAg being widely available and reliable.

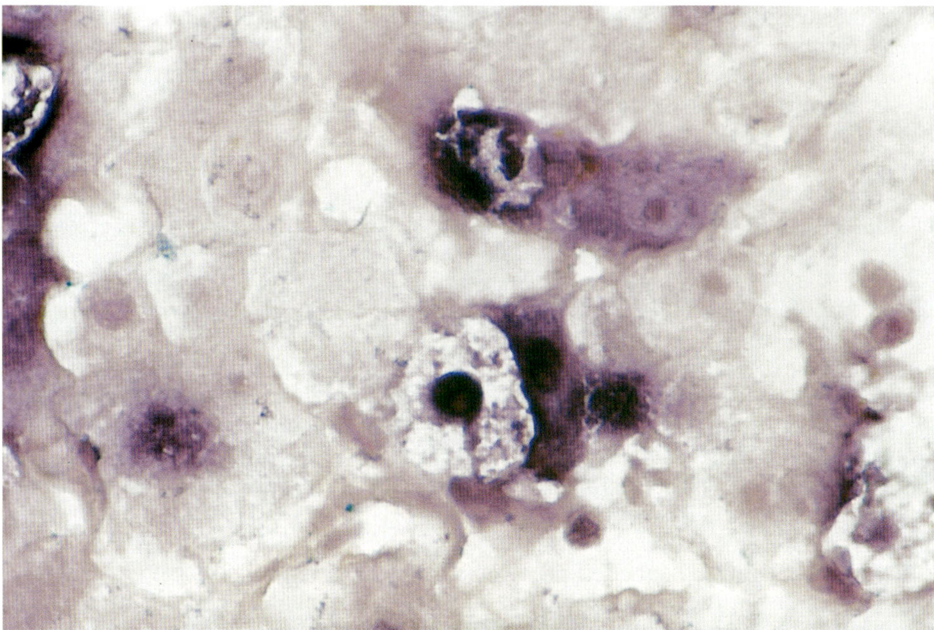

Fig 4.5   In situ hybridisation for hepatitis B virus. DNA showing granular positivity for both the cytoplasm and nuclei (digoxigenin-labelled hepatitis B virus with NBT/BCIP).

Hepatitis C virus

This recently described virus has been the subject of intense interest since its identification in 1989. This reflects its significance as a major cause of chronic hepatitis, cirrhosis and hepatocellular cancer. Accordingly, much effort has been expended trying to detect and localise the virus in the liver by immunohistochemistry, in situ hybridisation and electron microscopy. There are obviously many questions about the biology of the virus which these techniques can address, but some are of outstanding importance, namely the range of cells infected, the distribution of infected cells at different stages of infection, whether or not the virus is cytopathic, and the intracellular distribution of viral antigens. Of clinical importance, the ability to identify HCV reliably and sensitively in liver tissue would be a major diagnostic boon, as there are no pathognomonic histopathological criteria.

IMMUNOLOCALISATION OF HCV

Unfortunately, the demands of these techniques, when applied to HCV, have proved formidable. A range of polyclonal and monoclonal antibodies have been used for immunolocalisation (reviewed in Guido and Thung, 1996), but many of these antibodies suffer from false-positive artefacts. For example, we (as others) have tried many monoclonal and polyclonal antibodies, with various microwaving and enzymatic procedures, on formalin-fixed, paraffin-embedded tissue. We obtained (unpublished data) cytoplasmic granular staining in hepatocytes (Fig. 4.6). Occasional Kupffer cells were also positive. However, although 16 out of 19 HVC livers were positive, 11 out of 25 non-HCV livers were also positive. This included HBV, primary biliary cirrhotic, alcoholic and normal livers. Thus the signal is presumably false positive. However, given the apparent purity of the HCV antigen preparation used for antibody production, there are at least two other explanations. First, the signal may be genuine and HCV infection of the liver is more widespread than recognised, existing in the absence of seropositivity – this seems unlikely. Second, the signal is genuine but is a component of normal cells that is upregulated in damaged or inflamed tissue. It is not possible to exclude this latter possibility.

Despite the above, several publications have documented an apparent success in the cytological localisation of HCV. Of these, the most reproducible involves the use of immunofluorescence and immunoglobulin partially purified from high-titre human serum from HCV patients. This has produced a consistent granular, cytoplasmic staining of the hepatocytes in both infected humans and chimpanzees (Krawczynski *et al*, 1992; Ballardini *et al*, 1995). Recent publications have shown similar results with several monoclonal antibodies raised against a variety of viral antigens (Hiramatsu *et al*, 1992; Blight *et al*, 1994). However, these antibodies appear to work consistently only on frozen material. This is unfortunate, partly because of the poorer morphology resulting from the use of frozen sections, but also because of the complication of potential infectivity. These reports have highlighted another factor contributing to the difficulty of obtaining successful results, namely the sparseness of infected cells (at least in chronic hepatitis). Reported positivity ranges from less than 5% of lobular hepatocytes to only very occasional cells. The number of positive cells tends to increase with the stage of the disease.

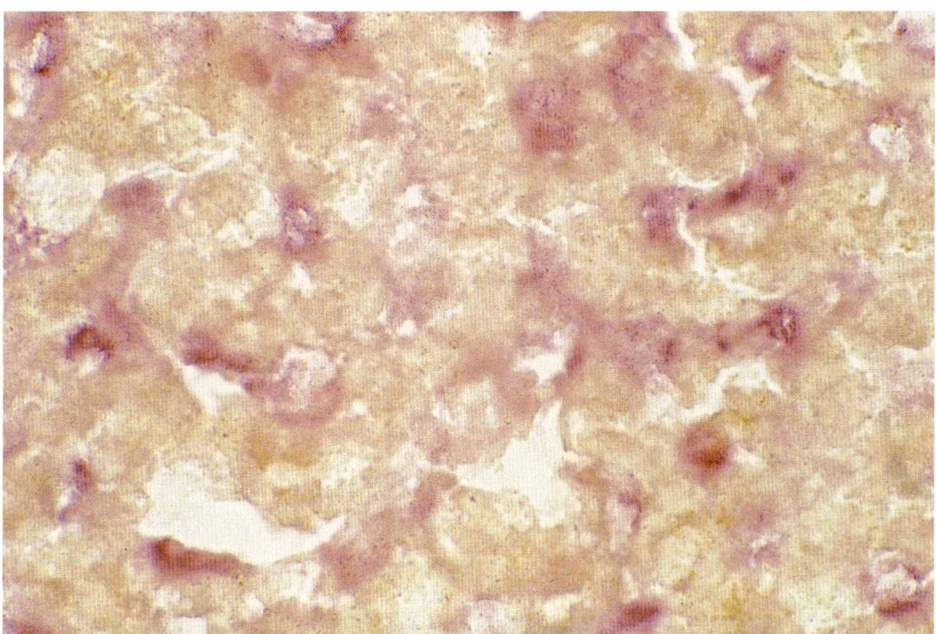

Fig 4.6   Indirect immunoperoxidase staining with DAB and polyclonal antibody for the C-100 antigen of hepatitis C virus, showing granular cytoplasmic positivity of the hepatocytes and Kupffer cells.

The results of the above experiments have shown viral antigen predominantly in hepatocytes. There has been the occasional demonstration of viral antigen in non-hepatocytic cells. The non-hepatocyte cells involved are intrasinusoidal mononuclear cells and bile duct epithelial cells (Nouri-Aria *et al*, 1995). The former may represent circulatory lymphoid and/or macrophage cells and provide a source of extrahepatic viral infection and replication (similar to that for HBV), and the latter may explain the mild bile duct damage and peribiliary lymphoid aggregates in HCV infection. Attempts to relate the virus-containing hepatocytes to evidence of liver cell death or inflammation have been inconclusive. Most reports have suggested that the virus can exist in hepatocytes without any consistent association with evidence of cell death or inflammation. Whether this reflects the true situation or the difficulties in detecting viral antigen in a sufficiently large series of patients is unclear. Finally, in the absence of a panel of antibodies that can reliably detect the various viral antigens, it has not yet been possible to analyse whether certain viral antigens are associated with different aspects of biology or pathology. All of these questions remain to be answered (Lau *et al*, 1996).

It is also interesting to note that HCV antigens have also been identified in lymphoid tissue, and it has been suggested that infection of lymphoid cells may play a role in the increased risk of lymphoma in patients with HCV (Nicoll *et al*, 1997).

IN SITU HYBRIDISATION FOR HCV

In situ hybridisation for viral genome has also been fraught with a relative lack of success. This again may reflect the relatively few infected cells found in chronically infected individuals, but may also suggest that infected cells contain few genomes, even when replicating. Accordingly, the polymerase chain reaction in situ may be of value, but this technique is still in development (Nuovo *et al*, 1993). While most publications have shown viral genome in the hepatocyte cytoplasm alone (Negro *et al*, 1992; Tanaka *et al*, 1993), some unresolved controversies exist. Several publications have shown virus in sinusoidal monocytes and in sinusoid-lining cells (Lamas *et al*, 1992; Nouri-Aria *et al*, 1993; Yamada *et al*, 1993). At least two publications have shown virus in hepatocyte nuclei (Haruna *et al*, 1993; Nouri-Aria *et al*, 1993), while others have also shown biliary epithelium to be infected (Nouri-Aria *et al*, 1993; Nuovo *et al*, 1993). A recent study combined in situ hybridisation and digital image analysis. This suggested that HCV viraemia depends on the number of infected hepatocytes and not on the relative viral load/infected cell (Gosalvez *et al*, 1998).

ELECTRON MICROSCOPY FOR HCV

In contrast to the above, descriptions of the putative electron microscopic features of HCV, namely the presence of swollen Golgi apparatus with tubules and vesicles in the hepatocyte cytoplasm, have been available for some years (Kamimura *et al*, 1983). However, it has been suggested that these structures may simply reflect IFN exposure. A recent publication has described the electron microscopic appearances of cell cultures infected with HCV (Shimizu *et al*, 1996). This paper described the appearance of 50 nm virus-like particles (which bound core and envelope antibody) in the cytoplasm and in perinuclear vesicular structures. These were related to amorphous material, the nature of which was unclear. Experiments on putative virus isolated from peripheral blood have shown 55 nm virus-like particles with a 33 nm core structure (Kaito *et al*, 1994). It is thus possible that the virus is a 50 nm enveloped structure that has a 33 nm core, and that the vesicles seen on conventional electron microscopy of infected liver are envelope material, analogous to the excess surface protein seen in HBV infection. Virus core is presumably synthesised in the cytosol and acquires an envelope by budding into tubules or vesicles.

An interesting observation in the paper from Shimizu *et al* (1996) is that immunofluorescence for core or envelope protein only detected infected hepatocytes abundant enough for electron microscopy in one out of 10 liver biopsies from experimentally infected chimpanzees biopsied during an episode of acute hepatitis. Virally infected cells were not abundant enough for electron microscopy in the livers from the eight humans with acute HCV hepatitis examined. These findings emphasise the sparsity of infected hepatocytes (*see* above) even in acute hepatitis.

In summary, immunohistology and in situ hybridisation for HCV are still under development and are not yet freely or reliably available. When they are achieved, they will provide a major contribution to both the diagnostic and scientific investigation of the virus (Lau *et al*, 1996).

Hepatitis D virus

IMMUNOHISTOCHEMISTRY OF HDV

Although HDV has characteristic histological features (including acidophilic degeneration not associated with a lymphoid infiltrate), these are not diagnostic and are not seen in every biopsy (*see* Chapter 3). Immunohistochemical means of identifying HDV in biopsies are therefore very useful diagnostically. Immunohistochemistry has also played an important role in understanding the pathobiology of HDV as well as in dissecting out the interactions between HBV and HDV. HDV superinfection is associated with an accelerated course of chronic HBV infection. Therefore in any case of chronic HBV in which the necroinflammatory activity is greater than expected, especially if there are features suggesting HDV, immunohistochemical staining is strongly recommended, particularly as the results are often available before those from virological studies (Goldin, 1994). Furthermore, it is considered that the demonstration of HDV antigen in the liver is the gold standard for the diagnosis of active infection.

HDV has been identified in tissue sections using a variety of immunohistochemical techniques. The most widely used antibody has been an IgG anti-HDV prepared from a patient's serum. Naturally, there are a number of potential problems with such an reagent, although in practice it has given satisfactory results. Drawbacks include the inevitable presence of HBV antigens and antibodies as well as autoantibodies, which are relatively common in patients with HDV (*see* Chapter 7). At the low dilutions used, on formalin fixed paraffin embedded tissue, it was shown that there were no detectable HBV antigens (or antibodies to them) and that, as assessed using a direct immunoperoxidase technique on human tissue, there were no recognisable autoantibodies (Kojima *et al*, 1990). We have used a rabbit polyclonal antibody prepared using the *E. coli*-expressed MS2 replicase HDVAg fusion product, that includes amino acids 13–76 of the open reading frame coding for HDVAg to detect the virus in tissue sections (Saldanha *et al*, 1990). In humans, chimpanzees and woodchucks, each of these antibodies gives predominantly nuclear staining with less marked cytoplasmic staining. As yet, no commercially available antibody to HDV is widely available.

The characteristic histological features of HDV have led to the suggestion that HDV is a cytopathic virus (*see* Chapter 7). In patients who were serologically positive for HDV, those cases expressing HDVAg in liver biopsies had more active disease as assessed biochemically and histologically (Lau *et al*, 1991). An Italian study demonstrated a strong positive correlation between the number of HDV-positive cells and the severity of the portal inflammation (Negro *et al*, 1988), but this has not been confirmed by the study carried out in the UK (Lau *et al*, 1991). Furthermore, when followed up, in neither group of patients did the outcome correlate with the severity of the initial pathology, and this led both groups of authors to suggest that individually determined immune mechanisms may also be important. If immune mechanisms are important, the HDV antigen (*see* Chapter 7) is the most likely immune target. However, this antigen is not detected on the cytoplasmic membrane by most immunohistochemical techniques, although it is present in the endoplasmic reticulum. This may relate to the insensitivity of the techniques used or to the presence of blocking, membrane-bound antibody. On the other hand, cells undergoing acidophilic degeneration infrequently contain HDVAg (*see* below). This makes it unlikely that this form of cell damage is immune mediated. HDVAg has been shown to be co-expressed with c-myc. This supports the suggestion, based on the observation that HDV-infected cells are often binucleate, that HDV infection triggers cell division.

While HDV requires HBV for its replication, it has been reported from both clinical and animal studies that co-infection with HDV inhibits HBV replication (*see* Chapter 7). Immunohistochemical support for the latter suggestion comes from the observation that, while HDVAg and HBsAg are not infrequently found in the same cell, HDVAg and HBcAg rarely co-localise (Facchetti *et al*, 1986; Ryley *et al*, 1992). However, the latter pattern of staining has been found more frequently in more recent studies, suggesting that the inhibition of HDV replication may only be relative and may be more marked in the acute phase of infection than in the later stages (Negro *et al*, 1988). Furthermore, this inhibition is less marked in HIV-positive patients (*see* Chapter 5). Cases expressing HBcAg as well as HDVAg tend to have more active disease. These studies have depended on double, and in one paper triple, immunohistochemical staining (Facchetti *et al*, 1986).

IN SITU HYBRIDISATION FOR HDV

A number of techniques based on in situ hybridisation have been employed. These have utilised both radioactive and non-radioactive probes. Negro *et al*, (1989), using ^{125}I-labelled oligonucleotide probes on frozen and paraffin-embedded tissues, detected HDV RNA in the nuclei of hepatocytes and detected RNAs of both polarities, with a marked preponderance of genomic species (Yamada *et al*, 1978). This group subsequently used digoxigenin-labelled oligonucleotide probes complementary to the viroid-like domain of HDV RNA. Other groups have used similar probes (Lopez Talavera *et al*, 1993). The use of non-radioactive labelled probes permitted better correlation between in situ hybridisation and histology (Negro *et al*, 1993). Infected nuclei were often giant or 'sanded' (*see* Chapter 3), and infected cells were frequently binucleate (*see* above). We have used 30 base-long DNA oligonucleotide probes to conserved regions to detect genomic HDV RNA in frozen tissue. Both genomic and antigenomic HDV RNA were found only in hepatocyte nuclei (Dourakis *et al*, 1991).

In situ hybridisation has proved to be more sensitive than immunohistochemistry, although this is not of diagnostic importance. However, a number of discrepancies between HDVAg and HDV RNA expression have been pointed out, which are of interest (Negro *et al*, 1989, 1993). For example, cells undergoing acidophilic degeneration express HDV

RNA but not HDVAg. This is somewhat surprising as HDVAg expression is a prerequisite for HDV RNA replication. It has been speculated that the accumulation of HDV RNA without HDVAg impairs the assembly of complete viral particles and that this in turn may lead to cell damage, as manifest by acidophilic degeneration.

Hepatitis E virus

Preliminary studies have demonstrated HEV in tissue from two patients with fulminant hepatitis (Lau *et al*, 1995). A recent paper used immunohistochemistry and non-isotopic in situ hybridisation to demonstrate viral antigens and RNA in tissue sections. Both were only found in hepatocytes, where they were localised to the cytoplasm. Furthermore, most of the cells in which virus could be demonstrated showed degenerative changes, supporting the suggestion that the virus is cytopathic.

References

Almeida, J.D., Rubenstein, D., Slott, E.J. 1971: New antigen–antibody system in Australia-antigen-positive hepatitis. *Lancet* **ii**, 1225–7.

Ballardini, G., Groff, P., Geostra, F. *et al*. 1995: Hepatocellular codistribution of c100, c33, c22 and NS5 hepatitis C virus antigen detected by using immunopurified polyclonal spontaneous human antibodies. *Hepatology* **21**, 730–4.

Barker, L.F., Chisari, F.V., McGrath, P.P. *et al*. 1973: Transmission of viral hepatitis type B to chimpanzees. *Journal of Infectious Diseases* **127**, 648–62.

Blight, K., Lesniewski, R.R., La Brooy, J.T., Gowans, E.J. 1994: Detection and distribution of hepatitis C-specific antigens in naturally infected liver. *Hepatology* **20**, 553–7.

Blum, H.E., Haase, A.T., Vyas, G.N. 1984: Molecular pathogenesis of hepatitis B virus infection: simultaneous detection of viral DNA and antigens in paraffin-embedded liver sections. *Lancet* **ii**, 771–5.

Burns, J. 1975: Immunoperoxidase localisation of hepatitis B antigen (HB) in formalin-paraffin processed liver tissue. *Histochemistry* **44**, 133–5.

Burrell, C.J., Gowans, E.J., Jilbert, A.R., Lake, J.R., Marmion, B.P., 1982: Hepatitis B virus DNA detection by in situ cytohybridisation: implication for viral replication strategy and pathogenesis of chronic hepatitis. *Hepatology* **2**, 855–915.

Burrell, C.J., Gowans, E.J., Marmion, B.P. 1985: High levels of cytoplasmic hepatitis B core antigens are reliable marker of HBV DNA replication. *Lancet* **i**, 454–5.

Chisari, F.V., Filippi, P., Buras, J. *et al*. 1987: Structural and pathological effects of synthesis of hepatitis B virus large envelope polypeptide in transgenic mice. *Proceedings of the National Academy of Sciences of the USA* **84**, 6909–13.

Chu, C.-M., Liau, Y.-F. 1987: Intra-hepatic distribution of hepatitis B surface and core antigens in chronic hepatitis B virus infection. Hepatocyte with cytoplasmic/membranous hepatitis B core antigen as a possible target for immune hepatolysis. *Gastroenterology* **92**, 220–5.

Chu, C.-M., Karayiannis, P., Fowler, M.J.F., Monjardino, J., Liaw, Y.F., Thomas, H.C. 1985: Natural history of chronic hepatitis B virus infection in Taiwan: studies of HBV-DNA in serum. *Hepatology* **5**, 431–4.

Dane, D.S., Cameron, C.H., Briggs, M. 1970: Virus-like particles in serum of patients with Australia-antigen-associated viral hepatitis. *Lancet* **i**, 695–8.

Dienes, H.P., Gerlich, W.H., Wörsdörfer, M. *et al*. 1990: Hepatic expression patterns of the large and middle hepatitis B virus surface proteins in viraemic and non-viraemic chronic hepatitis B. *Gastroenterology* **98**, 1017–23.

Dourakis, S., Karayiannis, P., Goldin, R., Taylor, M., Monjardino, J., Thomas, H.C. 1991: An in situ hybridisation, molecular biological and immunohistochemical study of hepatitis delta virus in woodchucks. *Hepatology* **14**, 534–9.

Facchetti, F., Tardanico, R., Bonetti, M.F., Guerini, A., Callea, F. 1986: HBsAg, HBcAg and Delta-Ag in liver tissue: simultaneous visualization in a single liver section by triple immunostaining. *Histology and Histopathology* **1**, 181–5.

Goldin, R.D., 1994: Viral hepatitis. *Current Diagnostic Pathology* **1**, 70–6.

Gosalvez, J., Rodriguez-Inigo, E., Ramira-Diaz, J.L. *et al*. 1998: Relative quantification and mapping of hepatitis C virus by in situ hybridization and digital image analysis. *Hepatology* **27**, 1428–34.

Gowans, E.J., Burrell, C.J., Jilbert, A.R., Marmion, B.P. 1981: Detection of hepatitis B virus DNA sequences in infected hepatocytes by in situ hybridisation. *Journal of Medical Virology*, **8**, 76–8.

Gudat, F., Bianchi, L., Sonnabend, W., Thiel, G., Aenishaenslin, W., Stalder, G.A. 1975: Pattern of core and surface expression in liver tissue reflects state of specific immune response in hepatitis B. *Laboratory Investigation* **32**, 1–9.

Guido, M., Thung, S.N. 1996: The value of identifying hepatitis C virus in liver pathology specimens. *Hepatology* **23**, 376–9.

Hadchuel, M., Pasquinelli, C., Fourrier, J.G. *et al*. 1988: Detection of mononuclear cells expressing hepatitis B virus in peripheral blood from HBsAg positive and negative patients by in situ hybridisation. *Journal of Medical Virology* **24**, 27–32.

Hadziyannis, S., Gerber, M., Vissoulis, C., Popper, H. 1973: Cytoplasmic hepatitis B antigen in 'ground glass' hepatocytes of carriers. *Archives of Pathology* **96**, 327–30.

Hadziyannis, S., Liebman, H.M., Karvountzis, G.G. *et al*. 1983: Analysis of liver disease nuclear HBcAg, viral replication and hepatitis B virus DNA in liver and serum of HBeAg vs. anti-HBe positive carriers of hepatitis B virus. *Hepatology* **3**, 656–62.

Han, K.H., Hollinger, F.B., Noonan, C.A. *et al*. 1993: Southern blot analysis and simultaneous in situ detection of hepatitis B virus-associated DNA and antigens in patient with end-stage liver disease. *Hepatology* **18**, 1032–8.

Haruna, Y., Hayashi, N., Hiramatsu, N. *et al*. 1993: Detection of hepatitis C virus RNA in liver tissue by an in situ hybridisation technique. *Journal of Hepatology* **18**, 96–100.

Hiramatsu, N., Hayashi, N., Haruma, Y. *et al*. 1992: Immunohistochemical detection of hepatitis C virus-infected hepatocytes in chronic liver disease with monoclonal antibodies to core, envelope and NS3 regions of the hepatitis C virus genome. *Hepatology* **16**, 306–11.

Hsu, H.C., Su, I.J., Lai, M.Y. *et al*. 1987: Biologic and prognostic significance of hepatocyte hepatitis B core antigen expressions in the natural course of chronic hepatitis B virus infection. *Journal of Hepatology* **5**, 45–50.

Hsu, H.C., Lai, M.Y., Su, I.J., *et al*. 1988: Correlation of hepatocyte HBsAg expression with virus replication and liver pathology. *Hepatology* **8**, 749–54.

Huang, S.N., Neurath, A.R. 1979: Immunohistologic demonstration of hepatitis B viral antigens in liver with reference to its significance in liver injury. *Laboratory Investigation* **40**, 1–17.

Kaito, M., Watanabe, S., Tsukiyama-Kohara, K. *et al*. 1994: Hepatitis C virus particles detected by immunoelectron microscopic study. *Journal of General Virology* **75**, 1755–60.

Kamimura, T., Ponzetto, A., Bonino, F., Feinstone, S.M., Gerin, J.L., Purcell, R.H. 1983: Cytoplasmic tubular structures in liver of HBsAg carrier chimpanzees infected with delta agent and comparison with cytoplasmic structures in non-A, non-B hepatitis. *Hepatology* **3**, 631–7.

Kojima, T., Callea, F., Desmyter, J., Sakurai, I., Desmet, V.J. 1990: Immuno-light and electron microscopic features of chronic hepatitis D. *Liver* **10**, 17–27.

Krawczynski, K., Beach, M.J., Bradley, D.W. *et al*. 1992: Hepatitis C virus antigen in hepatocytes: immunomorphologic detection and identification. *Gastroenterology* **103**, 622–9.

Kuroki, I., Russnak, R., Ganem, D. 1989: Novel N-terminal amino acid sequence required for retention of a hepatitis B virus glycoprotein in the endoplasmic reticulum. *Molecular Cell Biology* **9**, 4459–66.

Lamas, E. Baccarini, P., Housset, C., Kremsdorf, D., Bréchot, C. 1992: Detection of hepatitis C virus (HCV) RNA sequences in liver tissue by in situ hybridisation. *Journal of Hepatology* **16**, 219–23.

Lau, J.Y.N., Hansen, L.J., Bain, V.G., *et al.* 1991: Expression of intrahepatic hepatitis D viral antigen in chronic hepatitis D virus infection. *Journal of Clinical Pathology* **44**, 549–53.

Lau, J.Y.N., Davies, S., Bain, V.G. *et al.* 1992: High level expression of hepatitis B viral antigens in fibrosing cholestatic hepatitis. *Gastroenterology* **102**, 956–62.

Lau, J.Y., Bird, G.K., Nauomov, N.V., Williams, R. 1993: Hepatic HLA antigen display in chronic hepatitis B virus infection. Relation to hepatic expression of HBV genome/gene products and liver histology. *Digestive Diseases and Sciences* **38**, 888–95.

Lau, J.Y., Sallie, R., Fang, J.W.S. *et al.* 1995: Detection of hepatitis E virus genome and gene products in two patients with fulminant hepatitis E. *Journal of Hepatology* **22**, 605–10.

Lau, J.Y., Krawczynski, K., Negro, F., Gonzalez-Peralta, R.P. 1996: In situ detection of hepatitis C virus – a critical appraisal. *Journal of Hepatology* **24** (supplement 2), 43–51.

Lopez Talavera, J.C., Buti, M., Casacuberta, J. *et al.* 1993: Detection of hepatitis delta virus RNA in human liver tissue by non-radioactive in situ hybridisation. *Journal of Hepatology* **17**, 199–203.

McGarvey, M.J., Goldin, R.D., Karayiannis, P., Thomas, H.C. 1996: The expression of hepatitis B polymerase in hepatocytes during chronic HBV infection. *Journal of Viral Hepatitis* **3**, 67–73.

Mason, A., Wick, M., White, H., Pertillo, R. 1993: Hepatitis B virus replication in diverse cell types during chronic hepatitis B virus infection. *Hepatology* **18**, 781–9.

Millman, I., Zavatone, V., Gerstley, B.J.S., Blumberg, B. 1969: Australia antigen detected in the nuclei of liver cells of patients with viral hepatitis by the fluorescent antibody technique. *Nature* **222**, 181–4.

Mondelli, M., Tedder, R.S., Ferns, B., Portisso, P., Realdi, G., Alberti, A. 1988: Differential distribution of hepatitis B core and e antigens in hepatocytes: analysis by monoclonal antibodies. *Hepatology* **8**, 749–54.

Naoumov, N.V., Portman, B.C., Tedder, R.S., *et al.* 1990: Detection of hepatitis B virus antigens in liver tissue. A relation to viral replication and histology in chronic hepatitis B infection. *Gastroenterology* **99**, 1248–53.

Naoumov, N.V., Daniels, H.M., Davidson, F., Eddleston, A.L., Alexander, G.J., Williams, R. 1993: Identification of hepatitis B virus – DNA in the liver by in situ hybridisation using a biotinylated probe. Relation to HBcAg expression and histology. *Journal of Hepatology* **19**, 204–10.

Naoumov, N., Eddleston, A.L.W.F. 1994: Host immune response and variations in the virus genome: pathogenesis of liver damage caused by hepatitis B virus. *Gut* **35**, 1013–17.

Negro, F., Pacchioni, D., Shimizu, Y. *et al.* 1992: Detection of intrahepatic replication of hepatitis C virus RNA by in situ hybridisation and comparison with histopathology. *Proceedings of the National Academy of Sciences of the USA* **89**, 2247–51.

Negro, F., Bonino, F., Di Bisceglie, A., Hoofnagle, J.H., Gerin, J.L. 1989: Intrahepatic markers of hepatitis delta virus infection: a study by in situ hybridisation. *Hepatology* **10**, 916–20.

Negro, F., Baldi, M., Bonino, F., *et al.* 1988: Chronic HDV (hepatitis delta virus) hepatitis: intrahepatic expression of delta antigen, histologic activity and outcome of liver disease. *Journal of Hepatology* **6**, 8–14.

Negro, F., Pacchioni, D., Bussolati, G. *et al.* 1993: Pathobiology of hepatitis delta virus infection at the cell level. *Progress in Clinical and Biological Research* **382**, 155–60.

Nicoll, A.J., Angus, P.W., Chou, S.T., Luscombe, C.A., Smallwood, R.A., Locarnini, S.A. 1997: Demonstration of duck hepatitis B virus in bile duct epithelial cells: implications for pathogenesis and persistent infection. *Hepatology* **25**, 463–9.

Nouri-Aria, K.T., Sallie, R., Mizokami, M., Portmann, B.C., Williams, R. 1995: Intra-hepatic expression of hepatitis C virus antigens in chronic liver disease. *Journal of Pathology* **175**, 77–83.

Nouri-Aria, K.T., Sallie, R., Sangar, D. *et al.* 1993: Detection of genomic and intermediate replicative strands of hepatitis C virus in liver tissue by in situ hybridisation. *Journal of Clinical Investigation* **91** (5), 2226–34.

Nowoslawski, A., Brzosko, W., Madalinski, K., Krawczynski, K. 1970: Cellular localisation of Australia antigen in the liver of patients with lymphoproliferative disorders. *Lancet* **i**, 494–8.

Nuovo, G.J., Lidonnici, K., MacCownell, P., Lane, B. 1993: Intracellular localisation of polymerase chain reaction (PCR) – amplified hepatitis C cDNA. *American Journal of Surgical Pathology* **17**, 683–90.

Ray, M.B., Desmet, V.J., Bradburne, A.F., Desmyter, J., Fevery, J., de Groote, J. 1976: Differential distribution of hepatitis B surface antigen and hepatitis B core antigen in the liver of hepatitis B patients. *Gastroenterology* **71**, 462–7.

Roingeard, P., Romet-Lemonne, J., Leturcq, D., Goudeau, A., Essex, M. 1990: Hepatitis B virus core antigens (HBcAg) accumulation in a HBV non-producer clone of HepG2-transfected cells is associated with cytopathic effect. *Virology* **179**, 113–20.

Ryley, N.G., Heryet, A.R., Goldin, R., Monjardino, J., Saldanha, J., Fleming, K.A. 1992: Co-expression of markers for hepatitis delta and hepatitis B viruses in human liver. *Histopathology* **20**, 331–7.

Saldanha, J., Homer, E., Goldin, R., Thomas, H.C., Monjardino, J. 1990: Cloning and expression of an immunodominant region of the hepatitis delta antigen. *Journal of General Virology* **71**, 471–5.

Shimizu, Y.K., Feinstone, S.M., Kohara, M., Purcell, R.H., Yashihura, H. 1996: Hepatitis C virus: detection of intracellular virus particles by electron microscopy. *Hepatology* **23**, 205–9.

Su, Q., Schroder, C.H., Hofmann, W.J. *et al.* 1998: Expression of hepatitis B virus X protein in HBV-infected livers and hepatocellular carcinomas. *Hepatology* **27**, 1109–20.

Tanaka, Y., Enomoto, N., Kojima, S., *et al*, 1993: Detection of hepatitis C virus RNA in the liver by in situ hybridisation. *Liver* **13**, 203–8.

Taylor, G.M., Goldin, R.D., Karayiannis, P., Thomas, H.C. 1992: In situ hybridization studies in hepitiis A infection. *Hepatology* **16**, 642–8.

Taylor, M., Goldin, R.D., Ladva, S., Scheuer, P.J., Thomas, H.C. 1994: In situ hybridisation studies of hepatitis A viral RNA in patients with acute hepatitis A. *Journal of Hepatology* **20**, 380–7.

Yamada, G., Feinberg, L., Nakane, P. 1978: Hepatitis B: cytological localisation of virus antigens and the role of the immune response. *Human Pathology* **9**, 93–109.

Yamada, G., Nishimoto, H., Hisashi, E., *et al.* 1993: Localisation of hepatitis C viral RNA and capsid protein in human liver. *Digestive Diseases and Sciences* **38**(5), 882–7.

Yeh, C.T., Wong, S.W., Fung, Y.K., Ou, J.H., 1993: Cell cycle regulation of nuclear localisation of hepatitis B virus core protein. *Proceedings of the National Academy of Sciences of the USA* **90**, 6459–63.

CHAPTER 5

Viral hepatitis in immunosuppressed individuals

S G HÜBSCHER AND R D GOLDIN

Viral hepatitis in the liver allograft

S G HÜBSCHER

End-stage liver disease resulting from chronic viral hepatitis is one of the most common indications for liver transplantation. Infections with HBV and HCV frequently recur following transplantation and are important causes of graft dysfunction, sometimes resulting in graft failure or death. Many cases of post-transplant hepatitis occurring in patients transplanted for diseases of non-viral aetiology are also related to infection with HBV or HCV. These may be the result of the reactivation of latent virus in the recipient due to immunosuppression, or of acquired infection from the donor liver or blood products used during transplantation.

There are three important general factors related to liver transplantation that influence disease progression in the liver allograft infected with hepatitis B or C. These factors also have an important bearing on the histopathological assessment of specimens obtained from liver allograft recipients with HBV or HCV infection. First, the great majority of patients are maintained on long-term immunosuppression. In common with other immunocompromised individuals, this enables increased viral replication to occur, with possible direct cytopathic effects on infected hepatocytes. A second factor, unique to liver allograft recipients, is a disparity in MHC identity between the donor liver and recipient immune system. This prevents MHC-restricted viral clearance by T-lymphocytes and is another factor enabling uncontrolled viral replication to occur (*see* Chapter 7). A third problem concerns the relationship between viral hepatitis in the liver allograft and other complications of liver transplantation, especially rejection. For example, there are histological similarities between acute cellular rejection and hepatitis C infection, and the differential diagnosis between these two processes is often difficult in needle biopsy specimens. The synergistic actions of hepatitis viruses and rejection on common target structures (e.g. bile duct damage in hepatitis C and cellular rejection) is another possible factor to consider.

Liver transplantation is rarely carried out for other forms of viral hepatitis. A small number of people have been transplanted for fulminant hepatitis resulting from infection with HAV or HEV. Recent studies have identified HGV as a common infection in patients

Typical features of recurrent HBV infection

Three main phases of reinfection were identified in the studies by Demetris *et al* (1986) and Davies *et al* (1991). In the initial 'incubation phase' (the first 2–3 months post-transplant), serum HBsAg is typically negative or present in a falling titre. Biopsies obtained during this time show changes related to acute rejection or other early post-transplant complications of liver transplantation. There is some evidence to suggest that acute rejection is less common and less severe in patients transplanted for HBV cirrhosis than in those transplanted for non-viral cirrhosis (Adams *et al*, 1991; Farges *et al*, 1996). This may reflect immune 'paralysis' induced by HBV infection or the immunosuppressive effects of anti-HBs immunoglobulins. Histological changes directly attributable to HBV are rarely seen during the earliest stages of reinfection in conventionally stained sections (Fig. 5.1a). However, immunohistochemical staining for HBV-associated antigens is sometimes positive during this period, usually in the form of focal cytoplasmic or nuclear staining for core antigen (Demetris *et al*, 1990; Hopf *et al*, 1991) (Fig. 5.1b). In the study of Phillips *et al* (1992), the earliest indicator of recurrent infection was focal positive HBsAg staining, which was followed by nuclear HBcAg immunoreactivity. At this early stage, the liver appeared histologically normal or showed only a slight disarray of hepatocytes.

The second phase of 'early reinfection' (1–12 months post-transplant) is characterised serologically by the return of HBsAg or a rise in titre. Biopsies taken during this period typically show predominantly lobular changes characteristic of acute viral hepatitis (Fig. 5.2). These are generally mild and include spotty inflammation, scattered acidophil bodies, Kupffer cell hypertrophy and minor degrees of lobular disarray. More severe damage with prominent cholestasis and/or areas of confluent necrosis has been documented in occasional cases (Davies *et al*, 1991). Varying degrees of portal inflammation may also be present.

Portal inflammatory changes generally become more prominent as the disease progresses to the third stage of 'established (chronic) infection'. This is characterised serologically by HBsAg titres reaching a plateau level. Histological changes at this stage closely resemble those seen in chronic viral hepatitis involving the non-transplanted liver (Fig. 5.3). In addition to predominantly portal inflammation, there is variable interface hepatitis ('piecemeal necrosis') and progressive fibrosis, eventually leading in some cases to cirrhosis (Fig. 5.4).

Although histological features are generally similar to those occurring in the non-transplanted disease, severity and speed of progression are considerably greater in the liver allograft. In a combined series of 42 patients reinfected with HBV following transplantation, 41 developed acute hepatitis, 20 had histological features of chronic hepatitis and 8 had become cirrhotic within a period ranging from 7 to 70 months (Samuel *et al*, 1991; Todo *et al*, 1991).

Cases of apparent acquired infection, from either reactivation of latent infection in recipient liver or undetected infection in the donor, generally behave in a less aggressive manner than those with recurrent disease. The severity of the chronic hepatitic changes is less, fewer cases progress to cirrhosis and overall survival is better (Chazouillères *et al*, 1994a; Liu *et al*, 1996; Roche *et al*, 1997). The inoculum of the virus is generally much lower in these cases, which may account for their more favourable outcome.

Atypical features of recurrent HBV infection

Three main atypical patterns of reinfection have been identified: hepatocyte ballooning, fatty change and a distinctive cholestatic syndrome ('fibrosing cholestatic hepatitis').

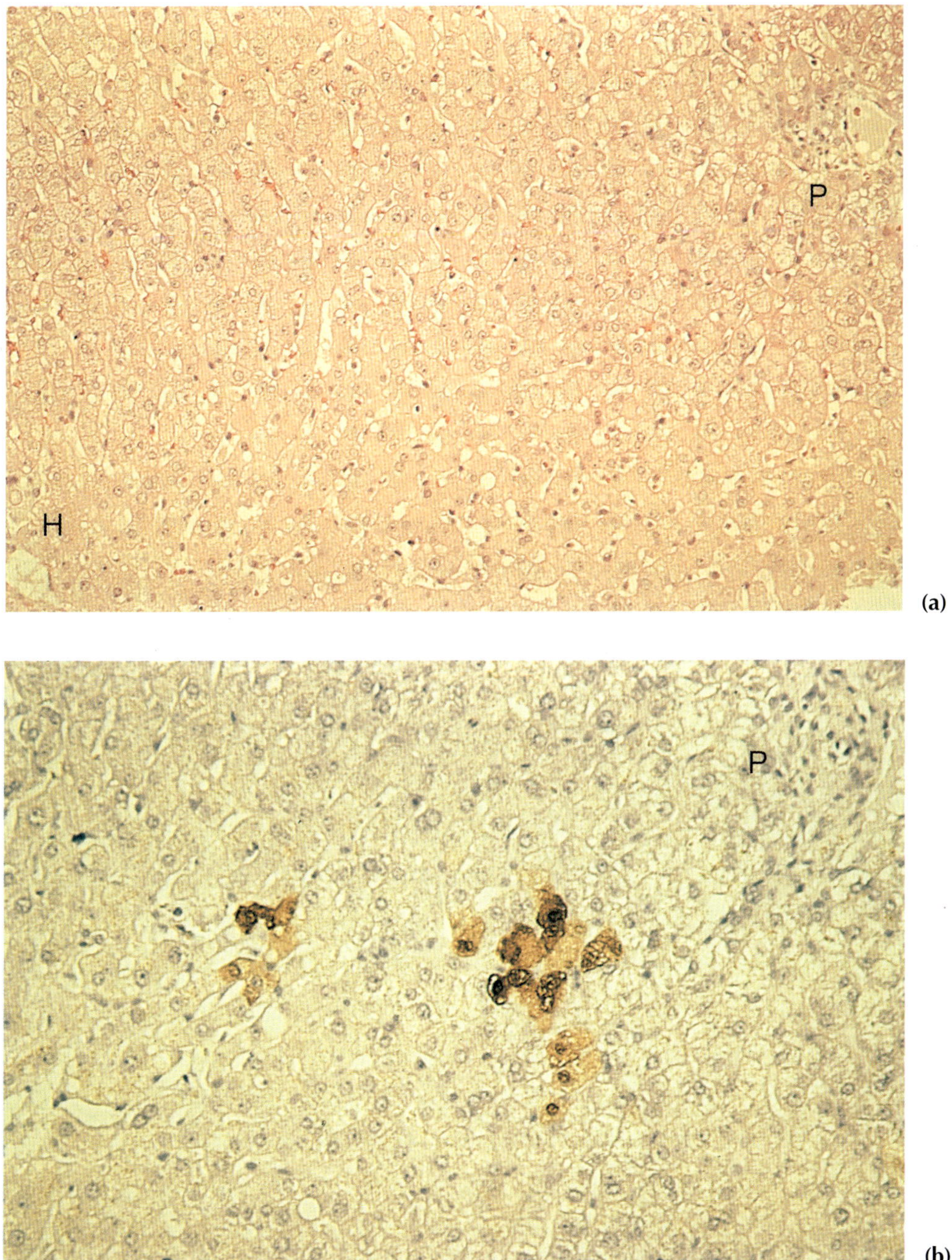

Fig 5.1 Early ('incubation phase') recurrent hepatitis B infection. (a) Liver biopsy, 5 weeks following liver transplantation, appears normal by conventional light microscopy (H&E). P, portal tract; H, hepatic venule. (b) Scattered hepatocytes show positive immunostaining for HBcAg (immunoperoxidase). P, portal tract.

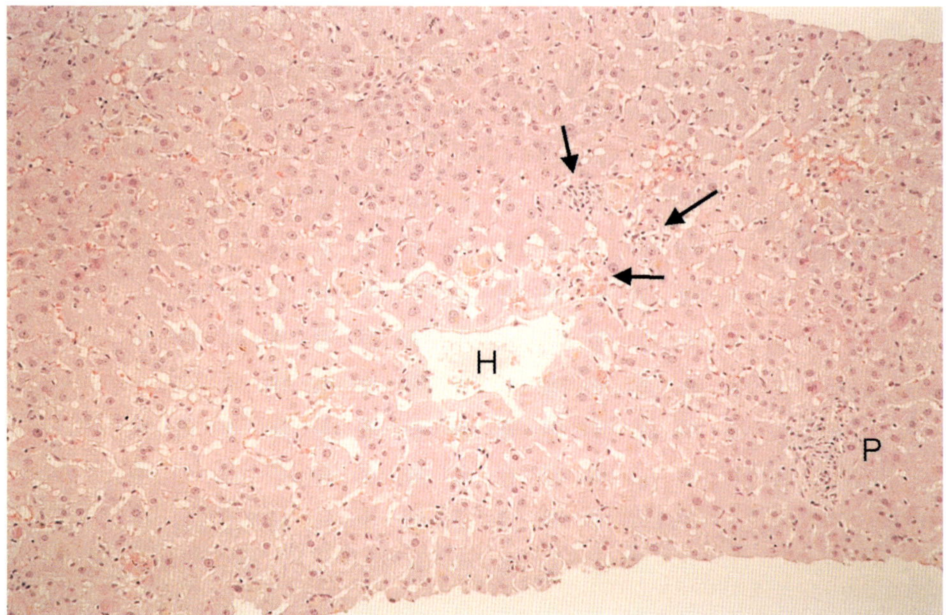

Fig 5.2   Early recurrent hepatitis B infection with mild lobular hepatitis. Needle biopsy, 3 months post-transplant, shows mild spotty inflammation (arrows) in parenchyma surrounding a terminal hepatic venule (H). Small portal tract (P) appears normal (H&E).

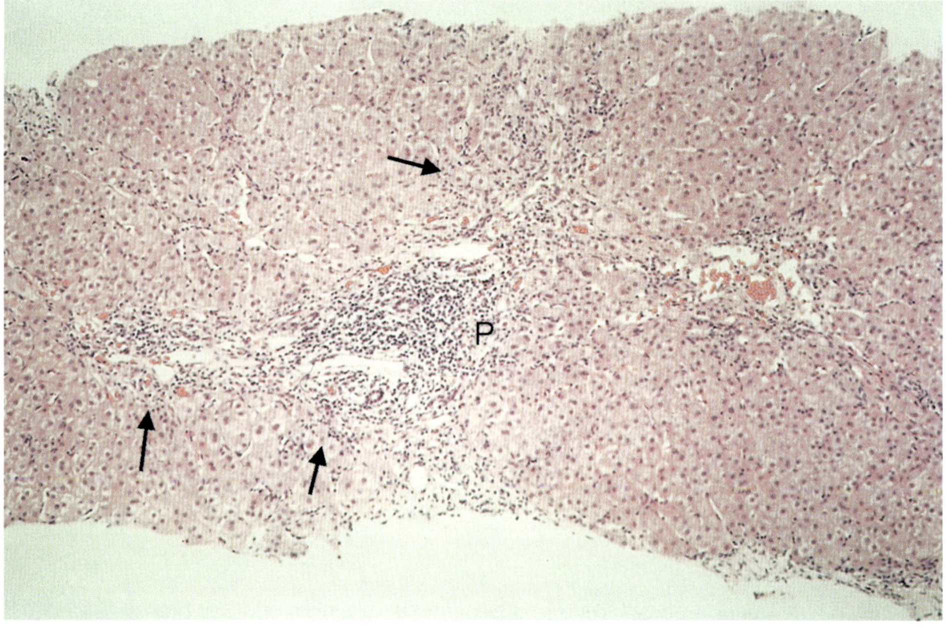

Fig 5.3   Chronic hepatitis in a liver allograft (recurrent hepatitis B infection). Needle biopsy, 25 months post-transplant. Portal tract (P) shows fibrous expansion and contains a moderately dense infiltrate of inflammatory cells. There is mild interface hepatitis (arrows) (H&E).

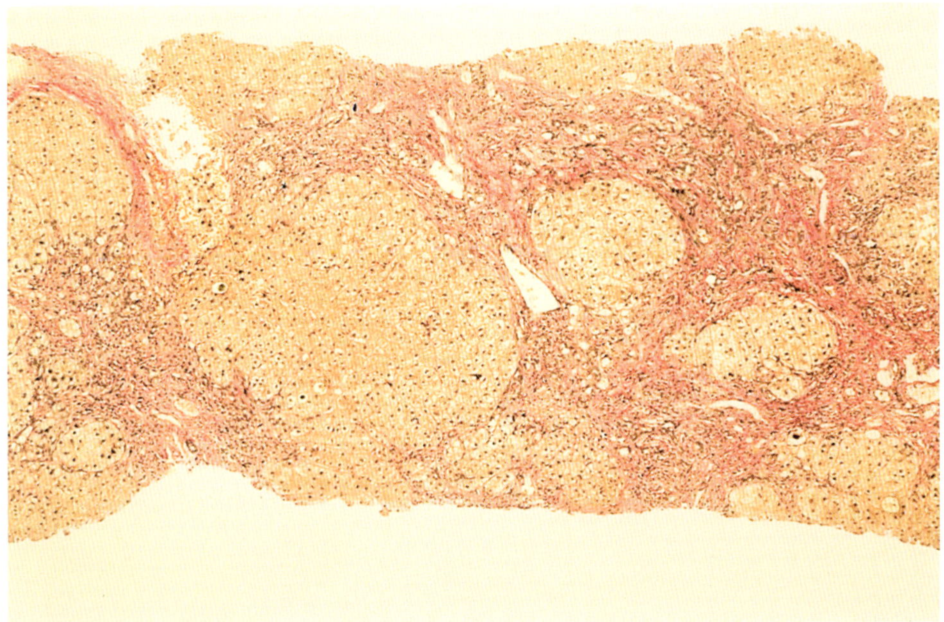

Fig 5.4   Recurrent hepatitis B with micronodular cirrhosis. Liver biopsy, 14 months post-transplant, shows an established micronodular cirrhosis. There is mild ongoing inflammatory activity (haematoxylin Van Gieson).

These frequently occur in combination and are probably part of a spectrum of HBV infection occurring in immunocompromised individuals.

Hepatocyte ballooning typically occurs without significant accompanying inflammation and is associated with diffuse (often panacinar) cytoplasmic and nuclear immunostaining for HBcAg (Fig. 5.5). A similar pattern of immunostaining has also been described for HBeAg (Harrison *et al*, 1993). These observations suggest massive viral replication resulting in direct cytopathic damage to hepatocytes.

Hepatocyte ballooning may be accompanied by varying degrees of fatty change. In cases where steatosis is particularly prominent, the term 'steatoviral hepatitis' has been used (Phillips *et al*, 1992). Ultrastructural studies by Phillips *et al* (1992) identified that changes related to ballooning, fat droplets and excess HBsAg frequently co-existed in the same cells, further supporting the idea that these hepatocellular degenerative changes have a common pathogenetic mechanism.

The term 'fibrosing cholestatic hepatitis' (FCH) was first used by Davies *et al* (1991) to describe a distinctive pattern of graft damage occurring in six out of 23 patients who developed recurrent HBV infection. Similar patterns of damage have been reported in other studies (Demetris *et al*, 1990; Todo *et al*, 1991; Benner *et al*, 1992; Lucey *et al*, 1992; Phillips *et al*, 1992; Harrison *et al*, 1993). Other terms that have been proposed for this condition are 'fibrosing cytolytic hepatitis' (Benner *et al*, 1992) and 'fibroviral hepatitis' (Phillips *et al*, 1992). FCH is characterised histologically by periportal fibrosis extending as thin perisinusoidal strands for varying distances into the liver acinus, accompanied by flat ductular structures without an identifiable lumen (Fig. 5.6). The liver parenchyma shows prominent hepatocyte ballooning and cholestasis. Inflammatory changes are generally mild or absent. The histological picture is suggestive of biliary

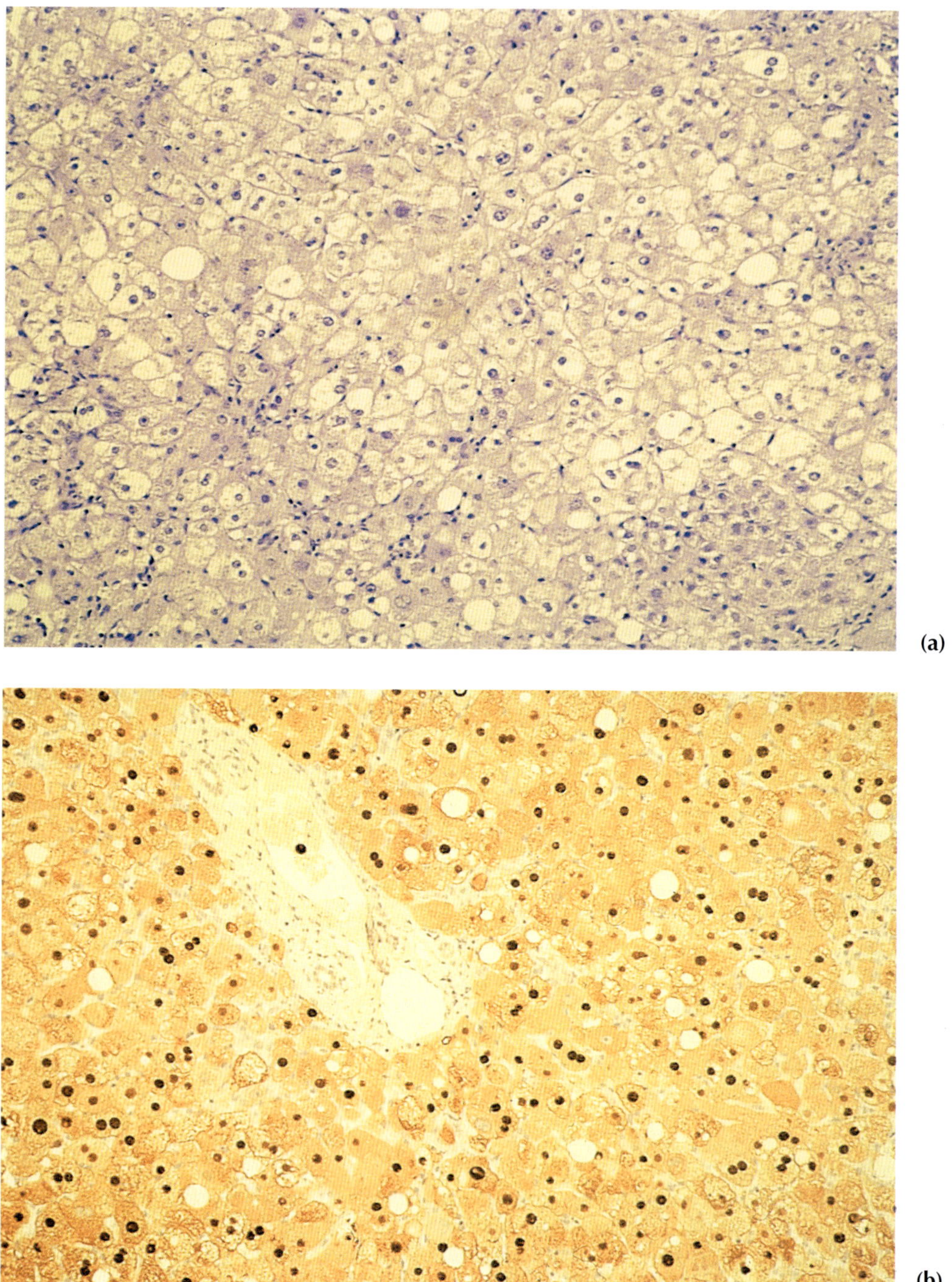

Fig 5.5   Recurrent hepatitis B associated with diffuse hepatocyte ballooning, focal mild steatosis and no obvious inflammatory infiltration. There is diffuse immunoreactivity for HBcAg (nuclear and cytoplasmic) (a, stained with H&E; b, stained with immunoperoxidase).

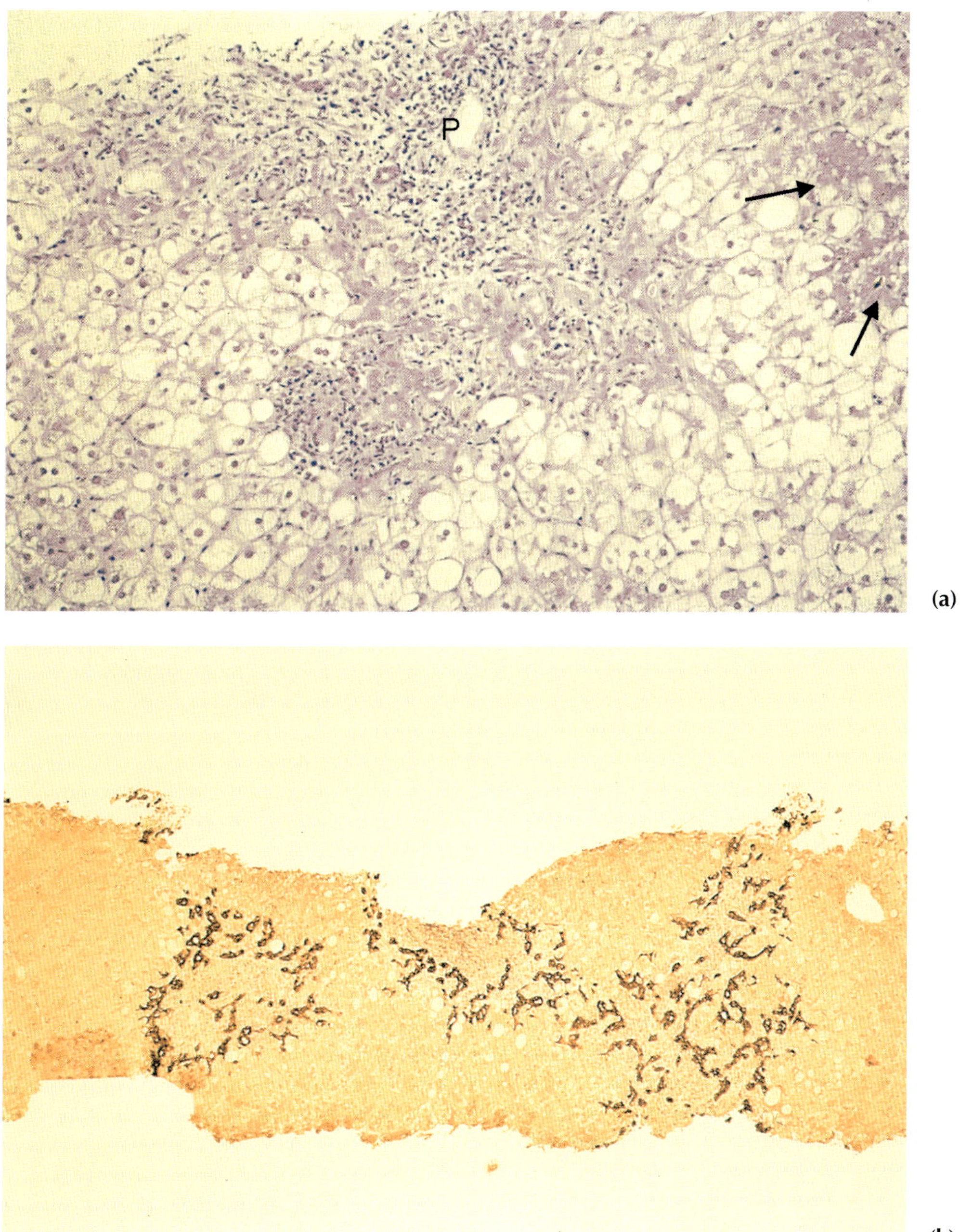

Fig 5.6 Fibrosing cholestatic hepatitis in recurrent hepatitis B infection. Portal tract (P) is expanded with prominent marginal ductular proliferation mimicking the changes seen in biliary obstruction. Liver parenchyma shows diffuse hepatocyte ballooning and focal bile plugging (arrows). Immunostaining for biliary cytokeratins (AE1) emphasises the extent of ductular proliferation (a, stained with H&E; b, stained with immunoperoxidase).

disease, and it is difficult to exclude biliary obstruction in some cases. Lack of portal oedema, well-preserved interlobular ducts and the radiological demonstration of a normal biliary tree help to exclude biliary obstruction and confirm a diagnosis of FCH. Immunohistochemical studies have produced variable results. In the study of Davies *et al* (1991), FCH was associated with extensive cytoplasmic HBsAg expression and variable HBcAg staining, mainly nuclear. Other studies have shown extensive nuclear and cytoplasmic expression of HBcAg in FCH (Benner *et al*, 1992; Lucey *et al*, 1992; Harrison *et al*, 1993). Most cases present during the first few months following transplantation. Once a diagnosis of FCH has been established, the clinical picture is one of rapidly progressive graft failure associated with prominent biochemical cholestasis. In cases where further specimens are available for histological examination, a distinctive pattern of extensive post-necrotic collapse with immature fibrosis and widespread ductular proliferation may be seen (Fig. 5.7)

In early studies of recurrent HBV infection, FCH was relatively common with a nearly universal poor outcome. In a combined series of 69 patients with recurrent HBV infection reported in five studies, 19 developed FCH and 18 of these progressed to death or graft failure (Davies *et al*, 1991; Todo *et al*, 1991; Benner *et al*, 1992; Lucey *et al*, 1992; Harrison *et al*, 1993). The one surviving patient was cirrhotic (Harrison *et al*, 1993). There is some evidence to suggest that FCH is becoming less common in recurrent HBV infection, possibly as a result of immunoprophylaxis and other measures used to reduce the incidence of recurrent HBV infection in general. Occasional patients with FCH have been successfully treated with antiviral agents such as lamivudine and ganciclovir (Woolf *et al*, 1995; Jamal *et al*, 1996).

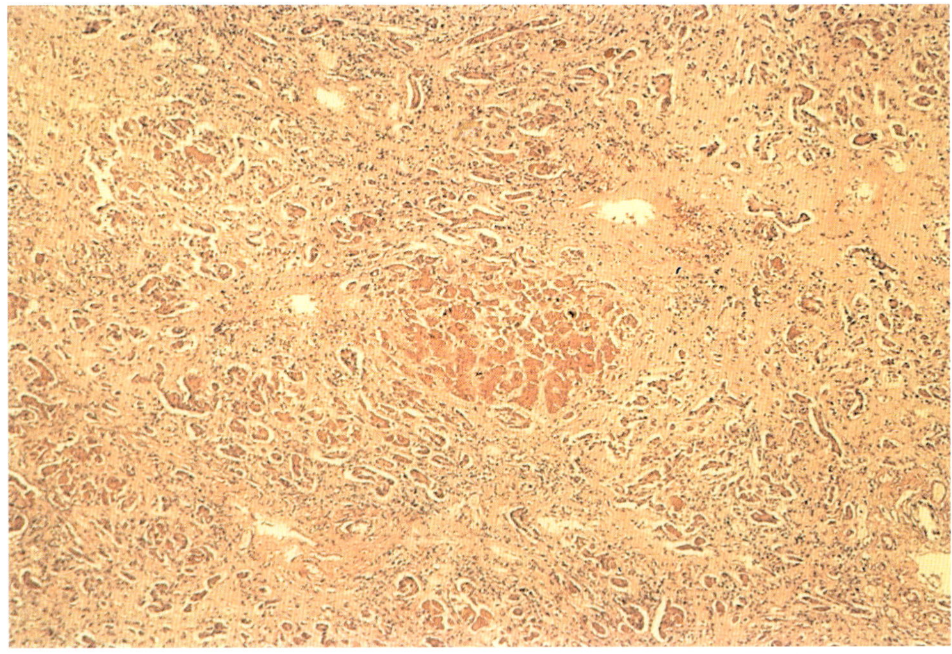

Fig 5.7 Fibrosing cholestatic hepatitis in recurrent hepatitis B infection. Post mortem liver, 18 months following liver transplantation. A solitary, small surviving hepatocyte nodule is surrounded by broad areas of post-necrotic collapse associated with extensive bile ductular proliferation (H&E).

Although FCH is generally regarded as a distinctive syndrome with histological features completely different from those of typical acute and chronic viral hepatitis, cases with combined or overlapping histological features do occur. We have also seen cases that initially presented with FCH-like features but then reverted to a more typical hepatitic picture following the withdrawal of immunosuppression.

Pathogenetic mechanisms

The mechanisms involved in liver allograft damage occurring with recurrent HBV infection are still not well understood. In immunocompetent individuals, damage to the liver is largely immune mediated (*see* Chapter 7). Viral peptides related to HBV nucleocapsid (HBcAg) are presented by class I MHC molecules on the surface of hepatocytes and are recognised by CD8+ cytotoxic T-cells expressing the same MHC antigens. It is possible that a similar mechanism may operate to some extent in the liver allograft. However, liver transplantation is associated with important effects both on the dynamics of the viral population and on the host immune system.

HBV-associated nucleic acids have been identified in peripheral blood mononuclear cells and several extrahepatic sites, including lymph nodes, spleen, kidney and various endocrine organs (Pontisso *et al*, 1984; Davison *et al*, 1987; Feray *et al*, 1990; Yoffe *et al*, 1990). It is likely that these are the source of reinfection in cases with recurrent HBV infection. Levels of HBV DNA increase markedly following liver transplantation, indicating increased viral replication (O'Grady *et al*, 1992). Two separate mechanisms related to immunosuppression are likely to be important in this respect. First, corticosteroids can directly activate HBV replication by acting on a steroid-responsive promotor in the HBV genome (Lam *et al*, 1981; Tur-Kapsa *et al*, 1986). Other immunosuppressive agents, including azathioprine, may also directly promote viral replication (McMillan *et al*, 1995). Second, the suppression of normal T-cell responses may have an indirect effect on viral replication. A similar mechanism has been postulated for the reactivation of HBV replication in cancer patients receiving chemotherapy (Lok *et al*, 1991).

HLA matching is not carried out routinely in liver transplantation, and host–viral interactions involving the recognition of class I MHC molecules by cytotoxic T-lymphocytes are thus likely to be impaired in most cases. Matching of class I antigens between donor and recipient would facilitate classical T-cell-mediated hepatocyte destruction, whereas mismatching would further promote uncontrolled viral replication.

Histological studies of recurrent HBV infection, as described above, suggest two main pathways of liver damage in recurrent HBV infection. Most cases have inflammatory infiltrates similar to those seen in viral hepatitis involving the non-transplanted liver. A minority have atypical features characterised by florid hepatocellular damage occurring without significant inflammation, suggesting the possibility of direct cytopathic damage. It would be tempting to postulate that cases of recurrent HBV with typical histological features of viral hepatitis have a partially intact MHC recognition system, while atypical histological patterns might be expected to reflect uncontrolled viral replication occurring in the face of complete mismatching for MHC class I antigens. While there are some limited observations in support of this hypothesis (Calmus *et al*, 1990; Demetris *et al*, 1990), no definite association has been demonstrated between HLA matching and graft hepatitis or survival in patients transplanted for HBV-related disease.

Further evidence for a direct cytopathic role for viral proteins is provided by experiments with transgenic mice, genetically manipulated to produce large amounts of cytoplasmic HBsAg with impaired secretion (Chisari *et al*, 1987). This results in direct cytopathic damage to the hepatocytes and a picture resembling FCH in human liver allografts (Lau *et al*, 1992).

In cases where there is complete mismatching for MHC class I antigens, class I-independent pathways of inflammatory liver damage have been postulated (Missale *et al*, 1993). These could involve the uptake of viral antigens by Kupffer cells, which are replaced by macrophages of recipient origin soon after transplantation (Gouw *et al*, 1987; Steinhoff *et al*, 1987), and subsequent class II-restricted presentation to CD4 T-cells. Activated CD4+ T-cells and macrophages release cytokines that are cytotoxic for HBV-positive and normal hepatocytes (Missale *et al*, 1993).

The possible role of HBV mutations in the pathogenesis of post-transplant liver disease has recently been investigated (*see* Chapter 1). The presence of the pre-core mutant is associated with more severe disease in the liver allograft, including FCH (Fang *et al*, 1993a; Angus *et al*, 1995; McMillan *et al*, 1996). It is possible that the lack of HBeAg expression that occurs with this mutation enables the virus to escape immune recognition and thus promotes uncontrolled viral replication. Mutations in the HBV genome have also been suggested as a possible mechanism for viral 'escape' in cases where reinfection occurs despite receiving HBsIg therapy (Carman *et al*, 1996; Hawkins *et al*, 1996). Mutations in the YMDD locus of the HBV polymerase gene have been identified in cases where viral 'escape' occurs on lamivudine therapy (Ling *et al*, 1996; Bartholomew *et al*, 1997). Similar changes have also been reported in drug-resistant HIV infection.

HEPATITIS C

Incidence and detection of recurrent infection

The great majority (more than 90%) of patients with chronic HCV infection who undergo liver transplantation have virological markers of recurrent infection post-transplant (Wright *et al*, 1992; Ascher *et al*, 1994; Feray *et al*, 1994; Weinstein *et al*, 1995). Conventional serological testing for anti-HCV antibodies is not reliable in this group of immunosuppressed individuals, and more sensitive techniques for detecting HCV RNA in serum are therefore required (Read *et al*, 1991; Poterucha *et al*, 1992; Shah *et al*, 1992; Caccamo *et al*, 1993; Hsu *et al*, 1994). The measurement of HCV RNA by the reverse transcription polymerase chain reaction (RT-PCR) has become the standard method of detecting disease recurrence. Using this technique, persistent HCV infection can be detected within the first few days following transplantation (Fukumoto *et al*, 1996; Gane *et al*, 1996a). HCV RNA can also be identified by signal amplification using a branched DNA assay technique developed by the Chiron Corporation (Chazouillères *et al*, 1994b; Davis *et al*, 1994). This technique is less sensitive than RT-PCR but provides quantitative measurements of HCV RNA. HCV RNA levels typically decrease immediately following transplantation but then rapidly increase, reaching up to 100 times the pre-transplant levels at 2–3 months post-transplantation (Chazouillères *et al*, 1994b; Gane *et al*, 1996a).

Risk factors for symptomatic or severe disease

Although recurrent infection is almost universal, not all patients develop symptomatic liver disease. Early studies, with relatively short follow-up periods, suggested that only about 50% of patients with recurrent infection developed symptomatic hepatitis during the first year following transplantation (Ferrell *et al*, 1992; Pereira *et al*, 1993; Knoop *et al*, 1994). However, more recent studies with longer periods of observation suggest that the majority of cases eventually develop the histological features of hepatitis (Feray *et al*, 1994; Shiffman *et al*, 1994; Gane *et al*, 1996b). In the study of Gane *et al* (1996b), only

15 (12%) out of 130 patients followed up for more than 6 months following transplantation had no evidence of hepatitis in their most recent biopsy.

A number of risk factors predisposing to more severe liver disease (usually defined according to severity of histological changes in post-transplant biopsies) have been identified (Table 5.2).

Several studies have identified HCV genotype 1b as a risk factor for the development of hepatitis and for the subsequent progression to fibrosis/cirrhosis (Feray *et al*, 1995a; Gane *et al*, 1996b; Alberti *et al*, 1997; Gordon *et al*, 1997), although other studies have failed to confirm this association (Zhou *et al*, 1996; Arnold *et al*, 1997). Genotype 1b has also been associated with more aggressive disease in the non-transplanted liver (Dusheiko *et al*, 1994; Pozzato *et al*, 1994; Qu *et al*, 1994) (*see* Chapter 7).

Levels of viraemia appear to correlate both with the onset of clinical episodes of acute graft hepatitis and with subsequent progression to chronic liver disease (Duvoux *et al*, 1995; Gretch *et al*, 1995; Gane *et al*, 1996a). Serial RNA measurements may be helpful in confirming a diagnosis of HCV hepatitis in cases where there is a problem distinguishing recurrent HCV infection from other causes of graft inflammation, especially acute cellular rejection (Duvoux *et al*, 1995).

Acute rejection in the early post-transplant period is a potentially important risk factor for the subsequent development of HCV-related graft damage. The severity of rejection, the number of episodes, the total amount of immunosuppression given and the use of potent immunosuppressive agents (e.g. OKT3 and FK 506) have all been associated with a higher risk of recurrent HCV hepatitis (Sheiner *et al*, 1995; Freeman *et al*, 1996; Johnson *et al*, 1996; Singh *et al*, 1996). Increased immunosuppression given to treat acute rejection episodes presumably permits the occurrence of increased viral replication, which predisposes to more severe HCV-related graft damage.

Experience with retransplantation for end-stage disease as a result of recurrent HCV infection is limited. Some studies have reported a poor outcome following retransplantation for HCV-related graft failure, including occasional cases with aggressive recurrent HCV infection (Dickson *et al*, 1996; Johnson *et al*, 1996; Schluger *et al*, 1996). However, it is not clear whether adverse outcome is related to recurrent HCV infection itself or is simply a manifestation of the problems associated with retransplantation in general (Rosen *et al*, 1996).

Histopathological features and natural history

As with recurrent HBV infection, histological findings in HCV infection of the liver allograft can be divided into two main categories. Typical features of HCV infection, as seen in the non-transplanted liver, occur in the majority of cases. More rarely, there are atypical patterns of liver damage, presumably related to other factors present in liver allograft recipients.

Table 5.2   Risk factors for symptomatic or severe hepatitis in recurrent hepatitis C infection

Genotype 1b
Early acute rejection
Severe rejection
Multiple episodes
Viral levels
Previous transplantation for hepatitis C

Typical features of recurrent HCV infection

As with recurrent HBV infection, three main phases can be identified. During the early stages of reinfection, when viral RNA levels are already high, histological features directly attributable to HCV are rarely seen. Acute cellular rejection is the most common histological diagnosis during the first month following transplantation. Although there are histological similarities between cellular rejection and HCV-related portal hepatitis (discussed further below), the differential diagnosis between these two conditions is rarely a problem in the early post-transplant period. In some cases, an initial episode of graft dysfunction, probably related to recurrent HCV infection, is characterised by a lack of inflammatory changes, including the absence of rejection (Petrovic *et al*, 1993; Greenson *et al*, 1996). Subsequent biopsies from these patients have shown progression to more typical features of HCV hepatitis. A recent study by pathologists contributing to the National Institute of Diabetes and Digestive and Kidney Disease Database suggested that histological abnormalities related to HCV could be seen as early as 1 week post-transplantation (Batts *et al*, presented at the AASLD Transplant course, Chicago, USA, 8 November 1996). These interesting observations clearly require further study.

The next stage is one of an acute lobular hepatitis, typically occurring 2–4 months post-transplant. Serial biopsies studied by Feray *et al* (1994), Gane *et al* (1996b) and Greenson *et al* (1996) showed median times to onset of acute lobular hepatitis of 4 months (range 30 days to 4 years), 77 days (range 23–469 days) and 135 days (range 39–279 days) respectively. Histological findings at this stage are generally mild and include lobular disarray, increased sinusoidal lymphocytes, hepatocellular ballooning, acidophil bodies and Kupffer cell enlargement (Fig. 5.8).

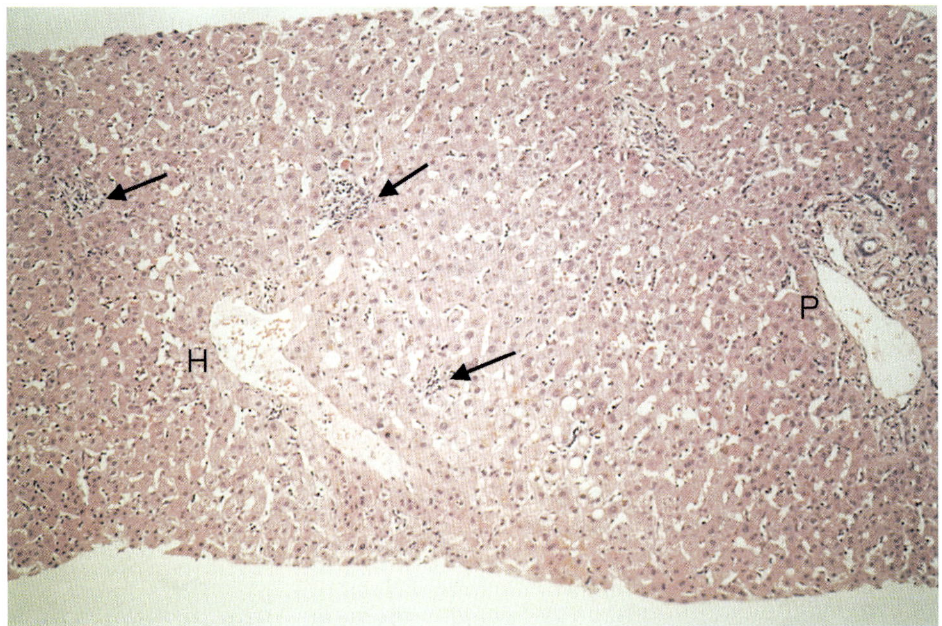

Fig 5.8   Early recurrent hepatitis C infection. Liver biopsy, 4 months post-transplant, shows mild spotty parenchymal inflammation (arrows). Portal tract (P) appears normal (H&E). H, hepatic venule.

The third stage is one of chronic hepatitis. This is typically seen more than 6 months post-transplant. Approximately 50% of patients have histological signs of chronic hepatitis at 1 year post-transplant, this figure rising with longer periods of follow-up (Feray *et al*, 1994; Gane *et al*, 1996b; Greenson *et al*, 1996). Histological features have been well documented (Ferrell *et al*, 1992; Randhawa and Demetris, 1995; Greenson *et al*, 1996) and resemble those seen in chronic HCV infection of the non-transplanted liver (Scheuer *et al*, 1991; Bach *et al*, 1992) (Fig. 5.9). There is a predominantly portal hepatitis with the formation of lymphoid aggregates and a focal lymphocytic infiltration of bile ducts. In cases where bile duct damage is conspicuous, distinction from acute cellular rejection can be difficult (*see* below). Variable interface hepatitis is seen. There is also commonly spotty lobular inflammation, fatty change (usually macrovesicular) and focal acidophil body formation.

Although histological features are generally similar to those seen in the non-transplanted liver, there is a general impression that the disease behaves more aggressively in the liver allograft. The majority of chronic HCV hepatitis occurring in the non-transplanted liver is associated with mild or minimal interface hepatitis ('piecemeal necrosis'). Progression to cirrhosis is slow, typically occurring over a period of 10–20 years. Precise comparison is difficult, but interface hepatitis is generally more conspicuous in post-transplant biopsies with recurrent HCV infection. Confluent and bridging necrosis (very uncommon in HCV in the non-transplant setting) may also be seen (Thung *et al*, 1993)

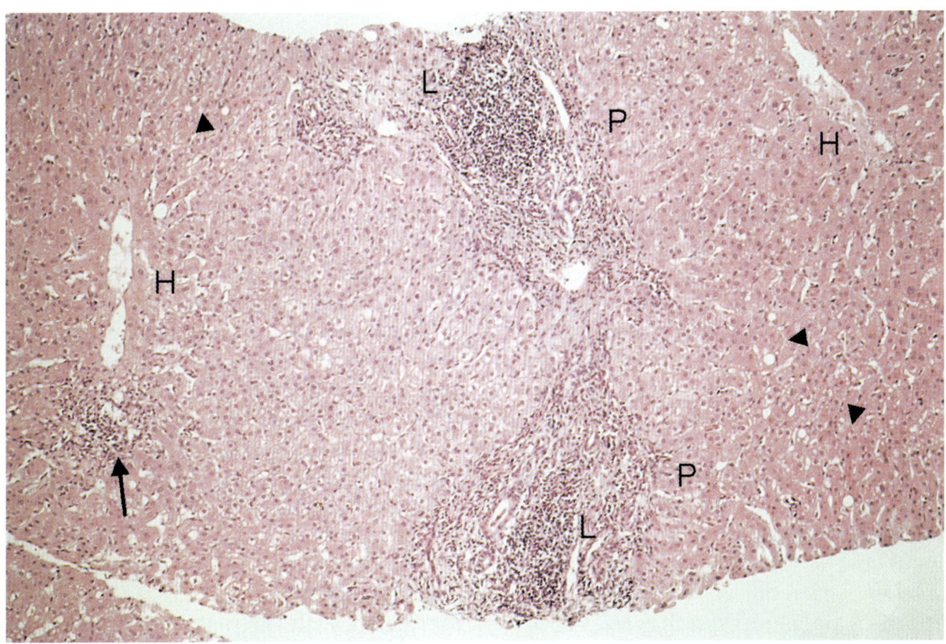

Fig 5.9   Chronic hepatitis in liver allograft (recurrent hepatitis C infection). Liver biopsy, 6 months post-transplant, shows characteristic features of chronic hepatitis C infection. Portal tracts (P) are expanded with a moderately dense infiltrate of inflammatory cells, including occasional lymphoid aggregates (L). An occasional small inflammatory aggregate (arrow) is present in the liver parenchyma along with focal mild fatty change (arrow heads). Also seen are hepatic venules (H) (H&E).

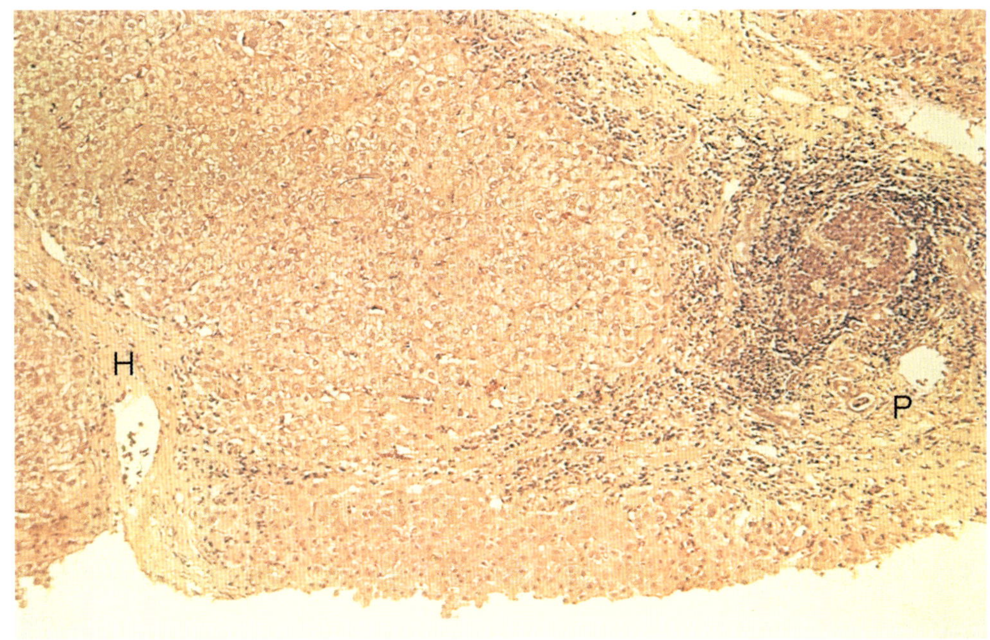

Fig 5.10 Recurrent hepatitis C infection with severe necroinflammatory activity. Liver biopsy, 3 years post-transplant. Portal tract (P) contains a moderately dense infiltrate of inflammatory cells including a lymphoid follicle with germinal centre. There is an area of bridging necrosis extending to a hepatic venule (H) (H&E).

(Fig. 5.10), and there appears to be more rapid progression to fibrosis and cirrhosis. In a study of 105 patients with chronic HCV hepatitis post-transplant, 70 (67%) had mild disease with cellular infiltrates mostly confined to portal areas, while the other 35 (33%) had moderate-to-severe disease associated with extensive interface hepatitis (Gane *et al*, 1996b). Ten (8%) out of 130 patients followed up for more than 6 months in this study had become cirrhotic at a median time of 51 months post-transplant. Cases of HCV-related cirrhosis occurring within 1 year of transplantation have been seen (Fig. 5.11).

There have been several studies describing techniques for specifically identifying HCV-related antigens (immunohistochemistry) or HCV RNA (in situ hybridisation, in situ polymerase chain reaction) in tissue sections (Hiramatsu *et al*, 1992; Krawczynski *et al*, 1992; Lamas *et al*, 1992; Blight *et al*, 1993; Chamlion *et al*, 1993; Nuovo *et al*, 1993) (*see* Chapter 4). These have shown much variation in the extent and distribution of HCV antigens and RNA in the non-transplanted liver. Limited immunohistochemical studies have been carried out on liver allograft specimens. In the study of Gretch *et al* (1995), the extent of cytoplasmic staining for HCV NS4 correlated with the histological severity of hepatitis. In serial biopsies examined by Gane *et al* (1996b), the initial appearance of the HCV core and NS4 antigens correlated with peak serum HCV RNA levels and the onset of lobular hepatitis. Immunohistochemistry is potentially a very valuable tool in augmenting conventional histological diagnoses and understanding pathogenetic mechanisms of HCV infection in liver allografts. Unfortunately, there are still considerable problems in obtaining reliable and reproducible results, especially in routinely processed paraffin-embedded tissues.

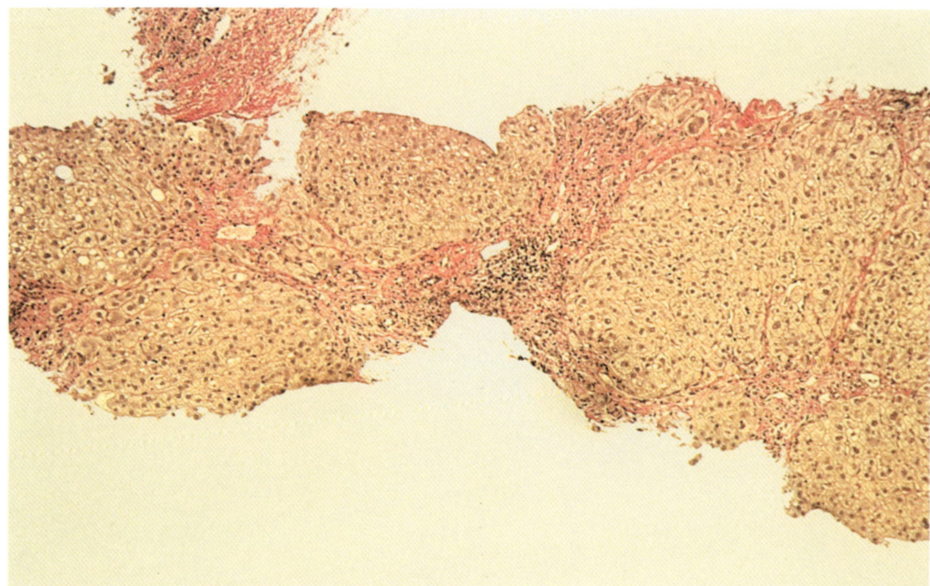

Fig 5.11 Recurrent hepatitis C infection with early cirrhosis. Liver biopsy, 1 year post-transplantation, showing periportal and bridging fibrosis with early nodule formation (H&E).

Atypical features of recurrent HCV infection

A number of atypical histological manifestations of recurrent HCV infection have been recognised. There are similarities between these and the atypical patterns of recurrent HBV infection described earlier.

Diffuse hepatocyte ballooning sometimes occurs without a conspicuous inflammatory reaction, raising the possibility of direct cytopathic damage (Ferrell *et al*, 1992) (Fig. 5.12). In cases where ballooning is confined to peripheral acinar regions, distinction from graft ischaemia or other causes of centrilobular ballooning (Goldstein *et al*, 1991; Hübscher, 1991; Ng *et al*, 1991) may be difficult.

A cholestatic syndrome resembling fibrosing cholestatic hepatitis B infection has also been seen in a small number of cases (Ferrell *et al*, 1992; Vargas *et al*, 1994; Dickson *et al*, 1996; Schluger *et al*, 1996). Histological features include portal expansion with prominent marginal zones of ductular proliferation, mimicking the changes seen in biliary obstruction (Ferrell *et al*, 1992; Randhawa and Demetris, 1995) (Fig 5.13). The liver parenchyma typically shows prominent hepatocyte ballooning, which may be the earliest histological manifestation of this condition (Dickson *et al*, 1996), and severe cholestasis. In some cases, cholestatic features are seen in conjunction with more typical hepatitic lesions. The outlook in cholestatic HCV hepatitis is poor. Most cases progress rapidly to graft failure or death within a few months of diagnosis. The examination of failed allografts obtained at retransplantation has shown varying histological changes including persistent severe cholestasis and hepatocyte ballooning, multiacinar necrosis, bridging fibrosis and cirrhosis (Dickson *et al*, 1996; Schluger *et al*, 1996).

An unusual pattern of recurrent HCV infection with granulomatous bile duct destruction, closely resembling the changes seen in primary biliary cirrhosis, has been noted in

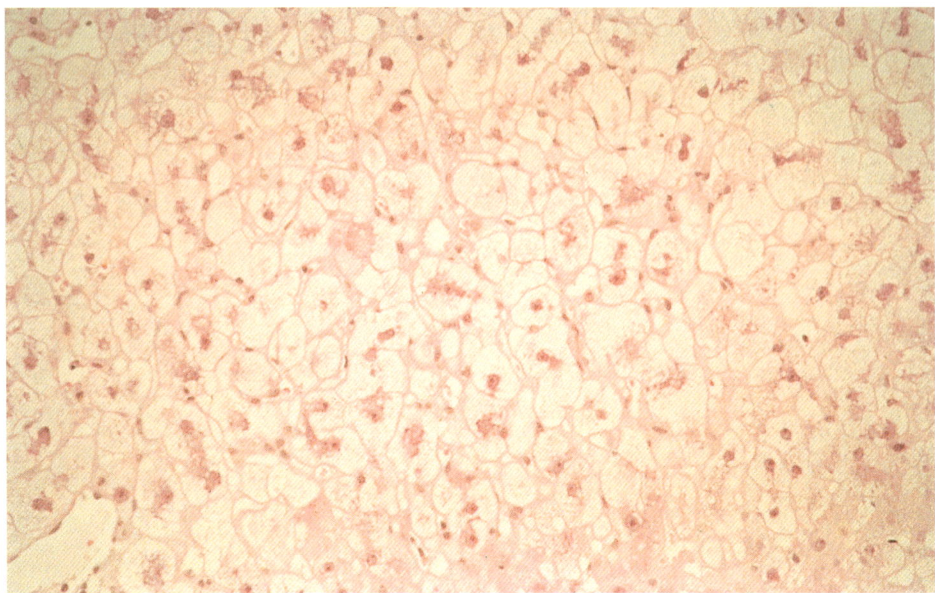

Fig 5.12 Recurrent hepatitis C infection associated with diffuse hepatocyte ballooning. Liver biopsy, 4 months post-transplant. Appearances resemble those of recurrent hepatitis B infection as seen in Figure 5.5. Note again the absence of inflammatory infiltration (H&E).

a single biopsy obtained 18 months post-transplant from a woman with recurrent HCV hepatitis (Sebagh *et al*, 1995). The original hepatectomy specimen from this patient contained parenchymal granulomas, which have recently been recognised as a histological feature of chronic HCV infection (Emile *et al*, 1993; Goldin *et al*, 1996a) (*see* Chapter 3).

Hepatitis C versus acute (cellular) rejection

A major problem in the assessment of post-transplant biopsies from patients transplanted for HCV-related liver disease is the distinction between recurrent HCV infection and acute cellular rejection. Acute rejection of the liver allograft is characterised by three main histological features: portal inflammation, bile duct damage and venous endothelial inflammation. All three of these features have also been identified in chronic HCV infection in the non-transplanted liver (Nonomura *et al*, 1991; Scheuer *et al*, 1991; Bach *et al*, 1992a; Zimmerman, 1994). Some of the features that may be helpful in distinguishing recurrent HCV hepatitis from acute cellular rejection are summarised in Table 5.3. However, none of the features listed here can be regarded as absolutely specific for either condition.

A recent study by Petrovic *et al* (1997) identified 11 histological variables showing a statistically significant difference between acute rejection and recurrent HCV. Ten of the 11 variables were rejection related, including portal eosinophils, bile duct inflammatory infiltration, bile duct necrosis, endothelialitis and cholestasis. Interestingly, the only significant feature associated with early recurrent HCV infection was sinusoidal dilatation. The pathogenesis of this lesion in the context of recurrent HCV infection is uncertain.

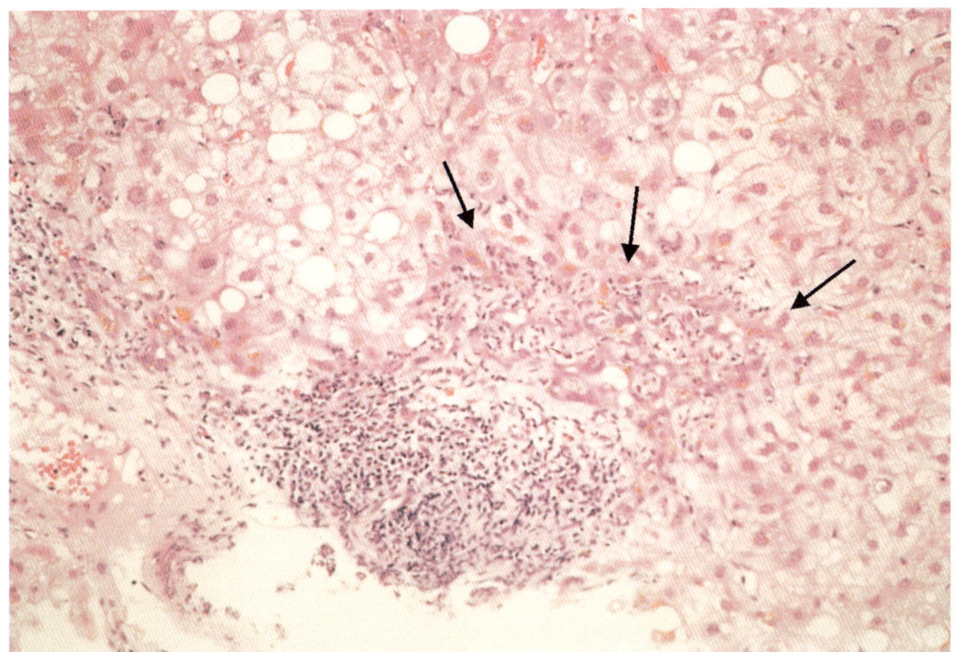

Fig 5.13 Fibrosing cholestatic hepatitis (recurrent hepatitis C infection). Liver biopsy, 11 months post-transplant. Portal tract contains a moderately dense infiltrate of inflammatory cells and has a prominent marginal area of ductular transformation (arrows). Adjacent liver parenchyma shows hepatocyte ballooning and fatty change without conspicuous inflammation (H&E).

The timing of events is probably most helpful in deciding whether cellular infiltrates in the liver are a result of rejection or hepatitis C. The majority of acute rejection episodes (approximately 90%) occur in the first month post-transplant (Anand *et al*, 1995). Although there is a suggestion that HCV-related inflammatory changes may occur during this period, a predominantly portal hepatitis usually takes several months to develop. The great majority of portal cellular infiltrates seen in the early post-transplant period can thus be ascribed to rejection. Problems exist in assessing later biopsies. There is a suggestion that late cellular rejection may have histological features different from those of early acute rejection, including hepatitis-like changes (Cakaloglu *et al*, 1995). A chronic hepatitis-like form of chronic rejection has also been postulated by Kemnitz *et al* (1989). Distinguishing rejection from HCV infection in these circumstances may be extremely difficult. The lack of a reliable method for identifying HCV antigens in tissue sections is a particular drawback in this situation.

In some cases where the distinction between cellular rejection and HCV hepatitis proves to be difficult histologically, it is likely that both conditions are present simultaneously. We have seen occasional cases with complex inflammatory changes suggesting both cellular rejection and HCV hepatitis. Following treatment with additional immunosuppression for presumed rejection, repeat biopsies obtained a few weeks later showed resolution of the rejection-like changes with a picture now typical of 'pure' chronic HCV hepatitis.

Table 5.3 Comparison of histological changes occurring in hepatitis C infection and acute cellular rejection of the liver allograft

	Hepatitis C	Acute rejection
Portal inflammation	Mononuclear	Mixed infiltrate
Lymphocytes	Yes	Yes
Lymphoid aggregates	Yes	No
Blast cells	No	Yes
Neutrophils	No	Yes
Eosinophils	No	Yes
Interface hepatitis	Variable (usually mild)	Mild (compared with density of portal infiltrate)
Bile duct damage/ inflammatory infiltration	Usually mild (lymphocytes)	More prominent (mixed infiltrate – mainly polymorphs)
Bile duct loss	Minimal/none	Possible (if progression to chronic rejection)
Venous endothelial inflammation	Mild/none	Yes
Fibrosis	Variable	No
Cholestasis	Mild/none (except rare cases of 'fibrosing cholestatic hepatitis')	Yes
Parenchymal inflammation	Mild (random distribution)	Minimal/mild (mainly perivenular) (more extensive in severe rejection)
Spotty necrosis	Common	Uncommon
Lobular disarray	Yes, usually mild	No
Fatty change	Yes (macrovesicular)	No

Recurrent HCV and chronic (ductopenic) rejection

A higher than expected incidence of chronic (ductopenic) rejection has been reported in some studies of recurrent HCV infection (Hoffmann *et al*, 1995; Loinaz *et al*, 1995; Charco *et al*, 1996). In the study of Hoffmann *et al*, chronic rejection was found in 4 out of 17 HCV-positive cases compared with 6 out of 103 HCV-negative cases. There are two possible reasons for this apparent association. First, bile ducts are targets for immune damage in HCV infection and rejection. Minor degrees of bile duct loss have been reported with chronic HCV infection in the non-transplanted liver (Goldin *et al*, 1996b). It is therefore possible that bile duct damage mediated by HCV is potentiated by additional immunological mechanisms in the liver allograft. An alternative explanation has been postulated in patients developing chronic rejection following IFN therapy for recurrent HCV infection (Dousset *et al*, 1994; Feray *et al*, 1995b). In these cases, it has been suggested that IFN stimulates the immune system in general, predisposing to more severe rejection.

HCV and acquired post-transplant hepatitis

Approximately 20–40% of patients biopsied as part of routine annual review have histological features of chronic hepatitis, not obviously related to recurrent viral disease (Hübscher, 1990; Nakhleh *et al*, 1990; Hübscher *et al*, 1993; Slapak *et al*, 1997). Early studies failed to demonstrate HCV infection in most cases, but these were carried out before the sensitive detection of HCV RNA was routinely available. Subsequent studies have identified HCV as the major cause of otherwise unexplained post-transplant hepatitis (Poterucha *et al*, 1992; Wright *et al*, 1992; Ascher *et al*, 1994; Vargas *et al*, 1994). One might expect acquired HCV hepatitis to behave less aggressively than recurrent disease, but this has not been convincingly demonstrated (Randhawa and Demetris, 1995).

Although several studies have identified HCV as the main cause of otherwise unexplained post-transplant hepatitis, this was not confirmed in a recent study from our centre. Only two (5%) out of 41 patients with chronic hepatitis were PCR-positive for HCV RNA (Ahmed *et al*, 1995). A higher than expected incidence of 'idiopathic' chronic hepatitis has been observed in patients with fulminant non-A, non-B, non-C hepatitis (Hübscher, 1990; Mohammed *et al*, 1997). This raises the possibility of another, as yet unidentified, virus in the aetiology of fulminant seronegative hepatitis and subsequent disease recurrence following liver transplantation.

Pathogenetic mechanisms

The pathogenesis of HCV-induced liver injury in the non-transplanted liver remains poorly understood (Gonzalez-Peralta *et al*, 1994; Gerber, 1995). Evidence exists both for immune-mediated mechanisms and for direct cytopathic damage. It is probable that both mechanisms are also present when HCV infects the liver allograft (*see* Chapter 7).

In common with recurrent HBV infection, reinfection of the liver allograft with HCV probably takes place via peripheral blood mononuclear cells (Bartolome *et al*, 1993; Pons, 1995).

In cases where there is diffuse hepatocellular damage occurring in the absence of significant inflammation, the possibility of direct cytopathic damage to hepatocytes should be considered. A similar mechanism has been proposed for hepatocellular degenerative changes such as ballooning and fatty change, which are sometimes seen in the non-transplanted liver without any conspicuous accompanying inflammation. One study of HCV-related FCH occurring in a heart allograft recipient showed the diffuse cytoplasmic expression of HCV RNA in more than 80% of the hepatocytes (Lim *et al*, 1994). The overall picture closely resembles the diffuse cytoplasmic immunostaining for HBcAg seen in cases of HBV-related FCH. This again supports the hypothesis of uncontrolled viral replication occurring in an immunocompromised individual resulting in direct cytopathic damage to liver cells.

In cases of recurrent HCV infection where there are prominent inflammatory changes, immune-mediated mechanisms are more likely to be present. The complex relationship that exists between recurrent HCV and rejection causing damage to the bile ducts further supports a concept of common immune pathways for damage to target structures in the liver allograft.

CO-INFECTION WITH HEPATITIS B AND C

Several patients transplanted for chronic viral hepatitis are co-infected with HBV and HCV (Loda *et al*, 1996). A few cases have also been reported in which transplantation was carried out for HBV or HCV disease alone and co-infection with the other virus occurred following transplantation (Huang *et al*, 1996).

Relatively little information exists on the interaction between HBV and HCV in the non-transplanted liver (Colombari *et al*, 1993; Crespo *et al*, 1994; Sato *et al*, 1994). There is some evidence to suggest that HCV may inhibit HBV replication. However, overall disease severity appears to be similar to or worse than that seen in single virus infection, suggesting that the two viruses may have synergistic actions in mediating hepatocellular damage.

The precise relationship between the two viruses in cases of co-infection undergoing liver transplantation is also not clear. In one study, cases that were HBV- and HCV-positive had a more favourable outcome than those with HBV infection alone (Huang *et al*, 1996). In particular, FCH was not seen in any of the seven patients with combined infection, compared with five out of 10 patients with HBV disease alone. This again raises the possibility of the HCV-induced inhibition of HBV replication as a mechanism for reducing the severity of post-transplant HBV infection. However, the number of cases examined in this study is small, and it is difficult to draw any clear conclusions. In patients with combined infection treated with HBIg, the predominant histological picture in post-transplant biopsies appears to be HCV related, again suggesting the effective inhibition of HBV replication. The severity of HCV hepatitis in these cases also appears to be less than in patients infected with HCV alone. It is possible that this is due to HBV inhibiting HCV replication or due to immunoglobulins used for HBV immunoprophylaxis also containing anti-HCV antibodies (Feray *et al*, 1993).

HEPATITIS DELTA

Co-infection with HDV is commonly present in patients undergoing liver transplantation for HBV-related liver disease. Studies of recurrent HDV infection in liver allografts have provided interesting new insights into the pathogenesis of liver damage caused by HDV and its relationship with HBV (*see* Chapter 7).

Patients with combined HDV/HBV infection are at a lower risk of developing recurrent HBV infection following liver transplantation than are those infected with HBV alone. In the study of Samuel *et al* (1993), the recurrence rate was 67% in patients with HBV cirrhosis compared with 32% in those with HDV cirrhosis. This is presumably related to the inhibitory effects of HDV on HBV replication (Mason and Taylor, 1991). Most patients co-infected with HDV have very low levels of HBV replication at the time of transplantation.

In the absence of immunoprophylaxis, patients co-infected with HBV and HDV still frequently develop recurrent HBV-related disease following liver transplantation. In a combined series of 38 patients (31 of whom received no immunoprophylaxis), 32 developed recurrent HBV and HDV infection (Ottobrelli *et al*, 1991; Davies *et al*, 1992). In contrast, only seven out of 68 patients receiving long-term immunoprophylaxis became HBsAg-positive after a mean follow-up period of 17 months (Samuel *et al*, 1995). This again supports the concept of immunoprophylaxis with anti-HBIg being most effective in patients with low levels of HBV replication.

Several studies have identified that reinfection with HDV can occur without HBV infection (Hopf *et al*, 1991; Ottobrelli *et al*, 1991; Davies *et al*, 1992; Samuel *et al*, 1995). HDV can be identified immunohistochemically in post-transplant biopsies as early as 1 week post-transplant (Davies *et al*, 1992). Northern blotting or polymerase chain reaction techniques can also identify HDV RNA in serum in the early post-transplant period and appear to be more sensitive than immunohistochemical detection in tissue sections. In Samuel *et al*'s study, 23 out of 26 patients tested during the first year after transplantation were HDV RNA-positive, compared with positive immunohistochemical staining in 13 out of 59 cases examined (Samuel *et al*, 1995). By itself, reinfection with HDV is not associated with clinically significant graft dysfunction or with histological signs of hepatitis, and markers of HDV infection eventually disappear. Only three out of the 59 patients studied by Samuel *et al* had serum markers of HDV infection more than 2 years post-transplant.

In many patients who eventually become HBV-positive, there is a latent period of several months in which HDV positivity alone is present. In other cases, markers of reinfection with HDV and HBV appear simultaneously. Reinfection with HBV is usually accompanied by clinical and histological signs of graft hepatitis. Morphological changes are similar to those described earlier for recurrent HBV infection. Recurrent hepatitis is generally less severe with combined HBV/HDV infection than with HBV infection alone. HBV-DNA levels are lower (O'Grady *et al*, 1992), there is a lower risk of progression to cirrhosis, and FCH is very uncommon (Pons, 1995). One recent study described two patients who developed fulminant recurrent HBV infection despite being HDV-positive (Marsman *et al*, 1997). Both had markers of active HBV replication at the time of transplantation, again emphasising the important role of viral load in determining the eventual outcome following liver transplantation for HBV cirrhosis.

HEPATITIS E

A small number of patients undergoing liver transplantation for fulminant non-A, non-B, non-C hepatitis are HEV-positive (Sallie *et al*, 1994). There is no evidence to suggest that infection with HEV recurs following transplantation.

HEPATITIS F

The term 'hepatitis F' has been tentatively suggested to describe a togavirus-like particle that was detected in the nuclei of hepatocytes in nine patients undergoing liver transplantation for fulminant hepatitis of unknown aetiology (Fagan *et al*, 1989, 1992). Five of these nine patients developed acute liver failure during the first week following transplantation, associated with massive haemorrhagic graft necrosis. Similar virus-like particles were also seen in all five failed allografts, suggesting the possibility of recurrent disease (Fagan *et al*, 1992). As yet, there have been no further studies confirming these interesting observations.

HEPATITIS G

HGV is a recently described RNA virus (Linnen *et al*, 1996) (*see* Chapter 1). In non-transplant patients, HGV infection is currently considered to be of limited significance (*see* Chapter 1).

Studies of HCV-positive patients undergoing liver transplantation have identified HGV infection in 10–25% of cases (Berg *et al*, 1996; Berenguer *et al*, 1996; Fried *et al*, 1997). One study reported a significantly higher incidence of hepatocellular carcinoma in patients who were HCV- and HGV-positive compared with those who were only

HCV-positive (Berg *et al*, 1996). Similar prevalence rates for HGV infection have also been observed in HBV-positive cases (Berg *et al*, 1996) and in patients undergoing liver transplantation for non-viral causes of liver disease (Fried *et al*, 1997; Haagsma *et al*, 1997). Prevalence rates of between 12% and 64% have been found in post-transplant samples (Berg *et al*, 1996; Berenguer *et al*, 1996; Dickson *et al*, 1997; Fried *et al*, 1997; Haagsma *et al*, 1997). Many of these cases presumably represent acquired infection. There is no evidence that HGV infection (recurrent or acquired) has any effect on graft function, histological changes or overall survival.

Viral hepatitis in other types of transplantation

S G HÜBSCHER

Liver disease due to chronic viral hepatitis is also an important problem in other organ transplant recipients. Many of the histological features and pathogenetic mechanisms are similar to those already described in liver allografts, and these will not be covered again in detail here.

The fundamental (and very obvious) difference between viral hepatitis occurring in liver allograft recipients and in other organ transplant patients is that the native liver is retained in the latter group. This has important implications for disease pathogenesis and histological diagnosis. The liver is the main site of replication of HBV and HCV, and immunosuppressed patients in whom the infected liver is retained would thus be expected to have more severe disease than those in whom it is removed. However, complete MHC matching of the liver is retained in non-liver transplant patients, which means that MHC-restricted T-cell responses are less severely inhibited in this group.

From a purely diagnostic point of view, there are none of the problems associated with distinguishing viral hepatitis from other causes of damage that occur in the liver allograft. This is one reason why liver biopsies are less frequently taken in non-liver transplant patients with chronic viral hepatitis, and there is thus less information on liver histology in these patients. One exception to this general rule applies in bone marrow graft recipients, where there are potential problems in distinguishing viral hepatitis from other hepatic complications of bone marrow transplantation (BMT) such as graft-versus-host disease (GVHD) and veno-occlusive disease (VOD). A possible role has also been suggested for HBV and HCV as risk factors for the development of VOD and GVHD post-BMT. In most cases, viral hepatitis is relatively easy to distinguish histologically from GVHD and VOD, and this matter will not be considered further here.

HEPATITIS B

The severity of HBV-related liver disease increases in HBsAg-positive patients following renal transplantation, presumably as a consequence of the immunosuppression permitting increased viral replication (Bang *et al*, 1995; Goffin *et al*, 1995; Fornairon *et al*, 1996). The incidence and histological severity of hepatitis increase, and there is more rapid progression to cirrhosis. Risk factors for the development of more severe disease following renal transplantation include active viral replication (Fairley *et al*, 1991) and severe histological abnormalities at the time of transplantation (Rao *et al*, 1993). In a large, single-centre study, the 10-year post-transplant survival was significantly lower in 107 HBsAg-positive patients (64%) than in 508 HBsAg-negative patients (80%) (Hillis *et al*, 1979).

There have been several case reports of fibrosing cholestatic hepatitis B infection in renal and other allograft recipients (Chen *et al*, 1994; McIvor *et al*, 1994; Booth *et al*, 1995; Cooksley and McIvor, 1995; Hung *et al*, 1995; Lam *et al*, 1996). Histological appearances and clinical outcome are similar to those seen in FCH involving liver allografts. Two of the cases reported in renal transplant patients (Chen *et al*, 1994; Booth *et al*, 1995) and one in a bone marrow transplant patient (McIvor *et al*, 1994) were associated with HBV pre-core mutants.

Liver disease related to acquired HBV infection in non-liver transplant patients has also been investigated (Wachs *et al*, 1995). The incidence and severity of acquired HBV appears to be less in renal and cardiac allograft recipients than in liver transplant patients. The most probable explanation is that the transplanted liver has a much higher viral load than other organs obtained from the same donors.

HEPATITIS C

Several studies have shown a high prevalence of HCV infection among patients undergoing renal transplantation (Roth, 1995), most cases probably being related to long-term haemodialysis (Goffin *et al*, 1995). High prevalence rates of HCV infection have also been reported in some studies of BMT, probably related to previous blood transfusion (Ribas and Gale, 1997). HCV infection is less commonly seen in cardiac allograft recipients (Zein *et al*, 1995).

HCV is the most common cause of chronic liver dysfunction in renal transplant patients (Allison *et al*, 1992; Pol *et al*, 1992; McCruden *et al*, 1994). In most cases, the disease appears to be mild with no obvious impact on graft survival or mortality (Stempel *et al*, 1993; Roth *et al*, 1994). Histological studies show the usual spectrum of changes associated with chronic hepatitis C infection. However, there is a suggestion that the disease may behave more aggressively than in the immunocompetent individual. Nineteen out of 39 HCV-positive renal transplant patients undergoing liver biopsy in the study of Cisterne *et al* (1996) had histological evidence of chronic hepatitis with prominent necroinflammatory activity, and in 12 of these, there was also bridging fibrosis. Three out of 28 patients studied by Brunson *et al* (1993) had cirrhosis 4 years following renal transplantation. There have also been occasional reports of a severe cholestatic form of HCV infection resembling FCH, two occurring in cardiac allograft recipients (Allison *et al*, 1992; Lim *et al*, 1994) and one in a renal transplant patient (Zylberberg *et al*, 1997).

Viral hepatitis in patients infected with HIV

R D GOLDIN

Patients with HIV suffer from an impaired immune function mainly related to a progressive loss of CD4+ T-lymphocytes. A wide range of liver pathology has been described in these patients (Schaffner, 1990; Wilkins *et al*, 1991; Bach *et al*, 1992b; McNair *et al*, 1994), falling into two main categories. The first of these comprises opportunistic infections and tumours that may involve the liver but are usually part of systemic disease. The second category is made up of hepatic diseases that are more common in HIV-positive patients because they share common risk factors with HIV. Viral hepatitis, of a number of types, falls into this group (Horvath and Raffanti, 1994). Their natural history is, however, modified by the concurrent immunodeficiency in a number of important ways.

HIV can directly infect the liver, and it has been suggested that the liver is an important reservoir of infection. It has been detected in the liver within lymphocytes (Housset *et al*, 1993), macrophages/Kupffer cells (Schmitt *et al*, 1990; Housset *et al*, 1993), endothelial cells (which in the liver express CD4; Scoazec and Feldmann, 1990) and hepatocytes but not in biliary epithelial cells. In one study, HIV-1 RNA was detected in the liver by the polymerase chain reaction in eight out of 13 patients, and in three of these HIV-1 RNA was demonstrated in hepatocytes by in situ hybridisation (Housset *et al*, 1993). It has been claimed that HIV is capable of producing a hepatitis itself. However, these claims have not always been well documented. In one study, a distinct syndrome of cholestasis and hepatitis was seen in infants with perinatally acquired HIV in whom no specific aetiological agent could be identified (Persaud *et al*, 1993). In none of these patients, however, could HIV mRNA be demonstrated in their liver tissue.

HEPATITIS A

Hepatitis A is common in homosexual men and consequently in patients who are HIV-positive (Corey and Holmes, 1980; Leentvaar Kuijpers *et al*, 1995). HIV appears to have no effect on the natural history of HAV infection.

HEPATITIS B

The routes of infection of HBV and HIV are very similar, and many patients have therefore been infected with both of these viruses. HBV is transmitted more efficiently than HIV by these routes. This is probably due to higher levels of HBV than HIV in blood and other body fluids (Stevens *et al*, 1986; Bhat *et al*, 1990). In one study of homosexual men who were initially HIV- and HBV-negative, it was calculated that HBV was transmitted over eight times more efficiently than HIV (Kingsley *et al*, 1990). Approximately 90% of patients with AIDS have evidence of previous or active infection with HBV (Rustgi *et al*, 1984; Lebovics *et al*, 1988). In a study from the Middle East, all multitransfused patients infected with HIV had evidence of infection with HBV (Brenner *et al*, 1994). HBV immunisation programmes are only beginning to decrease this figure (Rabeneck *et al*, 1993).

Interactions between HIV and HBV

There are a number of interesting similarities between these two viruses (Hilleman, 1994). For example, they are both hypermutable and exist as quasispecies, mainly as a result of errors in reverse transcription, while they have different survival mechanisms – HIV surviving mainly by antigenic variability, immune evasion and the impairment of immune function, HBV primarily by mutation of the e antigen/core genes, which impairs the cytotoxic T-cell activity. At the molecular level, there are a number of different direct and indirect mechanisms whereby HIV and HBV might interact.

A direct interaction would require the two viruses to infect the same cell. This is possible because HIV can infect hepatocytes (Housset *et al*, 1993), and, although HBV predominantly infects hepatocytes, HBV has also been isolated from lymphocytes. Using Southern blot hybridisation, HBV DNA was found in one-third of peripheral blood leukocytes and was identified in CD4+ lymphocytes in nine out of 11 patients (Calmus *et al*, 1994). There is conflicting evidence on the effect of co-infection with HIV on the frequency with which HBV DNA has been identified in peripheral blood mononuclear cells. In one study, it was found in 50% of HIV-negative controls but in 100% of patients who also had HIV (Noonan *et al*, 1986). However, a subsequent larger study failed to confirm this (Bartolome *et al*, 1990). This discrepancy can, at least partially, be explained by the different methodologies used in these papers.

Particular attention has been paid to the potential role of the HBV X protein, which has transactivating properties (Twu and Schloemer, 1987; Colgrove *et al*, 1989), on HIV expression. In both hepatocellular and lymphoblastoid cell lines that express the X protein, there is increased expression of both cellular and viral genes under the control of the HIV long terminal repeat (LTR) (Seto *et al*, 1988; Twu and Robinson, 1989). If the NF-κB binding sites on the LTR are disrupted, this is blocked. As it has been shown that the X protein does not directly bind DNA, it has been suggested that this effect is due to the binding of NF-κB (or other transcription factors) (Siddiqui *et al*, 1989). When transgenic mice carrying the X open reading frame, under the control of the antithrombin 3 regulatory sequence, were cross-bred with other transgenics carrying reporter genes under the control of HIV1-LPTR, the in vivo transactivating properties were demonstrated (Balsano *et al*, 1993).

Indirect interactions are also possible through the effect on HIV replication of the increased production of cytokines, such as tumour necrosis factor-α (TNF-α) and IFN, in patients co-infected with HBV. TNF-α increases HIV expression in chronically infected monocytes, probably through the induction of NF-κB (Poli *et al*, 1990). Although it has been shown that herpes viruses can increase HIV replication by inducing the production of TNF-α, it has not yet been directly demonstrated that HBV can interact with HIV via this route (Clouse *et al*, 1989). It has, however, been shown in a study of cytokine regulation of HIV-1 LTR transactivation in human hepatocellular cell lines that NF-κB plays an important role (Hsu *et al*, 1995). In this system, NF-κB may interact, either by itself or in conjunction with the 5′ proximal response elements, with cellular transactivating factors elicited by the cascade of transduction responses to cytokines. Infection by HBV can be associated with an increased endogenous production of IFN, and chronic infection with HBV is frequently treated with lymphoblastoid IFN. In vitro studies have demonstrated that IFN has an antiviral effect on HIV infection in T-lymphocytes and hepatocytes. On the other hand, HBV may, in certain circumstances, inhibit the production of IFN and its effect on individual cells (Foster *et al*, 1993).

There are therefore a number of potential molecular interactions whereby it has been suggested that HBV may increase HIV replication. However, a number of epidemiological studies have suggested that these interactions are not clinically significant. For example, in a cohort study, CD4+ T-cell counts did not fall more rapidly in patients who were HBV-positive (Solomon *et al*, 1990). Furthermore, clinical progression to AIDS was not accelerated. Although this is the consensus of most studies, there have been studies that have reached the opposite conclusion (Eskild *et al*, 1992). However, in conclusion, it appears that HBV does not have a significant effect on the evolution of infection with HIV.

Conversely, HIV does appear to have an important effect on the course of infection by HBV. HBV is considered not to be directly cytopathic (Hilleman, 1994). The infection of hepatocytes is followed by the expression of peptides derived from HBcAg on the surface of these cells. In association with HLA class I antigens on the cell membrane, this induces a cell-mediated humoral response involving mainly CD8+ T-cells but also CD4+ cells. This is important in both acute and chronic infections. The destruction of infected hepatocytes is therefore dependent on an intact T-cell response, and it could be predicted that in patients with HIV, especially those with significantly reduced CD4 counts, there would be an impaired elimination of HBV. This has been confirmed in both clinical and histological studies.

In one study into a group of men who became infected with HBV, HIV-positive individuals were three times more likely to develop chronic infection than HIV-negative individuals (Hadler *et al*, 1991). This was despite the fact that the average duration of HIV infection in the former group was less than 1 year and it was therefore unlikely that they were significantly immunosuppressed. In the acute phase, ALT levels were similar in the two groups, but at the end of 3 years of follow-up, enzyme levels were lower in the HIV-positive group. A second study also demonstrated an even greater risk of developing chronic infection in HIV-positive individuals (Bodsworth *et al*, 1989). Furthermore, the CD4 counts of those HIV-positive patients who cleared HBV were higher than in those who did not. In one study, six out of 57 patients with HIV who were initially HBV-negative acquired markers indicative of recent infection (Homann *et al*, 1991). Four out of the six developed chronic hepatitis, while the other two had acute subclinical hepatitis that resolved. In another study of patients who were chronically infected with HBV, HIV-positive patients were more likely to be HBeAg and HBV DNA-positive than were HIV-negative controls (Bodsworth *et al*, 1991). There was, however, no correlation between CD4 counts and the levels of HBeAg or HBV DNA. In the group of patients who were HBeAg-positive, concurrent HIV infection was associated with lower serum ALT levels, the level of which decreased with falling CD4 counts. We have studied the histopathological changes in liver biopsies in patients who were infected with both HIV and HBV, compared with controls with HBV alone. It was found that the severity of the histological changes, as assessed using the Knodell Histological Activity Index, was greater in the HIV-negative group but that there were higher levels of HBeAg and HBV polymerase staining in the HIV-positive group (Goldin *et al*, 1990a). This is again consistent with immune-mediated destruction of the HBV-infected hepatocytes being impaired in patients with HIV. All the above studies were carried out in Western populations and, unfortunately, only limited work has been carried out in the large population of African and Asian patients co-infected with these two viruses. In one study carried out in Central Africa, HIV-positive patients had lower titres of anti-HBs antibody and had more markers consistent with reactivated HBV (Kashala *et al*, 1994).

Reactivation of HBV

Reactivation of HBV infection under conditions of marked immunosuppression is well described (Davis and Hoofnagle, 1985), and cases have now been described in HIV-positive patients, related to progressive immunosuppression (Vandercam *et al*, 1990). In one study, in which patients with HIV were followed up for a median of 18 months, four out of 211 patients had serological evidence of hepatitis B reactivation (Homann *et al*, 1991). In patients who were anti-HBs-positive, following either infection (Waite *et al*, 1988) or immunisation (Loke *et al*, 1990), there is a progressive decline in titre as the CD4 count drops. Reactivation is associated with the reappearance of HBsAg, HBV DNA and, usually, HBeAg in the serum (Levy *et al*, 1990), sometimes despite the persistence of anti-Hbc (Waite *et al*, 1988). This has important implications for the virological screening of HIV-positive patients who have a hepatitic illness, who should always have their HBV DNA checked. Perhaps somewhat surprisingly, reactivation, even in patients with AIDS, is frequently associated with severe disease despite marked immunosuppression. This strongly suggests that there must be non-immune pathways via which HBV can cause liver cell damage, at least when there are very high levels of replicating virus. This is supported by isolated case reports of fibrosing cholestatic hepatitis (FCH) in HIV-positive patients with HBV, similar to those seen in some cases of recurrent HBV after transplantation (*see* above). One patient who had underlying cirrhosis was IgM HBc antibody-positive, suggesting that this was due to reactivated HBV (Fang *et al*, 1993b). The two cases we have seen, while having a histological picture consistent with FCH, both had relatively mild disease, as assessed histologically and clinically. In addition to reactivation, there is also evidence of an increased risk of reinfection with another sub type of HBV in patients who are also infected with HIV (Kashala *et al*, 1994).

The treatment of hepatitis B with lymphoblastoid IFN is increasingly widely used. Immunosuppression by, for example, HIV is, however, associated with decreased response rate. In the case of HIV, there may be a number of additional factors that impair the response to IFN (and which may also contribute to the increased carriage rates of HBV). These include higher viral load, the effects on cytokine production of high levels of acid labile IFN, reduced levels of IFN receptor expression and increased levels of anti-IFN antibodies. Pre-treatment with a short course of steroids has been shown to increase the probability of clearing HBV in patients with HIV who are subsequently given a course of IFN. It is unlikely that this will become a widely used treatment regimen. Reverse transcriptase inhibitors such as zidovudine have been used alone or in combination with IFN, but despite activity against HBV, these have not proved clinically useful.

HEPATITIS C

HCV is spread by parenteral routes and intravenous drug abuse, and blood products are the major risk factors (Alter *et al*, 1989). Although HCV may be transmitted by sexual intercourse, this is much less common than with HIV or HBV (Tedder *et al*, 1991). Co-infection with HCV and HIV is therefore less common than co-infection with HBV and HIV, and is seen in about 14% of HIV-positive patients (Hayashi *et al*, 1991; Botti *et al*, 1992). It is more often seen in drug abusers and haemophiliacs than in homosexuals, with up to 50% of HIV-positive drug abusers and up to 100% of HIV-positive haemophiliacs being HCV-positive (Kumar *et al*, 1993). In a French study, the prevalence of HCV in homosexual men, as assessed using the specific recombinant immunoblot assay (RIBA), was 5.3%, which fell to 3.8% when transfused patients were excluded (Marcellin *et al*, 1993). However, in an American study, over 10% of homosexuals had evidence of HCV infection as assessed by RIBA and/or polymerase chain reaction that apparently could not be ascribed to either blood transfusion or intravenous drug abuse (Wright *et al*, 1994). This suggests that, at least in some population groups, sexual transmission of HCV is more common than has previously been thought. In intravenous drug abusers, HCV infection occurs rapidly, 78% of patients becoming anti-HCV-positive within 2 years (Thomas *et al*, 1995). The transmission of HCV by sexual intercourse and from mother to child is more common in HIV-positive individuals, probably because they have higher titres of HCV RNA (Manzini *et al*, 1995). This, in contrast to a recent study, has failed to confirm higher HCV mRNA titres in patients who are HIV-positive (Berger *et al*, 1996), although HCV mRNA levels may be higher in patients with CD4 counts less than 200/mm^3 (Ghany *et al*, 1996).

Overall, these prevalence figures need to be interpreted with some caution. On one hand, HIV is associated with hypergammaglobulinaemia, which may lead to false positives when using the enzyme-linked immunosorbent assay (ELISA) test. For example, in the French study quoted above, out of 56 patients who were second-generation ELISA-positive, only six were RIBA-positive. On the other hand, the impaired immune response may lead to false-negative results. In one study of patients with an indeterminate RIBA, HCV viraemia was found more frequently in HIV-positive patients than in those who were HIV-negative. The use of the RIBA and polymerase chain reaction tests should, therefore, be used in evaluating HCV infection in patients who are HIV-positive (Marcellin *et al*, 1994). One further variable that has not always been taken into account has been the pattern of HCV genotype in patients co-infected with HIV. For example, the high incidence of genotype 1, which is associated with higher titres of HCV mRNA in HIV-negative patients, is relatively common in HIV-positive patients, and this may be a partial explanation of the higher titres seen in this group (Chambost *et al*, 1995). Yet another factor that may affect the detection of HCV is co-infection with HDV as well as HIV (Eyster *et al*, 1995). This study demonstrated that lower levels of HCV were found in patients also infected with HDV, HBV and HIV compared with those who were infected with HBV and HIV, although liver failure was relatively common (38% of patients).

Like HBV, HCV can infect lymphoid cells (Henin *et al*, 1994) and might therefore interact with HIV in both these cells and hepatocytes; few in vitro studies have explored this interaction. HCV is usually considered to be a cytopathic virus, and therefore HIV-induced immunosuppression would be predicted to increase liver damage by increasing viral replication. However, clinical studies have produced conflicting results. An early study described a small group of patients with HIV/HCV co-infection who progressed to symptomatic cirrhosis within three years, suggesting a more accelerated course (Martin *et al*, 1989). This was not confirmed in a larger study in which HIV positivity had no effect on ALT levels or on disease progression (Areias and Lopes, 1992). The discrepancy between these two studies may be explained by differences in the duration of the follow-up. In one study with a 15-year follow-up, 25% of HCV/HIV co-infected patients developed cirrhosis compared with 6.5% of patients infected with HCV alone (Sanchez Quijano *et al*, 1995). Similar incidences of cirrhosis were found in both patient groups within five and 10 years; most of the HIV-positive patients developed cirrhosis in a time interval longer than 15 years. These results suggest that HIV does alter the natural history of HCV.

Perhaps surprisingly, no difference was found in the histological features seen in the liver biopsies at the start of the study. Contradictory results came from a study of liver biopsies from patients with HCV and HIV (Guido *et al*, 1994). This found that there was a correlation between the CD4 counts and the grade of the liver inflammation. There was no difference between biopsies from HIV-negative patients and HIV-positive patients with CD4 counts over 400/mm³. However, with CD4 counts less than 400/mm³, the HIV-positive patients had less severe portal and periportal inflammation. The authors concluded that, contrary to the widely accepted suggestion that HCV is a cytopathic virus, it can under certain conditions be immunopathic. There is a single case report claiming that co-infection with HIV and HCV was associated with a histological picture resembling an autoimmune hepatitis, although with a response to α-IFN (Berk *et al*, 1991). Although widely quoted, this observation has not been made by other workers (Fischer *et al*, 1996). It is interesting, however, that in patients with marked HIV-associated immunodeficiency, both HBV and HCV appear to display pathogenic mechanisms apparently less important in immunocompetent individuals. Overall, those studies which have depended on the biochemical measurement of disease activity have tended to show that HIV has relatively little effect on HCV, while those based on histology have tended to reach the opposite conclusion. This is, perhaps, not surprising given the observation that, in HIV-negative patients who are HCV-positive, there is no good correlation between biochemical and histological changes. It is increasingly observed that HCV is an important cause of mortality in patients who are co-infected with HCV and HIV (*see*, for example, Fischer *et al*, 1996).

The effect of HCV on disease progression in patients with HIV has also been examined. An American study of HIV-infected patients with and without AIDS failed to demonstrate disease progression patients co-infected with HCV (Wright *et al*, 1994), and this has been confirmed in an Italian study (Dorrucci *et al*, 1995). However, an earlier, relatively small, study carried out in children had demonstrated that the presence of liver disease (of which HCV was the cause in five out of 18) was associated with a relatively poor prognosis (Nigro *et al*, 1993). Interferon is less effective in the treatment of HCV than HBV; co-infection with HIV and HCV appears further to decrease this. In one study, in which the E2/NS1 first hypervariable region of HCV was sequenced, it was shown that there was an increased accumulation of envelope variants in HCV/HIV co-infected patients (Sherman *et al*, 1996). The authors suggested that this could be a result of less efficient viral clearance and might explain decreased responsiveness to interferon in this group of patients.

HEPATITIS DELTA

HDV, like HCV, is not efficiently transmitted by sexual intercourse, and therefore co-infection with HIV is also most common in intravenous drug abusers and haemophiliacs. The presence of HIV is, however, associated with persistent HDV antigen positivity (Roingeard *et al*, 1992). Among homosexuals, different prevalence figures have been described (Goldin *et al*, 1990b). Also, like HCV, there are some difficulties in the diagnosis of HDV in patients with HIV (Lake-Bakaar *et al*, 1994). It has been shown that, in HIV-positive patients who are intravenous drug abusers, there is a significant reduction in the incidence of IgG and IgM anti-HDV in the serum. It has been suggested that the low prevalence of anti-HDV in these patients is probably a result of defective anti-HDV production rather than decreased HDV replication.

HDV, also like HCV, is considered to be a cytopathic virus, and it does appear that co-infection with HIV, with its associated immunosuppression, causes more severe disease (Farci *et al*, 1988). The situation is complicated because HDV can only infect patients in association with HBV. Infection with HDV usually inhibits HBV replication. Co-infection with HIV appears to reverse this inhibition, and 23% of patients infected with all three viruses have detectable HBV DNA in the serum, whereas it is usually undetectable in patients with only HBV and HDV (Cassidy *et al*, 1989). This has been supported by a more recent study concluding that, although HIV infection counters the inhibitory effect of HDV superinfection on HBV replication (with a virtually identical percentage of patients infected with all three viruses having detectable HBV DNA in their serum), markers of HDV replication were found equally frequently in HIV-positive and negative patients (Pol *et al*, 1989). Furthermore, histological activity, as assessed using the Knodell Histological Activity Index, was similar in these two groups of patients. Contradictory evidence came from another study, concluding that, although the persistence of HBV replication is a major determinant of severe liver damage in chronic delta hepatitis, HIV infections do not influence the natural history of chronic delta hepatitis (Lozano *et al*, 1994). A third study found that co-infection with HIV inhibited the antibody response to HDV, and this resulted in episodes of activation and liver damage. As described above, co-infection with HCV and HDV in HIV-positive patients is associated with severe disease (Eyster *et al*, 1995).

HEPATITIS E

There are no data on the interaction between HEV and HIV. HEV is most common in Africa and Asia and, although usually self-limiting, has a mortality rate of 20% in pregnant women (Myint *et al*, 1985). This suggests that HIV-associated immunosuppression may also result in increased mortality.

References

Adams, D.H., Hübscher, S.G., Neuberger, J.M., McMaster, P., Elias, E., Buckels, J.A. 1991: Reduced incidence of rejection in patients undergoing liver transplantation for chronic hepatitis B. *Transplantation Proceedings* **23**, 1436–7.

Ahmed, M., Mutimer, D.J., Elias, E., Hübscher, S.G. 1995: Hepatitis C virus (HCV) infection is not frequently related to chronic hepatitis in liver allografts. *Hepatology* **22**, 136A.

Alberti, A.B., Belli, L.S., Silini, E. *et al.* 1997: Hepatitis C virus genotypes and severe hepatitis C virus recurrence after liver transplantation. *Transplantation Proceedings* **29**, 522–3.

Allison, M.C., Mowat, A., McCruden, E.A. *et al.* 1992: The spectrum of chronic liver disease in renal transplant recipients. *Quarterly Journal of Medicine* **83**, 355–67.

Alter, H.J., Purcell, R.H., Shih, J.W. *et al.* 1989: Detection of antibody to hepatitis C virus in prospectively followed transfusion recipients with acute and chronic non-A and non-B hepatitis. *New England Journal of Medicine* **321**, 1394–500.

Anand, A.C., Hübscher, S.G., Gunson, B.K., McMaster, P., Neuberger, J.M. 1995: Timing, significance, and prognosis of late acute liver allograft rejection. *Transplantation* **60**, 1098–103.

Angus, P.W. 1997: Review: Hepatitis B and liver transplantation. *Journal of Gastroenterology and Hepatology* **12**, 217–23.

Angus, P.W., Locarnini, S.A., McCaughan, G.W., Jones, R.M., McMillan, J.S., Bowden, D.S. 1995: Hepatitis B virus precore mutant infection is associated with severe recurrent disease after liver transplantation. *Hepatology* **21**, 14–18.

Areias, J., Lopes, I. 1992: Influence of HIV infection in chronic hepatitis C in intravenous drug addicts. *Hepatology* **16**, 295A.

Arnold, J.C., Tox, U., Goeser, T. *et al.* 1997: Recurrent hepatitis C virus infection after liver transplantation – long term follow up with respect to the HCV genotypes/subtypes. *Zeitschrift für Gastroenterologie* **35**, 255–61.

Ascher, N.L., Lake, J.R., Emond, J., Roberts, J. 1994: Liver transplantation for hepatitis C virus-related cirrhosis. *Hepatology* **20**, 24S–27S.

Bach, N., Thung, S.N., Schaffner, F. 1992a: The histological features of chronic hepatitis C and autoimmune chronic hepatitis: a comparative analysis. *Hepatology* **15**, 572–7.

Bach, N., Theise, N.D., Schaffner, F. 1992b: Hepatic histopathology in the acquired immunodeficiency syndrome. *Seminars in Liver Disease* **12**, 205–12.

Balsano, C., Billet, O., Bennoun, M. *et al.* 1993: The hepatitis B virus X gene product transactivates the HIV-LTR in vivo. *Archives of Virology* **8** (supplement), 63–71.

Bang, B.K., Yang, C.W., Yoon, S.A. *et al.* 1995: Prevalence and clinical course of hepatitis B and hepatitis C liver disease in cyclosporine treated renal allograft recipients. *Nephron* **70**, 397–401.

Bartholomew, M.M., Jansen, R.W., Jeffers, L.J. *et al.* 1997: Hepatitis B virus resistance to lamivudine given for recurrent infection after orthotopic liver transplantation. *Lancet* **349**, 20–2.

Bartolome, F., Moraleda, G., Castillo, I. *et al.* 1990: Presence of HBV DNA in the peripheral blood mononuclear cells from anti-HIV symptomless carriers. *Journal of Hepatology* **10**, 186–90.

Bartolome, J., Castillo, I., Quiroga, J.A., Navas, S., Carreno, V. 1993: Detection of hepatitis C virus RNA in serum and peripheral blood mononuclear cells. *Journal of Hepatology* **17**, S90–S93.

Benner, K.G., Lee, R.G., Keeffe, E.B. *et al.* 1992: Fibrosing cytolytic liver failure secondary to recurrent hepatitis B after liver transplantation. *Gastroenterology* **103**, 1307–12.

Berenguer, H., Terrault, N.A., Piatak, M. *et al.* 1996: Hepatitis G virus infection in patients with hepatitis C virus infection undergoing liver transplantation. *Gastroenterology* **111**, 1569–75.

Berg, T., Naumann, U., Fukumoto, T. *et al.* 1996: GB virus-C infection in patients with chronic hepatitis B and hepatitis C before and after liver transplantation. *Transplantation* **62**, 711–14.

Berger, A., von Depka Prondzinski, M., Doerr, H.W., Rabenau, H., Weber, B. 1996: Hepatitis C plasma viral load is associated with HCV genotype but not with HIV coinfection. *Journal of Medical Virology* **148**, 339–43.

Berk, L., Schalm, S.W., Heijtink, R.A. 1991: Severe chronic active hepatitis (autoimmune type) mimicked by coinfection of hepatitis C and human immunodeficiency viruses. *Gut* **32**, 1198–200.

Bhat, A.R., Ulrich, P.P., Vyas, G.N. 1990: Molecular characterisation of a new variant of hepatitis B virus in a persistently infected homosexual man. *Hepatology* **11**, 271–6.

Blight, K., Rowland, R., Hall, P.D. *et al.* 1993: Immunohistochemical detection of the NS4 antigen of hepatitis C virus and its relation to histopathology. *American Journal of Pathology* **143**, 1568–73.

Bodsworth, N., Donovan, B., Nightingale, B. 1989: The effect of concurrent human immunodeficiency virus infection on chronic hepatitis B: a study of 150 homosexual men. *Journal of Infectious Diseases* **160**, 577–82.

Bodsworth, N.J., Cooper, D.A., Donovan, B. 1991: The influence of human immunodeficiency virus type 1 on the development of the hepatitis B virus carrier state. *Journal of Infectious Diseases* **163**, 1138–40.

Booth, J.C., Goldin, R.D., Brown, J.L., Karayiannis, P., Thomas, H.C. 1995: Fibrosing cholestatic hepatitis in renal transplant recipient associated with the hepatitis B virus precore mutant. *Journal of Hepatology* **22**, 500–3.

Botti, P., Pistelli, A., Gambassi, F. *et al.* 1992: HBV and HCV infection in i.v. drug addicts; coinfection with HIV. *Archives of Virology*, **4** (supplement), 329–32.

Brenner, B., Back, D., Ben-Porath, E., Hazani, A., Martinowitz, U., Tatarsky, I. 1994: Co-infection with hepatitis viruses and human immunodeficiency virus in multiply transfused patients. *Israeli Journal of Medical Sciences* **30**(12) 886–90.

Brunson, M.E., Lau, J.Y., Davis, G.L., Scornik, J., Howard, R.J., Pfaff, W.W. 1993: Non-A, non-B hepatitis and elevated serum aminotransferases in renal transplant patients. Correlation with hepatitis C infection. *Transplantation* **56**, 1364–7.

Caccamo, L., Colledan, M., Gridelli, B. *et al.* 1993: Hepatitis C virus infection in liver allograft recipients. *Archives of Virology* **8**(supplement), 291–304.

Cakaloglu, Y., Devlin, J., O'Grady, J. *et al.* 1995: Importance of concomitant viral infection during late acute liver allograft rejection. *Transplantation* **59**, 40–5.

Calmus, Y., Hannoun, L., Dousset, B. *et al.* 1990: HLA class 1 matching is responsible for the hepatic lesions in recurrent viral hepatitis B after liver transplantation. *Transplantation Proceedings* **22**, 2311–13.

Calmus, Y., Marcellin, P., Beaurain, G., Chatenoud, L., Brechot, C. 1994: Distribution of hepatitis B virus DNA sequences in different peripheral blood mononuclear cell subsets in HBs antigen-positive and negative patients. *European Journal of Clinical Investigation* **24**, 548–52.

Carman, W.F., Trautwein, C., Van Deursen, F.J. *et al.* 1996: Hepatitis B virus envelope variation after transplantation with and without hepatitis B immune globulin prophylaxis. *Hepatology* **24**, 489–93.

Cassidy, W., Govindarajan, S., Gupta, S. *et al.* 1989: Influence of HIV on chronic hepatitis B and D infection. *Hepatology* **10**, 690.

Chambost, H., Gerolami, V., Halfon, P. *et al.* 1995: Persistent hepatitis C virus RNA replication in haemophiliacs: role of co-infection with human immunodeficiency virus. *British Journal of Haematology* **91**, 703–7.

Chamlion, A., Benkoel, L., Sahel, J. *et al.* 1993: Nuclear immunostaining of hepatitis C infected hepatocytes with monoclonal antibodies to C100-3 nonstructural protein. Comparison of immunogold silver staining with other immunohistochemical methods. *Cellular and Molecular Biology* **39**, 243–51.

Charco, R., Vargas, V., Allende, H. *et al.* 1996: Is hepatitis C virus recurrence a risk factor for chronic liver allograft rejection? *Transplantation International* **9**, 195–7.

Chazouillères, O., Mamish, D., Kim, M. *et al.* 1994a: 'Occult' hepatitis B virus as source of infection in liver transplant recipients. *Lancet* **343**, 142–6.

Chazouillères, O., Kim, M., Combs, C. *et al.* 1994b: Quantitation of hepatitis C virus RNA in liver transplant recipients. *Gastroenterology* **106**, 994–9.

Chen, C.H., Chen, P.J., Chu, J.S., Yeh, K.H., Lai, M.Y., Chen, D.S. 1994: Fibrosing cholestatic hepatitis in a hepatitis B surface antigen carrier after renal transplantation. *Gastroenterology* **107**, 1514–18.

Chisari, F.V., Filippi, P., Buras, J. *et al.* 1987: Structural and pathological effects of synthesis of hepatitis B virus large envelope polypeptide in transgenic mice. *Proceedings of the National Academy of Sciences of the USA* **84**, 6909–13.

Cisterne, J.M., Rostaing, L., Izopet, J. *et al.* 1996: Epidemiology of HCV infection – disease and renal transplantation. *Nephrology Dialysis–Transplantation* **11**, 46–7.

Clouse, K.A., Robbins, P.B., Fernie, B., Ostrove, J.M., Fauci, A.S. 1989: Viral antigen stimulation of the production of human monokines capable of regulating HIV1 expression. *Journal of Immunology* **143**, 470–5.

Colgrove, R., Simon, G., Ganem, D. 1989: Transcriptional activation of homologous and heterologous genes by the hepatitis B virus X gene product in cells permissive for viral replication. *Journal of Virology* **63**, 4019–26.

Colombari, R., Dhillon, A.P., Pizzola, E. *et al.* 1993: Chronic hepatitis in multiple virus infection: histopathological evaluation. *Histopathology* **22**, 319–25.

Cooksley, W.G.E., McIvor, C.A. 1995: Fibrosing cholestatic hepatitis and HBV after bone marrow transplantation. *Biomedicine and Pharmacotherapy* **49**, 117–24.

Corey, L., Holmes, K. 1980: Sexual transmission of hepatitis A in homosexual men: incidence and mechanism. *New England Journal of Medicine* **4**, 415–21.

Crespo, J., Lozano, J.L., De la Cruz, F. *et al.* 1994: Prevalence and significance of hepatitis C viremia in chronic active hepatitis. *American Journal of Gastroenterology* **89**, 1147–51.

Davies, S.E., Portmann, B.C., O'Grady, J.G. *et al.* 1991: Hepatic histological findings after transplantation for chronic hepatitis B virus infection, including a unique pattern of fibrosing cholestatic hepatitis. *Hepatology* **13**, 150–7.

Davies, S.E., Lau, J.Y.N., O'Grady, J.G., Portmann, B.C., Alexander, G.J.M., Williams, R. 1992: Evidence that hepatitis D virus needs hepatitis B virus to cause hepatocellular damage. *American Journal of Clinical Pathology* **98**, 554–8.

Davis, G.L., Hoofnagle, J.H. 1985: Reactivation of chronic type B hepatitis presenting as a viral hepatitis. *Annals of Internal Medicine* **102**, 762–5.

Davis, G.L., Lau, J.Y.N., Urdea, M.S. *et al.* 1994: Quantitative detection of hepatitis C virus RNA with a solid phase signal amplification method: definition of optimal conditions for specimen collection and clinical application of interferon-treated patients. *Hepatology* **19**, 1337–41.

Davison, F., Alexander, G.J.M., Trowbridge, R., Fagan, E.A., Williams, R. 1987: Detection of hepatitis B virus DNA in spermatozoa, urine, saliva and leucocytes, of chronic HBsAg carriers: a lack of relationship with serum markers of replication. *Journal of Hepatology* **4**, 37–44.

Demetris, A.J., Jaffe, R., Sheahal, D.B. *et al.* 1986: Recurrent hepatitis B in liver allograft recipients. Differentiation between viral hepatitis B and rejection. *American Journal of Pathology* **125**, 161–72.

Demetris, A.J., Todo, S., Van Thiel, D.H. *et al.* 1990: Evolution of hepatitis B virus liver disease after hepatic replacement. *American Journal of Pathology* **137**, 667–76.

Dickson, R.C., Caldwell, S.H., Ishitani, M.B. *et al.* 1996: Clinical and histologic patterns of early graft failure due to recurrent hepatitis C in 4 patients after liver transplantation. *Transplantation* **61**, 701–5.

Dickson, R.C., Qian, K.P., Lau, J.Y.N. 1997: High prevalence of GB virus-C hepatitis G virus infection in liver transplant recipients. *Transplantation* **63**, 1695–7.

Dorrucci, M., Pezzotti, P., Phillips, A.N., Lepri, A.C., Rezza, G. 1995: Coinfection of hepatitis C virus with human immunodeficiency virus and progression to AIDS. Italian Seroconversion Study. *Journal of Infectious Diseases* **172**, 1503–8.

Douglas, D.D., Rakela, J., Taswell, H.F., Krom, R.A.F., Wiesner, R.H. 1993: Hepatitis B virus replication patterns after orthotopic liver transplantation: de novo versus recurrent infection. *Transplantation Proceedings* **25**, 1755–7.

Dousset, B., Conti, F., Houssin, D., Calmus, Y. 1994: Acute vanishing bile duct syndrome after therapy for recurrent HCV infection in liver transplant recipients. *New England Journal of Medicine* **330**, 1160–1.

Dusheiko, G., Schmilovitz-Weiss, H., Brown, D. *et al.* 1994: Hepatitis C virus genotypes: an investigation of type-specific differences in geographic origin and disease. *Hepatology* **19**, 31–8.

Duvoux, C., Pawlotsky, J.M., Cherqui, D. *et al.* 1995: Serial quantitative determination of hepatitis C virus RNA levels after liver transplantation – a useful test for diagnosis of hepatitis C virus reinfection. *Transplantation* **60**, 457–61.

Emile, J.F., Sebagh, M., Feray, C., David, F., Reynes, M. 1993: The presence of epithelioid granulomas in hepatitis C virus-related cirrhosis. *Human Pathology* **24**, 1095–7.

Eskild, A., Magnus, P., Petersen, G. *et al.* 1992: Hepatitis B antibodies in HIV-infected homosexual men are associated with more rapid progression to AIDS. *AIDS* **6**, 571–4.

Eyster, M.E., Sanders, J.C., Battegay, M., Di Bisceglie, A.M. 1995: Suppression of hepatitis C virus (HCV) replication by hepatitis D virus (HDV) in HIV-infected hemophiliacs with chronic hepatitis B and C. *Digestive Diseases and Sciences* **40**, 1583 8.

Fagan, E.A., Ellis, D.S., Tovey, G.M. *et al.* 1989: Toga-like virus as a cause of fulminant hepatitis attributed to sporadic non-A, non-B. *Journal of Medical Virology* **28**, 150–5.

Fagan, E., Yousef, G., Braham, J. *et al.* 1990: Persistence of hepatitis A in fulminant hepatitis and after liver transplantation. *Journal of Medical Virology* **30**, 131–6.

Fagan, E.A., Ellis, D.S., Tovey, G.M. *et al.* 1992: Toga virus-like particles in acute liver failure attributed to sporadic non-A, non-B hepatitis and recurrence after liver transplantation. *Journal of Medical Virology* **38**, 71–7.

Fairley, K.C., Mijch, A., Gust, I.D., Nichilson, S., Dimitrakakis, M., Lukas, C.R. 1991: The increased risk of fatal liver disease in renal transplant patients who are hepatitis B antigen and/or HBV DNA positive. *Transplantation* **52**, 497–500.

Fang, J.W.S., Tung, F.Y.T., Davis, G.L., Dolson, D.J., Van Thiel, D.H., Lau, J.Y.N. 1993a: Fibrosing cholestatic hepatitis in a transplant recipient with hepatitis B virus precore mutant. *Gastroenterology* **105**, 901–4.

Fang, J.W., Wright, T.L., Lau, J.Y. 1993b: Fibrosing cholestatic hepatitis in patient with HIV and hepatitis B. *Lancet* **342**, 1175.

Farci, P., Croxson, T.S., Taylor, M.B. *et al.* 1988: Effect of human immunodeficiency virus on the increased severity of liver disease associated with delta hepatitis. *Gastroenterology* **94**, A578.

Farges, O., Saliba, F., Farhamant, H. *et al.* 1996: Incidence of rejection as a function of the primary disease: possible influence of alcohol and polyclonal immunoglobulins. *Hepatology* **3**, 240–8.

Feray, C., Zignegno, A.L., Samuel, D. *et al.* 1990: Persistent hepatitis B virus infection of mononuclear blood cells without concomitant liver infection. The liver transplantation model. *Transplantation* **49**, 1155–8.

Feray, C., Samuel, D., Gigon, M., David, M.F., Reynes, M., Arulnaden, J.L. 1993: Low incidence of hepatitis due to hepatitis C virus after liver transplantation for cirrhosis type B and C. Oral presentation at the 6th Congress of the European Society for Organ Transplantation, Rodos, Greece, October.

Feray, C., Gigou, M., Samuel, D. *et al.* 1994: The course of hepatitis C virus infection after liver transplantation. *Hepatology* **20**, 1137–43.

Feray, C., Gigou, M., Samuel, D. *et al.* 1995a: Influence of the genotypes of hepatitis C virus on the severity of recurrent liver disease after liver transplantation. *Gastroenterology* **108**, 1088–96.

Feray, C., Samuel, D., Gigou, M. *et al.* 1995b: An open trial of interferon-alfa recombinant for hepatitis C after liver transplantation. Antiviral effects and risk of rejection. *Hepatology* **22**, 1084–9.

Ferrell, L.D., Wright, T.L., Roberts, J., Ascher, N., Lake, J. 1992: Hepatitis C viral infection in liver transplant recipients. *Hepatology* **16**, 865–76.

Fischer, H.P., Willsch, E., Bierhoff, E., Pfeifer, U. 1996: Histopathological findings in chronic hepatitis C. *Journal of Hepatology* **2**, 35–42.

Fornairon, S., Pol, S., Legendre, C. *et al.* 1996: The long term virologic and pathologic impact of renal transplantation on chronic hepatitis B virus infection. *Transplantation* **62**, 297–9.

Foster, G.R., Goldin, R.D., Hay, A., McGarvey, M.J., Stark, G.R., Thomas, H.C. 1993: Expression of the terminal protein of hepatitis B virus is associated with failure to respond to interferon therapy. *Hepatology* **17**, 757–62.

Freeman, R.B., Tran, S., Lee, Y.M., Rohrer, R.J., Kaplan, M.M. 1996: Serum hepatitis C RNA titers after liver transplantation are not correlated with immunosuppression or hepatitis. *Transplantation* **61**, 542–6.

Fried, M.W., Khudyakov, Y.E., Smallwood, G.A. *et al.* 1997: Hepatitis G virus co-infection in liver transplantation recipients with chronic hepatitis C and non-viral chronic liver disease. *Hepatology* **25**, 1271–5.

Fukumoto, T., Berg, T., Ku, Y. *et al.* 1996: Viral dynamics of hepatitis C early after orthotopic liver transplantation – evidence for rapid turnover of serum virions. *Hepatology* **24**, 1351–4.

Gane, E., Sallie, R., Saleh, M., Portmann, B., Willians, R. 1995: Clinical recurrence of hepatitis A following liver transplantation for acute liver failure. *Journal of Medical Virology* **45**, 35–9.

Gane, E.J., Naoumov, N.V., Qian, K.P. *et al.* 1996a: A longitudinal analysis of hepatitis C virus replication following liver transplantation. *Gastroenterology* **110**, 167–77.

Gane, E.J., Portmann, B.C., Naoumov, N.V. *et al.* 1996b: Long-term outcome of hepatitis C infection after liver transplantation. *New England Journal of Medicine* **334**, 815–20.

Gerber, M.A. 1995: Pathobiologic effects of hepatitis C. *Journal of Hepatology* **22**, 83–6.

Ghany, M.G., Leissinger, C., Lagier, R., Sanchez Pescador, R., Lok, A.S. 1996: Effect of human immunodeficiency virus infection on hepatitis C virus infection in hemophiliacs. *Digestive Diseases and Sciences* **41**, 1265–72.

Goffin, E., Pirson, Y., Van Ypersele de Strihou, C. 1995: Implications of chronic hepatitis B or hepatitis C infection for renal transplant candidates. *Nephrology Dialysis and Transplantation* **10**, 88–92.

Goldin, R.D., Fish, D.E., Hay, A. *et al.* 1990a: Histological and immunohistochemical study of hepatitis B virus in human immunodeficiency virus infection. *Journal of Clinical Pathology* **43**, 203–5.

Goldin, R., Saldanha, J., Thomas, H. 1990b: Hepatitis delta virus infection in human immunodeficiency virus-positive patients. *Hepatology* **11**, 903–4.

Goldin, R.D., Levine, T.S., Foster, G.R., Thomas, H.C. 1996a: Granulomas and hepatitis C. *Histopathology* **28**, 265–7.

Goldin, R.D., Patel, N.K., Thomas, H.C. 1996b: Hepatitis C and bile duct loss. *Journal of Clinical Pathology* **49**, 836–8.

Goldstein, N., Hart, J., Lewin, K. 1991: Diffuse hepatocyte ballooning in liver biopsies from orthotopic liver transplant patients. *Histopathology* **18**, 331–8.

Gonzalez-Peralta, R.P., Davis, G.L., Lau, J.Y.N. 1994: Pathogenetic mechanisms of hepatocellular damage in chronic hepatitis C virus infection. *Journal of Hepatology* **21**, 255–9.

Gordon, F.D., Poterucha, J.J., Germer, J. *et al.* 1997: Relationship between hepatitis C genotype and severity of recurrent hepatitis C after liver transplantation. *Transplantation* **63**, 1419–23.

Gouw, A.S., Houthoff, H.J., Huitema, S., Beelen, J.M., Gips, C.H., Poppema, S. 1987: Expression of major histocompatibility complex antigens and replacement of donor cells by recipient ones in human liver grafts. *Transplantation* **43**, 291–6.

Greenson, J.K., Svoboda-Newman, S.M., Merion, R.M., Frank, T.S. 1996: Histologic progression of recurrent hepatitis C in liver transplantation allografts. *American Journal of Surgical Pathology* **20**, 731–8.

Grellier, L., Mutimer, D., Ahmed, M. *et al.* 1996: Lamivudine prophylaxis against reinfection in liver-transplantation for hepatitis-B cirrhosis. *Lancet* **348**, 1212–15.

Gretch, D.R., Bachhi, C.E., Corey, L. *et al.* 1995: Persistent hepatitis C virus infection after liver transplantation: clinical and virological features. *Hepatology* **22**, 1–9.

Gugenheim, J,, Baldini, E., Ouzan, D., Mouiel, J. 1997: Absence of initial viral replication and long term high dose immunoglobulin administration improve results of hepatitis B virus recurrence prophylaxis after liver transplantation. *Transplantation Proceedings* **29**, 517–18.

Guido, M., Rugge, M., Rocchetto, P. *et al.* 1994: Human immunodeficiency virus infection and hepatitis C pathology. *Liver* **14**, 314–19.

Haagsma, E.B., Cuypers, H.T.M., Gouw, A.S.H. *et al.* 1997: High prevalence of hepatitis G virus after liver transplantation without apparent influence on long-term graft function. *Journal of Hepatology* **26**, 921–5.

Hadler, S.C., Judson, F.N., O'Malley, P.M. *et al.* 1991: Outcome of hepatitis B virus infection in homosexual men and its relation to prior human immunodeficiency virus infection. *Journal of Infectious Diseases* **163**, 454–9.

Harrison, R.F., Davies, M.H., Goldin, R.D., Hübscher, S.G. 1993: Recurrent hepatitis B in liver allografts: a distinctive form of rapidly developing cirrhosis. *Histopathology* **23**, 21–8.

Hawkins, A.E., Gilson, R.J.C., Gilbert, N. *et al.* 1996: Hepatitis B virus surface mutations associated with infection after liver transplantation. *Journal of Hepatology* **24**, 8–14.

Hayashi, P.H., Flynn, N., McCurdy, S.A., Kuramoto, I.K., Holland, P.V., Zeldis, J.B. 1991: Prevalence of hepatitis C virus antibodies among patients infected with human immunodeficiency virus. *Journal of Medical Virology* **33**, 177–80.

Henin, C., Makris, M., Brown, J., Peake, I.R., Preston, E.F. 1994: Peripheral mononuclear cells of haemophiliacs with chronic liver disease are infected with replicating hepatitis C virus. *British Journal of Haematology* **87**, 215–17.

Hilleman, M.R. 1994: Comparative biology and pathogenesis of AIDS and hepatitis B viruses: related but different. *Aids Research and Human Retroviruses* **10**, 1409–19.

Hillis, W.D., Hillis, A., Walter, W.G. 1979: Hepatitis B surface antigenemia in renal transplant recipients. Increased mortality risk. *Journal of the American Medical Association* **242**, 329–32.

Hiramatsu, N., Hayashi, N., Haruna, Y. *et al.* 1992: Immunohistochemical detection of hepatitis C virus-infected hepatocytes in chronic liver disease with monoclonal antibodies to core, envelope and NS3 regions of the hepatitis C virus genome. *Hepatology* **16**, 306–11.

Ho, B.M., So, S.K., Esquivel, C.O., Keeffe, E.B. 1997: Liver transplantation in Asian patients with chronic hepatitis B. *Hepatology* **25**, 223–5.

Hoffmann, R.M., Gunther, C., Diepolder, H.M. *et al.* 1995: Hepatitis C virus infection as a possible risk factor for ductopenic rejection (vanishing bile duct syndrome) after liver transplantation. *Transplantation International* **8**, 353–9.

Holt, C.D., Millis, J.M., Busuttil, R.W. 1995: Role of liver transplantation in patients with hepatitis B infection. *Clinical Transplantation* **9**, 269–76.

Homann, C., Krogsgaard, K., Pedersen, C., Andersson, P., Nielsen, J.O. 1991: High incidence of hepatitis B infection and evolution of chronic hepatitis B infection in patients with advanced HIV infection. *Journal of Acquired Immune Deficiency Syndrome* **4**, 416–20.

Hopf, U., Neuhaus, P., Lobeck, H. *et al.* 1991: Follow-up of recurrent hepatitis B and delta infection in liver allograft recipients after treatment with recombinant interferon-α. *Hepatology* **13**, 339–46.

Horvath, J., Raffanti, S.P. 1994: Clinical aspects of the interactions between human immunodeficiency virus and the hepatotropic viruses. *Clinics in Infectious Diseases* **18**, 339–47.

Housset, C., Lamas, E., Courgnaud, V. *et al.* 1993: Presence of HIV-1 in human parenchymal and non-parenchymal liver cells in vivo. *Journal of Hepatology* **19**, 252–8.

Hsu, H.H., Wright, T.L., Tsao, S.C. *et al.* 1994: Antibody response to hepatitis C virus infection after liver transplantation. *American Journal of Gastroenterology* **89**, 1169–74.

Hsu, M.L., Chen, S.W., Lin, K.H., Liao, S.K., Chang, K.S.S. 1995: Cytokine regulation of HIV-1 LTR transactivation in human hepatocellular carcinoma cell lines. *Cancer Letters* **94**(1), 41–8.

Huang, E.J., Wright, T.L., Lake, J.R., Combs, C., Ferrell, L.D. 1996: Hepatitis B and C coinfections and persistent hepatitis B infections: clinical outcome and liver pathology after transplantation. *Hepatology* **23**, 396–404.

Hübscher, S.G., 1990: Chronic hepatitis in liver allografts. *Hepatology* **12**, 1257–8.

Hübscher, S.G., 1991: Histological findings in liver allograft rejection – new insights into the pathogenesis of hepatocellular damage in liver allografts. *Histopathology* **18**, 377–83.

Hübscher, S.G., Elias, E., Buckels, J.A.C., Mayer, A.D., McMaster, P., Neuberger, J.M. 1993: Primary biliary cirrhosis: histological evidence of disease recurrence after liver transplantation. *Journal of Hepatology* **18**, 173–84.

Hung, Y.B., Liang, J.T., Chu, J.S., Chen, K.M., Lee, C.S. 1995: Fulminant hepatic failure in a renal transplant recipient with positive hepatitis B surface antigens – a case report of fibrosing cholestatic hepatitis. *Hepato-Gastroenterology* **42**, 913–18.

Jacobs, J.M., Martin, P., Munoz, S.J. *et al.* 1993: Liver transplantation for chronic hepatitis B in Asian males. *Transplantation Proceedings* **25**, 1904–6.

Jamal, H., Regenstein, F., Farr, G., Perrillo, R.P. 1996: Prolonged survival in fibrosing cholestatic hepatitis with long term ganciclovir therapy. *American Journal of Gastroenterology* **91**, 1027–30.

Johnson, M.W., Washburn, W.K., Freeman, R.B. *et al.* 1996: Hepatitis C viral infection in liver transplantation. *Archives of Surgery* **313**, 284–91.

Jurim, O., Martin, P., Shaked, A. *et al.* 1994: Liver transplantation for chronic hepatitis B in Asians. *Transplantation* **57**, 1393–411.

Kashala, O., Mubikayi, L., Kayembe, K., Mukeba, P., Essex, M. 1994: Hepatitis B virus activation among Central Africans infected with human immunodeficiency virus (HIV) type 1: pre-s2 antigen is predominantly expressed in HIV infection. *Journal of Infectious Diseases* **169**(3), 628–32.

Kemnitz, J., Gubernatis, G., Bunzendahl, H., Ringe, B., Pichlmayr, R., Georgii, A. 1989: Criteria for the histological classification of liver allograft rejection and their clinical relevance. *Transplantation Proceedings* **21**, 2208–10.

Kingsley, L.A., Rinaldo, C.R., Lyter, D.W., Valdiserri, R.O., Bell, S.H., Ho, M. 1990: Sexual transmission efficiency of hepatitis B virus among homosexual men. *Journal of the American Medical Association* **264**, 230–4.

Knoop, M., Lüsebrink, R., Langrehr, J.M. *et al.* 1994: Incidence and clinical relevance of recurrent hepatitis C infection after orthotopic liver transplantation. *Transplantation International* **7**, S221–S223.

Krawczynski, K., Beach, M.J., Bradley, D.W. *et al.* 1992: Hepatitis C virus antigen in hepatocytes. Immunomorphologic detection and identification. *Gastroenterology* **103**, 622–9.

Kumar, A., Kulkarni, R., Murray, D.L. *et al.* 1993: Serological markers of viral hepatitis A, B, C and D in patients with hemophilia. *Journal of Medical Virology* **41**, 205–9.

Lake-Bakaar, G., Bhat, K., Govindarajan, S. 1994: The effect of HIV disease on serum markers of hepatitis delta infection in intravenous drug abusers. *Laboratory and Clinical Medicine* **124**(4), 564–8.

Lam, K.C., Lai, C.L., Ng, R.P., Trepo, C., Wu, P.C. 1981: Deleterious effect of prednisolone in HBsAg-positive chronic active hepatitis. *New England Journal of Medicine* **304**, 380–6.

Lam, P.W., Wachs, M.E., Somberg, K.A., Vincenti, F., Lake, J.R., Ferrell, L.D. 1996: Fibrosing cholestatic hepatitis in renal transplant recipients. *Transplantation* **61**, 378–81.

Lamas, E., Baccarini, P., Housset, C., Kremsdorf, D., Brechot, C. 1992: Detection of hepatitis C virus RNA in the liver using in situ hybridisation: evidence for infection of both hepatocytes and mononuclear cells. *Journal of Hepatology* **16**, 219–23.

Lau, J.Y.N., Bain, V.G., Davies, S.E. *et al.* 1992: High-level expression of hepatitis B viral antigens in fibrosing cholestatic hepatitis. *Gastroenterology* **102**, 956–62.

Lebovics, E., Dworkin, B., Heier, S., Rosenthal, W. 1988: The hepatobiliary manifestations of human immunodeficiency virus infection. *American Journal of Gastroenterology* **83**, 1–7.

Leentvaar Kuijpers, A., Kool, J.L., Veugelers, P.J., Coutinho, R.A., van Griensven, G.J. 1995: An outbreak of hepatitis A among homosexual men in Amsterdam, 1991–1993. *International Journal of Epidemiology* **24**, 218–22.

Lei, D.H., Wu, J.W., Sullivan, D.E., Dash, S., Gerber, M.A. 1995: Detection of hepatitis-B virus sequences in liver tissues of seronegative organ donors. *International Hepatology Communications* **3**, 145–60.

Levy, P., Marcellin, P., Martinot, P.M., Degott, C., Nataf, J., Benhamou, J.P. 1990: Clinical course of spontaneous reactivation of hepatitis B virus infection in patients with chronic hepatitis B. *Hepatology* **12**, 570–4.

Lim, H.L., Lau, G.K.K., Davis, G.L., Dolson, D.J., Lau, J.Y.N. 1994: Cholestatic hepatitis leading to hepatic failure in a patient with organ-transmitted hepatitis C virus infection. *Gastroenterology* **106**, 248–51.

Ling, R., Mutimer, D., Ahmed, N. *et al.* 1996: Selection of mutations in the hepatitis B virus polymerase during therapy of transplant recipients with lamivudine. *Hepatology* **24**, 711–13.

Linnen, J., Wages, J., Zhang-Keck, Z.Y. *et al.* 1996: Molecular cloning and disease association of hepatitis G virus: a transfusion-transmissible agent. *Science* **271**, 505–8.

Liu, P.P., Chen, C.L., Chen, Y.S., Tai, D.I. 1996: De-novo hepatitis-B virus infection after orthotopic liver transplantation. *Transplantation Proceedings* **28**, 1684–6.

Loda, M., Fiorentino, M., Meckler, J. *et al.* 1996: Hepatitis C virus reinfection in orthotopic liver transplant patients with or without concomitant hepatitis B infection. *Diagnostic Molecular Pathology* **5**, 81–7.

Loinaz, C., Lumbreras, C., Gonzalex-Pinto, I. *et al.* 1995: High incidence of post transplant hepatitis and chronic rejection associated with hepatitis C virus infection in liver transplant recipients. *Transplantation Proceedings* **27**, 1217–18.

Lok, A.S.F., Liang, R.H.S., Chiu, E.K.W., Wong, K.L., Chan, T.K., Todd, D. 1991: Reactivation of hepatitis B virus replication in patients receiving cytotoxic therapy. *Gastroenterology* **100**, 182–8.

Loke, R., Murray-Lyon, I., Coleman, J. *et al.* 1990: Diminished response to recombinant hepatitis B vaccine in homosexual men with HIV antibody: an indicator of poor prognosis. *Journal of Medical Virology* **31**, 109–11.

Lowell, J.A., Howard, T.K., White, H.M. *et al.* 1995: Serological evidence of past hepatitis B infection in liver donor and hepatitis B infection in liver allograft. *Lancet* **345**, 1084–5.

Lozano, J.L., Crespo, J., de la Cruz, F. *et al.* 1994: Correlation between hepatitis B viremia and the clinical and histological activity of chronic delta hepatitis. *Medical Microbiology and Immunology* **183**(3), 159–67.

Lucey, M.R., Graham, D.M., Martin, P. *et al.* 1992: Recurrence of hepatitis B and delta hepatitis after orthotopic liver transplantation. *Gut* **33**, 1390–6.

Lugassy, C., Bernuau, J., Thiers, V. *et al.* 1987: Sequences of hepatitis B virus DNA in the serum and liver of patients with acute benign and fulminant hepatitis. *Journal of Infectious Diseases* **155**, 64–71.

McCruden, E.A., Welch, S., Batchelor, B. *et al.* 1994: Hepatitis C virus infection detected by antibody tests and the polymerase chain reaction as a cause of liver dysfunction in renal transplant recipients. *Journal of Medical Virology* **42**, 158–63.

McDonald, G.S.A., Courtney, M.G., Shattock, A.G., Weir, D.G. 1989: Prolonged IgM antibodies and histopathological evidence of chronicity in hepatitis A. *Liver* **9**, 223–8.

McIvor, C., Morton, J., Bryant, A., Cooksley, W.K., Durrant, S., Walker, N. 1994: Fatal reactivation of precore mutant hepatitis B virus associated with fibrosing cholestatic hepatitis after bone marrow transplantation. *Annals of Internal Medicine* **121**, 274–5.

McMillan, J.S., Shaw, T., Angus, P.W., Locarnini, S.A. 1995: Effect of immunosuppressive and antiviral agents on hepatitis B virus replication in vitro. *Hepatology* **22**, 36–43.

McMillan, J.S., Bowden, D.S., Angus, P.W., McCaughan, G.W., Locarnini, S.A. 1996: Mutations in the hepatitis B virus precore/core gene and core promoter in patients with severe recurrent disease following liver transplantation. *Hepatology* **24**, 1371–8.

McNair, A., Main, J., Goldin, R. *et al.* 1994: Liver disease and AIDS. In Broder, S., Merigan, T.C., Bolognesi, D. (eds) *Textbook of AIDS Medicine*. Baltimore: Williams & Wilkins, 581–96.

Manzini, P., Saracco, G., Cerchier, A. *et al.* 1995: Human immunodeficiency virus infection as risk factor for mother-to-child hepatitis C virus transmission: persistence of anti-hepatitis C virus in children is associated with the mother's anti-hepatitis C virus immunoblotting pattern. *Hepatology* **21**, 328–32.

Marcellin, P., Colin, J., Martinot-Peignoux, M. *et al.* 1993: Hepatitis C virus infection in anti-HIV positive and negative French homosexual men with chronic hepatitis: comparison of second and third generation anti-HCV testing. *Liver* **13**, 319–22.

Marcellin, P., Martinot-Peignoux, M., Elias, A. *et al.* 1994: Hepatitis C virus (HCV) viremia in human immunodeficiency virus seronegative and seropositive patients with indeterminate HCV recombinant immunoblot assay. *Journal of Infectious Diseases* **170**, 433–5.

Marsman, W.A., Wiesner, R.H., Batts, K.P. *et al.* 1997: Fulminant hepatitis B virus: recurrence after liver transplantation in two patients also infected with hepatitis delta virus. *Hepatology* **25**, 434–8.

Martin, P., Di Bisceglie, A.M., Kassianides, C., Lisker Melman, M., Hoofnagle, J.H. 1989: Rapidly progressive non-A, non-B hepatitis in patients with human immunodeficiency virus infection. *Gastroenterology* **97**, 1559–61.

Masada, C.T., Shaw, B.W., Zetterman, R.K., Kaufman, S.S., Markin, R.S. 1993: Fulminant hepatic failure with massive necrosis as a result of hepatitis A infection. *Journal of Clinical Gastroenterology* **17**, 158–62.

Mason, W.S., Taylor, J.M., 1991: Liver transplantation: a model for the transmission of hepatitis delta virus. *Gastroenterology* **101**, 1741–3.

Missale, G., Brems, J.J., Takiff, H., Pockros, P.J., Chisari, F.V. 1993: Human leukocyte antigen class I-independent pathways may contribute to hepatitis B virus-induced liver disease after liver transplantation. *Hepatology* **18**, 491–6.

Mohammed, R., Hübscher, S.G., Mirza, D.F., Gunson, B.K., Mutimer, D.J. 1997: Post transplantation chronic hepatitis in fulminant hepatic failure. *Hepatology* **25**, 1003–7.

Myint, H., Soe, M.M., Khin, T. *et al.* 1985: A clinical and epidemiological study of an epidemic of non-A, non-B hepatitis in Rangoon. *American Journal of Tropical Medicine and Hygiene* **34**, 1183–9.

Nakhleh, R.E., Schwarzenberg, S.J., Bloomer, J., Payne, W., Snover, D.C. 1990: The pathology of liver allografts surviving longer than one year. *Hepatology* **11**, 465–70.

Ng, I., Burroughs, A., Rolles, K., Belli, L., Scheuer, P. 1991: Hepatocellular ballooning after liver transplantation; a light and electronmicroscopic study with clinicopathological correlation. *Histopathology* **18**, 323–30.

Nigro, G., Taliani, G., Krzysztofiak, A. *et al.* 1993: Multiple viral infections in HIV-infected children with chronically-evolving hepatitis. *Archives of Virology* **8** (supplement), 237–48.

Nonomura, A., Mizukami, Y., Matsubara, F., Kobayashi, K. 1991: Clinicopathological study of lymphocyte attachment to endothelial cells (endothelialitis) in various liver diseases. *Liver* **11**, 78–88.

Noonan, C., Yoffe, B., Mansell, P., Melnich, J., Hollinger, F. 1986: Extra-chromosomal sequences of hepatitis B virus DNA in peripheral blood mononuclear cells of acquired immune deficiency syndrome patients. *Proceedings of the National Academy of Sciences of the USA* **835**, 698–702.

Nuovo, G.J., Lidonnici, K., MacConnell, P., Lane, B. 1993: Intracellular localization of polymerase chain reaction (PCR)-amplified hepatitis C cDNA. *American Journal of Surgical Pathology* **17**, 683–90.

O'Grady, J.G., Smith, H.M., Davies, S.E. *et al.* 1992: Hepatitis B virus reinfection after orthotopic liver transplantation. *Journal of Hepatology* **14**, 104–11.

Ottobrelli, A., Marzano, A., Smedile, A. *et al.* 1991: Patterns of hepatitis delta virus reinfection and disease in liver transplantation. *Gastroenterology* **101**, 1649–55.

Pereira, B.J.G., Milford, R.L., Kirkman, R.L. *et al.* 1993: Liver disease and HCV infection after transplantation of organs from hepatitis C antibody positive donors. *Transplantation Proceedings* **25**, 1458–9.

Persaud, D., Bangaru, B., Greco, M.A. *et al.* 1993: Cholestatic hepatitis in children infected with the human immunodeficiency virus. *Pediatric Infectious Disease Journal* **12**, 492–8.

Petrovic, L.M., Villamil, F.G., Elashoff, J.D., Vierling, J.M., Makowka, L., Geller, S.A. 1993: Histopathologic features that differentiate acute rejection from early recurrent hepatitis C after liver transplantation. *Gastroenterology* **104**, A972.

Petrovic, L.M., Villamil, F.G., Vierling, J.M., Makowka, L., Geller, S.A. 1997: Comparison of histopathology in acute allograft rejection and recurrent hepatitis C infection after liver transplantation. *Liver Transplantation and Surgery* **3**, 398–406.

Phillips, M.J., Cameron, R., Flowers, M.A. *et al.* 1992: Post transplant recurrent hepatitis B viral liver disease. *American Journal of Pathology* **140**, 1295–308.

Pol, S., Dubois, F., Roingeard, P. 1989: Hepatitis delta virus infection in French male HBsAg-positive homosexuals. *Hepatology* **10**(3), 342–5.

Pol, S., Legendre, C., Saltiel, C. *et al.* 1992: Hepatitis C virus in kidney recipients. Epidemiology and impact on renal transplantation. *Journal of Hepatology* **15**, 202–6.

Poli, G., Kinter, A.L., Justement, J.S. *et al.* 1990: Tumor necrosis factor alpha functions in an autocrine manner in the induction of HIV expression. *Proceedings of the National Academy of Sciences of the USA* **87**, 782–5.

Pons, J.A. 1995: Role of liver transplantation in viral hepatitis. *Journal of Hepatology* **22**, 146–53.

Pontisso, P., Poon, M.C., Tiollais, P., Brechot, C. 1984: Detection of hepatitis B virus DNA in mononuclear blood cells. *British Medical Journal* **288**, 1563–6.

Poterucha, J.J., Rakela, J., Lumeng, L., Lee, C.H., Taswell, H.F., Wiesner, R.H. 1992: Diagnosis of chronic hepatitis C after liver transplantation by the detection of viral sequences with polymerase chain reaction. *Hepatology* **14**, 42–5.

Pozzato, G., Kaneko, S., Moretti, M. *et al.* 1994: Different genotypes of hepatitis C virus are associated with different severity of chronic liver disease. *Journal of Medical Virology* **43**, 291–6.

Qu, D., Li, J.S., Vitvitski, L. *et al.* 1994: Hepatitis C virus genotypes in France: comparison of clinical features of patients infected with HCV type I and type II. *Journal of Hepatology* **21**, 70–5.

Rabeneck, L., Risser, J.M.H., Murray, N.G.B., McCabe, B.K., Lacke, C.E., Lucco, L.J. 1993: Failure of providers to vaccinate HIV-infected men against hepatitis B: a missed opportunity. *American Journal of Gastroenterology* **88**(12), 2015–18.

Randhawa, P.S., Demetris, A.J., 1995: Hepatitis C virus infection in liver allografts. *Pathology Annual* **2**, 203–26.

Rao, V.K., Anderson, W.R., Kasiske, B.L., Dahl, D.C. 1993: Value of liver biopsy in the evaluation and management of chronic liver disease in renal transplant recipients. *American Journal of Medicine* **94**, 241–50.

Read, A.E., Donegan, E., Lake, J. *et al.* 1991: Hepatitis C in patients undergoing liver transplantation. *Annals of Internal Medicine* **114**, 282–4.

Ribas, A., Gale, R.P., 1997: Should people with hepatitis C virus infection receive a bone marrow transplant? *Bone Marrow Transplantation* **19**, 97–9.

Roche, B., Samuel, D., Gigou, M. *et al.* 1997: De-novo and apparent de novo hepatitis B virus infection after liver transplantation. *Journal of Hepatology* **26**, 517–26.

Roingeard, P., Dubois, F., Marcellin, P. 1992: Persistent delta antigenaemia in chronic delta hepatitis and its relation with human immunodeficiency virus infection. *Journal of Medical Virology* **38**, 191–4.

Rosen, H.R., O'Reilly, P.M., Shackleton, C.R. *et al.* 1996: Graft loss following liver transplantation in patients with chronic hepatitis C. *Transplantation* **62**, 1773–6.

Roth, D., Zucker, K., Cirocco, R. *et al.* 1994: The impact of hepatitis C virus infection on renal allograft recipients. *Kidney International* **45**, 238–44.

Roth, D. 1995: Hepatitis C virus infection and the renal allograft recipient. *Nephron* **71**, 249–53.

Rustgi, V.K., Hoofnagle, J.H., Gerin, J.L. *et al.* 1984: Hepatitis B infection in the acquired immunodeficiency syndrome. *Annals of Internal Medicine* **101**, 795–7.

Sallie, R., Silva, A.E., Purdy, M. *et al.* 1994: Hepatitis C and hepatitis E in non-A and non-B fulminant hepatic failure – a polymerase chain reaction and serological study. *Journal of Hepatology* **20**, 580–8.

Samuel, D., Bismuth, A., Mathieu, D. *et al.* 1991: Passive immunoprophylaxis after liver transplantation in HBsAg-positive patients. *Lancet* **337**, 813–15.

Samuel, D., Muller R., Alexander, G. *et al.* 1993: Liver transplantation in European patients with the hepatitis B surface antigen. *New England Journal of Medicine* **329**, 1842–7.

Samuel, D., Zignego, A.L., Reynes, M. *et al.* 1995: Long-term clinical virological outcome after liver transplantation for cirrhosis caused by chronic delta hepatitis. *Hepatology* **21**, 333–9.

Sanchez Quijano, A., Andreu, J., Gavilan, F. *et al.* 1995: Influence of human immunodeficiency virus type I infection on the natural course of chronic parenterally acquired hepatitis C. *European Journal of Clinical Microbiology and Infectious Diseases* **14**, 949–53.

Sato, S., Fujiyama, S., Tanka, M. *et al.* 1994: Coinfection of hepatitis C virus in patients with chronic hepatitis B infection. *Journal of Hepatology* **21**, 159–66.

Schaffner, F. 1990: The liver in HIV infection. *Progress in Liver Disease* **9**, 505–22.

Scheuer, P.J., Ashrafzadeh, P., Sherlock, S., Brown, D., Dusheiko, G.M. 1991: The pathology of hepatitis C. *Hepatology* **15**, 567–71.

Schluger, L.K., Sheiner, P.A., Thung, S.N. *et al.* 1996: Severe recurrent cholestatic hepatitis C following orthotopic liver transplantation. *Hepatology* **23**, 971–6.

Schmitt, M.P., Gendrault, J.L., Schweitzer, C. *et al.* 1990: Permissivity of primary cultures of human Kupffer cells for HIV-1. *Aids Research and Human Retroviruses* **6**(8), 987–91.

Scoazec, J.Y., Feldmann, G. 1990: Both macrophages and endothelial cells of the human hepatic sinusoid express the CD molecule, a receptor for the human immunodeficiency virus. *Hepatology* **12**, 505–10.

Sebagh, M., Farges, O., Emile, J.F., Bismuth, H., Reynes, M. 1995: An unusual pattern of hepatitis C virus infection in a liver allograft. *Histopathology* **27**, 190–2.

Seto, E., Yen, T., Peterlin, B., Ou, J. 1988: Transactivation of the human immunodeficiency virus long terminal repeat by the hepatitis B virus X protein. *Proceedings of the National Academy of Sciences of the USA* **85**, 8286–90.

Shah, G., Demetris, A.J., Cavaler, J.S. *et al.* 1992: Incidence, prevalence and clinical course of hepatitis C following liver transplantation. *Gastroenterology* **103**, 323–9.

Sheiner, P.A., Schwartz, M.E., Mor, E. *et al.* 1995: Severe or multiple rejection episodes are associated with early recurrence of hepatitis C after orthotopic liver transplantation. *Hepatology* **21**, 30–4.

Sherman, K.E., Andreatta, C., O'Brien, J., Gutierrez, A., Harris, R. 1996: Hepatitis C in human immunodeficiency virus-coinfected patients: increased variability in the hypervariable envelope coding domain. *Hepatology* **23**, 688–94.

Shiffman, M.L., Contos, M.J., Luketic, V.A. *et al.* 1994: Biochemical and histologic evaluation of recurrent hepatitis C following orthotopic liver transplantation. *Transplantation* **57**, 526–53.

Siddiqui, A., Gaynor, R., Srinivasan, A. *et al.* 1989: Trans-activation of viral enhancers including long terminal repeat of the human immunodeficiency virus by the hepatitis B virus X protein. *Virology* **16**, 9479–84.

Singh, N., Gayowski, T., Ndimbie, O.K., Nedjar, S., Wagener, M.M., Yu, V. 1996: Recurrent hepatitis C virus hepatitis in liver transplant recipients receiving tacrolimus – association with rejection and increased immunosuppression after transplantation. *Surgery* **119**, 452–6.

Slapak, G.I., Saxena, R., Portmann, B. *et al.* 1997: Graft and systemic disease in long-term survivors of liver transplantation. *Hepatology* **25**, 195–202.

Solomon, R.E., VanRaden, M., Kaslow, R.A. *et al.* 1990: Association of hepatitis B surface antigen and core antibody with acquisition and manifestations of human immunodeficiency virus type 1 (HIV-1) infection. *American Journal of Public Health* **80**, 1475–8.

Steinhoff, G., Wonigeit, K., Happrecht, J., Johnson, J.P., Pichlmayr, R. 1987: Expression of donor and recipient class I and class II major histocompatibility complex antigens in human liver grafts. *Transplantation Proceedings* **19**, 3561–4.

Stempel, C.A., Lake, J., Kuo, G., Vincenti, F. 1993: Hepatitis C – its prevalence in end stage renal failure patients and clinical course after kidney transplantation. *Transplantation* **55**, 273–6.

Stevens, C.E., Taylor, P.E., Zang, E.A. *et al.* 1986: Human T cell lymphotropic virus type III infection in a cohort of homosexual men in New York City. *Journal of the American Medical Association* **225**, 2167–72.

Tedder, R.S., Gilson, R.J.C., Briggs, M. *et al.* 1991: Hepatitis C virus: evidence for sexual transmission. *British Medical Journal* **302**, 1299–302.

Terrault, N.A., Wright, T.L. 1997: Hepatitis B virus infection and liver transplantation. *Gut* **40**, 568–71.

Thomas, D.L., Vlahov, D., Solomon, L. *et al.* 1995: Correlates of hepatitis C virus infections among injection drug users. *Medicine (Baltimore)* **74**, 212–20.

Thung, S.N., Shim, K.-S., Shieh, C. *et al.* 1993: Hepatitis C in liver allografts. *Archives of Pathology* **117**, 145–9.

Tibbs, C., Williams, R. 1995: Viral causes and management of acute liver failure. *Journal of Hepatology* **22** (suppl 1), 68–73.

Todo, S., Demetris, A., Van Thiel, D., Teperman, L., Fung, J.J., Starzl, T.E. 1991: Orthotopic liver transplantation for patients with hepatitis B virus related liver disease. *Hepatology* **13**, 619–26.

Tur-Kapsa, R., Burk, R.D., Shaul, Y., Shafritz, D.A. 1986: Hepatitis B virus contains a glucocorticoid-responsive element. *Proceedings of the National Academy of Sciences of the USA* **83**, 1627–31.

Twu, J.S., Schloemer, R.H. 1987: Transcriptional trans-activating function of hepatitis B virus. *Journal of Virology* **61**, 3488–93.

Twu, J.S., Robinson, W. 1989: Hepatitis B virus X gene can transactivate heterologous viral sequences. *Proceedings of the National Academy of Sciences of the USA* **86**, 2046–50.

Vandercam, B., Cornu, C., Gala, J. *et al.* 1990: Reactivation of hepatitis B virus infection in a previously immune patient with HIV infection. *European Journal of Clinical Microbiology and Infectious Diseases* **9**, 701–2.

Vargas, V., Comas, P., Castells, L.I. *et al.* 1994: Incidence and outcome of hepatitis C virus infection after liver transplantation. *Transplantation International* **1**, S216–S220.

Wachs, M.E., Amend, W.J., Ascher, N.L. *et al.* 1995: The risk of transmission of hepatitis B from HBsAg(−), HBcAb(+), HBIgM(−) organ donors. *Transplantation* **59**, 230-4.

Waite, J., Gilson, R.J.C., Weller, I.V.D. *et al.* 1988: Hepatitis B virus reactivation or reinfection associated with HIV-1 infection. *AIDS* **2**, 443–4.

Weinstein, J.S., Poterucha, J.J., Zein, N., Wiesner, R.H., Persing, D.H., Rakela, J. 1995: Epidemiology and natural history of hepatitis C infection in liver transplant recipients. *Journal of Hepatology* **22**, 154–9.

Wilkins, M.J., Lindley, R., Dourakis, S.P., Goldin, R.D. 1991: Surgical pathology of the liver in HIV infection. *Histopathology* **18**, 459–64.

Woolf, G.M., Villamil, F.G., Petrovic, L.M. *et al.* 1995: Lamivudine therapy of fibrosing cholestatic hepatitis (FCH) due to recurrent hepatitis B virus (HBV) post-liver transplantation. *Hepatology* **22**, 1615.

Wright, T.L., Donegan, E., Hsu, H.H. *et al.* 1992: Recurrent and acquired hepatitis C viral infection in liver transplant recipients. *Gastroenterology* **103**, 317–22.

Wright, T.L., Hollander, H., Pu, X. *et al.* 1994: Hepatitis C in HIV-infected patients with and without AIDS: prevalence and relationship to patient survival. *Hepatology* **20**, 1152–5.

Yoffe, B., Burns, D.K., Bhatt, H.S., Combes, B. 1990: Extrahepatic hepatitis B virus DNA sequences in patients with acute hepatitis B infection. *Hepatology* **12**, 187–92.

Zein, N.N., McGreger, C.G.A., Wendt, N.K. *et al.* 1995: Prevalence and outcome of hepatitis C infection among heart transplant recipients. *Journal of Heart and Lung Transplantation* **14**, 865–9.

Zhou, S., Terrault, N.A., Ferrell, L. *et al.* 1996: Severity of liver disease in liver transplantation recipients with hepatitis C virus infection – relationship to genotype and level of viremia. *Hepatology* **24**, 1041–6.

Zimmerman, A. 1994: Endothelitis-like changes in chronic hepatitis C viral infection: are small portal vein branches a site of immune attack? Paper presented at the International Symposium on Hepatitis C Viral Infection and Liver Transplantation, Brussels, Belgium, 20 October.

Zylberberg, H., Carnot, F., Mamzer, M.F., Blancho, G., Legendre, C., Pol, S. 1997: Hepatitis C virus related fibrosing cholestatic hepatitis after renal transplantation. *Transplantation* **63**, 158–60.

CHAPTER 6

Hepatitis from non-hepatotropic viruses

R S MARKIN

Many different viral infections affect the liver. These effects may be both structural and functional, the liver being both the primary target and/or significantly involved as a secondary target. Viral infections of the liver can be divided into two general types:

1. *hepatotropic* – those viruses that specifically infect the liver, including hepatitis A, B, C, D, E and possibly HGV (GVC); see Chapter 1.
2. *non-hepatotropic viruses* – such as those listed in Table 6.1, which may infect and damage a wide variety of tissues including the liver.

A brief discussion of the clinical and histological changes associated with each viral infection is presented. Table 6.2 summarises the characteristics of each virus, its geographical distribution, the natural reservoir/vector and the key clinical and histological features of each infection.

Herpes viruses

There are four members of the herpes virus group. The herpes virus group contains double-stranded DNA and includes the following well-known viruses: herpes virus hominis (herpes simplex I and II, Herpes virus varicellae (varicella–zoster virus), cytomegalovirus and Epstein–Barr virus (EBV).

HERPES SIMPLEX I AND II

The primary infection with herpes simplex is characterised by dermatitis, superficial vesicle formation and mucosal ulceration. These lesions are typically associated with a fever of variable intensity that may last for up to 10 days. A primary infection with herpes simplex may resolve, however, recurrent attacks of variable intensity and duration may occur for many years.

There are two strains of herpes simplex virus: types I and II. Herpes simplex virus type I is usually responsible for generalised infections in both adults and older children. Herpes simplex virus type II is primarily associated with genital tract lesions and is usually the viral strain that affects newborns. There is some overlap between the diseases and disorders caused in both populations as a result of either virus (Fakan, 1977).

Table 6.1 Major families of non-hepatotropic viruses and the most frequent viruses associated with each category

Herpes viruses
  Herpes simplex I and II
  Varicella–zoster
  Cytomegalovirus
  Epstein–Barr virus
Adenovirus
Enteroviruses
  Coxsackie B
  Echovirus
Paramyxovirus
  Measles
Togavirus
  Rubella
Arboviruses
  Yellow fever
  Crimean–Congo fever
  Dengue fever
  Rift Valley fever
  Kyasaur Forest disease
  Korean haemorrhagic fever
Arenaviruses
  Lassa fever
  Argentinian/Bolivian haemorrhagic fever
Filoviruses
  Marburg virus
  Ebola virus
  Parvovirus
  Hantavirus

Infection in the neonate is usually by herpes simplex type II and may be a widely disseminated disease (Watanabe *et al*, 1984). In disseminated herpes simplex infections, extensive hepatic involvement may occur (Fakan, 1977). Similar clinical and histological changes are seen in patients who are immunocompromised as a result of chemotherapy for lymphoma or other malignancies. Patients undergoing solid organ and bone marrow transplantation are also immunosuppressed, either functionally (as a result of the transplant) or chemically, as a result of post-transplant anti-rejection therapy (Haagsma *et al*, 1987; Singh *et al*, 1988; Markin *et al*, 1990a). In the absence of immunosuppression, however, disseminated herpes simplex infections in an adult are rare (Fakan, 1977).

The changes present, both macroscopically and microscopically, are characteristic of this infection. Grossly, the liver is enlarged, and multiple yellow foci of necrosis surrounded by congestion and haemorrhage are present. These areas may be large enough to become confluent.

Microscopically, foci of coagulative necrosis that involves hepatocytes, vascular structures and other hepatic components is prominent. Inflammation is conspicuously absent. Prominent congestion and haemorrhage are present, along with individual hepatocyte necrosis. Prominent intranuclear inclusions are present. Both Cowdry type A (halo lesions) and Cowdry type B (Feulgen-positive inclusions) may be present (Fig. 6.1). The

Table 6.2

Virus	Disease	Nuclear material	Virus family	Geographical distribution	Natural reservoir	Clinical features	Key hepatic histological features	Other system/organ involvement
Herpes simplex I and II (HSV)	Herpes stomatitis 'cold sores' and genital lesions	DNA	Herpes viridae	Worldwide	Mammals, including humans	Adults–Superficial vesicular formation on the skin followed by recrudescent attacks at variable intervals. Generalised infections usually due to herpes simplex I, Genital infections usually due to herpes simplex II, usually a disseminated disease in neonates with extensive hepatic involvement. Fulminant hepatic disease in imunosuppressed/ immunocompromised individuals	Enlarged liver with numerous yellow foci of necrosis surrounded by haemorrhagic rings. Focal areas of coagulative necrosis, which may or may not be confluent. Minimal inflammatory response, prominent characteristic inclusions within the nucleii of hepatocytes (Cowdry type B). Giant cell transformation of hepatocytes in the neonate	May involve CNS (encephalitis) and respiratory tract
Varicella–zoster (VZV)	Chickenpox and shingles	DNA	Herpes viridae	Worldwide	Human (species specific)	Vesicular eruption with dermatomal distribution of skin lesions. May become disseminated in immunocompromised patients, especially those with lymphoma or undergoing chemotherapy	Enlarged liver with numerous yellow foci of necrosis surrounded by haemorrhagic rings. Focal areas of coagulative necrosis which may or may not be confluent, minimal inflammatory response, prominent characteristic inclusions within the nuclei of hepatocytes (Cowdry type B). Giant cell transformation with prominent multinucleated cells at the limiting plate or at the periphery of necrosis in the neonate	Lungs/oesophagus and cornea
Cytomegalo-virus (CMV)	Cytomegalic inclusion disease	DNA	Herpes viridae	Worldwide	Human (species specific)	*Congenital infections* – may result in abortion/stillbirth. In some cases, children may excrete virus at birth but, however, be normal. In cytomegalic inclusion disease, there are a variety of pathological changes, including cerebral, occular, respiratory, cardiac, hepatic and splenic lesions associated with thrombocytopenia and haemolytic anaemia. CMV has been implicated in obliterative cholangitis biliary atresia. *Older children and adults –* unexplained pyrexia, liver disease; may mimic infectious mononucleosis. Post-transfusion syndrome, prominent in organ transplant recipients or those receiving chemotherapy, may be due to CMV	Prominent cytomegalic cells present in the liver with 'owl's eye' nuclear inclusions. Giant cell transformation and areas of necrosis may be seen. Cholestasis may also be present. In some cases, non-necrotic hepatic granulomas are present. Inclusions may also occur within endothelial cells or bile duct endothelium	Spleen, central nervous system, lung, heart and eye

Table 6.2 *Continued*

Virus	Disease	Nuclear material	Virus family	Geographical distribution	Natural reservoir	Clinical features	Key hepatic histological features	Other system/organ involvement
Epstein–Barr virus (EBV)	Infectious mononucleosis (IM)/lympho-proliferative disorder (LPD)	DNA	*Herpesviridae*	Worldwide	Human – transmitted via saliva	Primarily endemic disease that affects between 40% and 90% of young adults. Infects lymphoreticular tissue, B-cells in particular. Infection may be transmitted by oral contact or by transfusion. Features of a clinically overt infection include fever, fatigue, sore throat, splenomegaly and lymphadenopathy. Liver involvement occurs in approximately 15% of those patients who are not immunosuppressed	Small foci of necrosis with an infiltrate of large atypical lymphocytes and a prominent cellular infiltrate of atypical lymphocytes in the portal areas. Cholestasis in severe cases of IM. Fulminant hepatic failure with massive hepatic necrosis may result in IM and LPD	Burkitt's lymphoma, nasopharyngeal carcinoma and chronic fatigue syndrome. Associated with X-linked lympho-proliferative disease (XLP; Duncan's disease)
Adenovirus (AV)	Upper respiratory tract infections/conjunctivitis	DNA	*Adenoviridae*	Worldwide	Human (for human adenovirus strains	Far reaching but including respiratory tract infections, conjunctivitis or diarrhoea	Prominent focal collections of necrosis throughout liver. Characteristic 'smoky' or 'blueberry' intranuclear inclusions at the periphery of necrotic areas in the liver. Minimal inflammatory infiltrate	CNS – meningo-encephalitis; gastrointestinal colitis
Coxsackie B	Coxsackie B infection	RNA	*Picornaviridae*, *Enterovirus* genus	Worldwide	Human (human strains)	Monocytosis, aseptic meningitis and myocarditis	*Children* – haemorrhagic necrosis and prominent portal and parenchymal inflammatory infiltrates. *Adults* – small foci of neutrophilic infiltrates and bile stasis in the perivenular areas. Prominent inflammatory cell infiltrates in the portal tracts in patients with myocarditis	Myocardium, CNS and skin
Echovirus	Aseptic meningitis/pneumonia	RNA	*Echoviridae*, species specific multiple subtypes	Worldwide	Human (for species-specific strains)	Most frequently associated with fever, aseptic meningitis or respiratory illness	Not defined	Not defined
Measles	Measles	RNA	*Paramyxoviridae*, *Morbilli virus* genus	Worldwide	Human	Catarrhal prodrome, sneezing, runny nose, cough and high fever. Elevated liver function tests suggestive of minor hepatic involvement	Non-specific findings including nuclear vacuolisation and leukocytic infiltrate in the sinusoids. Ten cases of paramyxovirus infection with identification of viral particles showed prominent syncytial giant cell hepatitis (Phillips *et al*, 1991)	CNS – encephalitis – gastrointestinal – enteritis; lungs – pneumonia

Table 6.2 *Continued*

Virus	Disease	Nuclear material	Virus family	Geographical distribution	Natural reservoir	Clinical features	Key hepatic histological features	Other system/organ involvement
Rubella	Rubella	RNA	*Toga viridae*	Worldwide	Primates and humans	Childhood rubella infections are not usually associated with liver disease. Neonatal disease may be associated with liver disease	Giant cell transformation with or without cholestasis. Prominent chronic inflammatory infiltrate and rarely massive hepatic necrosis	Skin, maculopapular rash, lymph node, joints (arteritis) and CNS (encephalitis). Association with biliary atresia or paucity of bile ducts
Yellow fever virus	Yellow fever	RNA	*Arboviridae, Flavivirus* genus	South America and tropical Africa	*Aedes aegypti* mosquitoes	Acute infectious disease, sudden onset characterised by fever, jaundice, haemorrhagic manifestations and albuminuria. Incubation time 3–6 days	Mid-zonal necrosis with prominent cholestasis. Occasionally, confluent necrosis. Prominent acidophilic degeneration and distinct eosinophilic intranuclear inclusions (Torres bodies). Prominent steatosis	Haemorrhage. Death later in the course of the disease is usually due to acute renal failure
Crimean–Congo haemorrhagic fever virus	Nairovirus fever	RNA	*Arboviridae, Flavivirus* genus	Pakistan, Soviet Middle Asia, Europe and Africa	*Hyalomma* ticks	Rigors, muscle pains, headache and vomiting. Profound systemic shock associated with haemorrhagic state	Extensive pericentral (zone III) necrosis. Occasionally massive hepatic necrosis and collapse	Heart and CNS
Rift Valley fever virus	Rift Valley fever	RNA	*Arboviridae, Bunyaviridus* genus	Africa	Sheep and cattle, transmitted by *Aedes/Culex* mosquitoes	Backache, limb pain, myalgia, diarrhoea and vomiting. May be associated with hallucinations, chorea, stupor and coma	Focal haemorrhagic necrosis in acinar zones II and III. Prominent Councilman bodies in a mild inflammatory infiltrate. Electron microscopy shows characteristic spiral particles and other system/organ involvement	CNS – encephalitis; retinitis
Dengue virus	Dengue fever	RNA	*Arboviridae, Flavivirus* genus	South East Asia	Mosquito – *Aedes egypti*	Mild, self-limiting disease with some haemorrhagic manifestations	Focal necrosis in zone III which may form horseshoe-shaped areas of necrosis, a prominent inflammatory infiltrate consisting of lymphocytes and neutrophils and occasionally acidophilic bodies	Cause of death is usually associated with shock due to haemorrhagic diathesis
Kyasanur Forest virus	Kyasanur Forest virus	RNA	*Arboviridae, Flavivirus* genus	India	Tick – *Haemaphysalis spinigera*	Fever, headache, myalgia, cough, bradycardia and haemorrhage	Focal hepatocellular necrosis. No residual findings upon recovery	Gastrointestinal – diarrhoea. 3–5% case fatality rate

Table 6.2 *Continued*

Virus	Disease	Nuclear material	Virus family	Geographical distribution	Natural reservoir	Clinical features	Key hepatic histological features	Other system/organ involvement
Hantaan virus	Korean haemorrhagic fever	RNA	*Aborviridae, Bunyavirus* genus	Korea, Siberia and China	Field mouse – *Apodemus agrarius*	Haemorrhagic fever with renal insufficiency	Focal coagulative necrosis with prominent parenchymal haemorrhage	Death usually associated with renal failure and muroid virus nephropathy
Lassa fever virus	Lassa fever	RNA	*Arenaviridae*	Central and West Africa	Rodent – *Mastomys natalensis*	Fever, exudative pharyngitis, diarrhoea and haemorrhagic diathesis. Hepatic pain and tenderness, jaundice and elevated transaminases	Prominent acidophilic bodies, some Kupffer cell hyperplasia and focal coagulative necrosis, which may be bridging. Prominent lipofuscin pigment deposition in hepatocytes. Histological features may be similar to those of yellow fever	Albuminuria with casts – renal failure develops terminally
Machepo/ Junin virus	Argentinian/ Bolivian haemorrhagic fever	RNA	*Arenaviridae*	Argentina and Bolivia (South America)	Rodents – *Calomys musculinus/ callosus*	Shock and disseminated intravascular coagulation	Include focal coagulative necrosis with associated apoptotic bodies, intranuclear inclusions (one reported case), Kupffer cell hyperplasia and erythrophagocytosis	Features associated with shock
Marburg virus	Marburg disease	RNA	*Filoviridae*	Marburg, West Germany and Yugoslavia	African vervet monkeys – *Circopithecus, Aethiops*	Sudden onset of fever, including rigor with headache, myalgia, diarrhoea and vomiting. Macropapular skin rash, lymphadenopathy, conjunctivitis and pharyngitis	Steatosis with spotty focal necrosis and apoptosis. Prominent glycogen depletion (by PAS staining) may progress to focal necrosis that occurs in all parts of the lobule. Prominent nuclear debris and minimal inflammatory infiltrate	Direct person-to-person transmission can be demonstrated. Mortality rate as high as 25%. Terminal events related to liver disease and haemorrhagic diathesis
Ebola fever virus	Ebola fever	RNA	*Filoviridae*	Sudan and Zaire	African monkeys	Sudden onset of fever, including rigors with headache, myalgia, diarrhoea and vomiting. Macropapular skin rash, lymphadenopathy, conjunctivitis and pharyngitis	Steatosis with spotting necrosis and apoptosis. Prominent glycogen depletion may progress to focal necrosis which occurs in all parts of the acinus/lobule, prominent nuclear debris and minimal inflammatory infiltrate	Direct person-to-person transmission can be demonstrated. Mortality rate as high as 80% (range 50–80%). Terminal events related to liver disease and haemorrhagic diathesis
Parvovirus	Parvovirus hepatitis	DNA	*Parvovirus*	Worldwide	Mammals, including humans and dogs (subtype dependent)	Increased liver enzymes in liver involvement associated with acute liver failure in adults and children. Liver involvement may occur in B19 infection following some marrow transplantations or immunosuppression	Submassive-to-massive geographical necrosis and individual cell necrosis	Bone marrow suppression, including anaemia, leukopenia and thrombocytopenia. Chronic rheumatoid-like arthritis, non-immune fetal hydrops and chronic and recurrent bone marrow suppression in immunocompromised hosts

viral inclusions present in herpes simplex, varicella–zoster and cytomegalovirus infections may be difficult to differentiate.

Giant hepatocyte transformation may also be present, usually occurring in newborns. Herpes virions may be demonstrated within the hepatocytes by electron microscopy. Immunoperoxidase stains and molecular probes for herpes simplex are very useful tools for identifying inclusions in infected cells (Lopez *et al*. 1990). The most reliable method for determining the presence of herpes virus is culture of the affected tissue.

VARICELLA–ZOSTER

Varicella–zoster virus usually affects children, presenting clinically as chickenpox. Adults infected with varicella–zoster usually develop shingles. Dissemination of varicella–zoster virus is rare; however, it may occur in association with chickenpox lesions in healthy children (Fakan, 1977). Adults are more frequently immunosuppressed as a result of chemotherapy or malignancy and may initially present their underlying malignancy as a case of shingles (Markin *et al*, 1990a).

The hepatic involvement results in massive necrosis and is usually fatal (Watanabe *et al*, 1984). Gross and microscopic changes present in livers infected with varicella virus are almost indistinguishable from those of patients infected with herpes simplex virus.

CYTOMEGALOVIRUS

Cytomegalovirus is named after the enlarged appearance of the infected cells. Histological features including increased cell size, prominent 'owl's eye' intranuclear inclusion and square-to-amorphous cytoplasmic inclusions are usually seen.

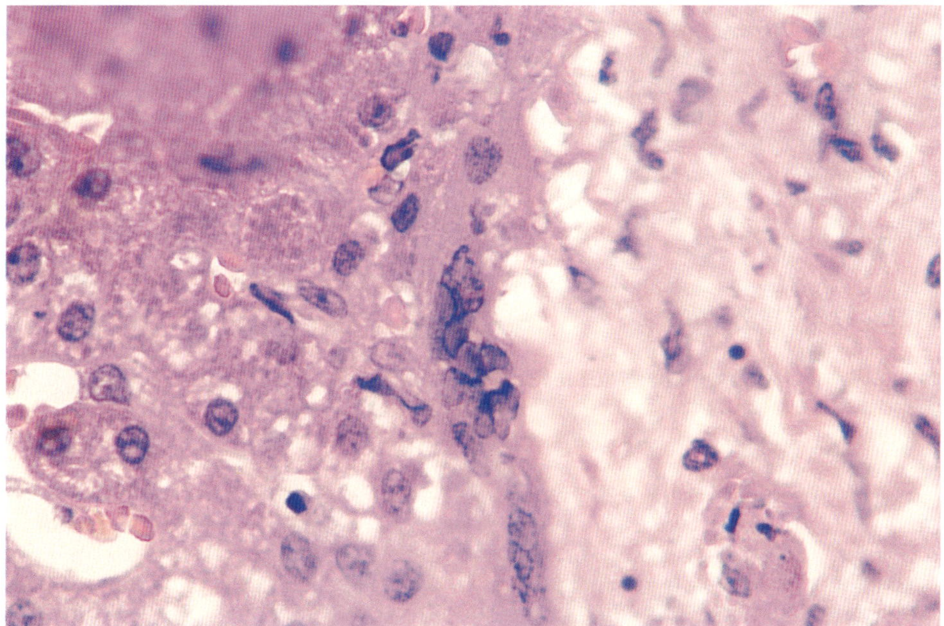

Fig 6.1   Photomicrograph of liver showing features of varicella–zoster infection (H&E, ×100).

Cytomegalovirus infection occurs in a variety of clinical settings (Breinig *et al*, 1987; Aschan *et al*, 1992; Chang *et al*, 1992; Climent *et al*, 1992; Frank *et al*, 1992). Congenital infections in others are frequently asymptomatic but may be associated with spontaneous abortion or stillbirth. Neonates born excreting the virus may be normal at birth and develop normally. Neonatal cytomegalic inclusion disease, which includes cerebral, ocular, respiratory, cardiac, hepatic and splenic lesions, may develop as a result of congenital infection (Kosai *et al*, 1991). The prognosis for neonatal cytomegalic inclusion disease is poor (Makkonen *et al*, 1992). When patients survive, they are usually left with permanent brain damage, microcephaly and periventricular calcifications (Matveev *et al*, 1992).

Older children and adults may present with unexplained fever, liver disease or the clinical features of infectious mononucleosis. Cytomegalovirus has also been shown to be responsible for post-transfusion syndrome. Cytomegalovirus is a common opportunistic organism in the immunocompromised patient, including those who have undergone solid organ transplantation or bone marrow transplantation, or have received chemotherapy for malignancy (Singh *et al*, 1988). Although it is one of the most common opportunistic viruses reported in the literature, cytomegalovirus infection can be thwarted by the use of intravenous and immune globulin (concentrated immunoglobulin, Sandoz Inc., East Hanover, New Jersey) (Pan *et al*, 1992; Stratta *et al*, 1992). Fatal massive necrosis of the liver has been reported in non-immunosuppressed patients as a result of cytomegalovirus infection (Sano and Izumi, 1991). Cytomegalovirus infection has been implicated in the development of neonatal hepatitis and the development of biliary atresia (Hart *et al*, 1991; Arnold *et al*, 1992).

A variety of changes are present in the liver of patients with the clinical symptoms of cytomegalovirus disease. Changes vary from individual hepatocytes transformed into cytomegalic cells with prominent inclusions, through to cholestasis and associated viral hepatitis-like features. Giant cell transformation is commonly seen in biopsies from neonates. The intranuclear and cytoplasmic inclusions may be present in biliary epithelial cells and endothelial cells in addition to liver cells (Fig. 6.2). The absence of typical intranuclear inclusions or cytoplasmic inclusions does not exclude the possibility of cytomegalovirus infection. Immunoperoxidase staining using a monoclonal antibody directed against cytomegalovirus-encoded proteins is useful for identifying inclusions in tissue sections (Hondo *et al*, 1982). Bile duct damage similar to that seen in allograft rejection (Wright, 1992) in graft-versus-host disease may lead to difficulty in diagnosing cytomegalovirus infection (Arnold *et al*, 1992).

EPSTEIN–BARR VIRUS

EBV is historically associated with infectious mononucleosis. EBV is spread by direct or indirect oral contact via the exchange of saliva (*Lancet* Editorial, 1973a). It may also be transmitted by blood transfusion and theoretically via contaminated needles and instruments (Enck *et al*, 1979).

The virus specifically infects B-lymphocytes (*Lancet* Editorial, 1973b). The involvement of other organs, in particular the liver, may be evident clinically as the result of T-cell-directed B-cell destruction (*Lancet* Editorial, 1973b). The frequency of hepatic involvement in EBV infection depends heavily upon the state of the patient at the time of infection or reactivation. In young adults, the infection is endemic, affecting up to 90% of the populations examined using serological assays for EBV antibodies (*Lancet* Editorial, 1973b).

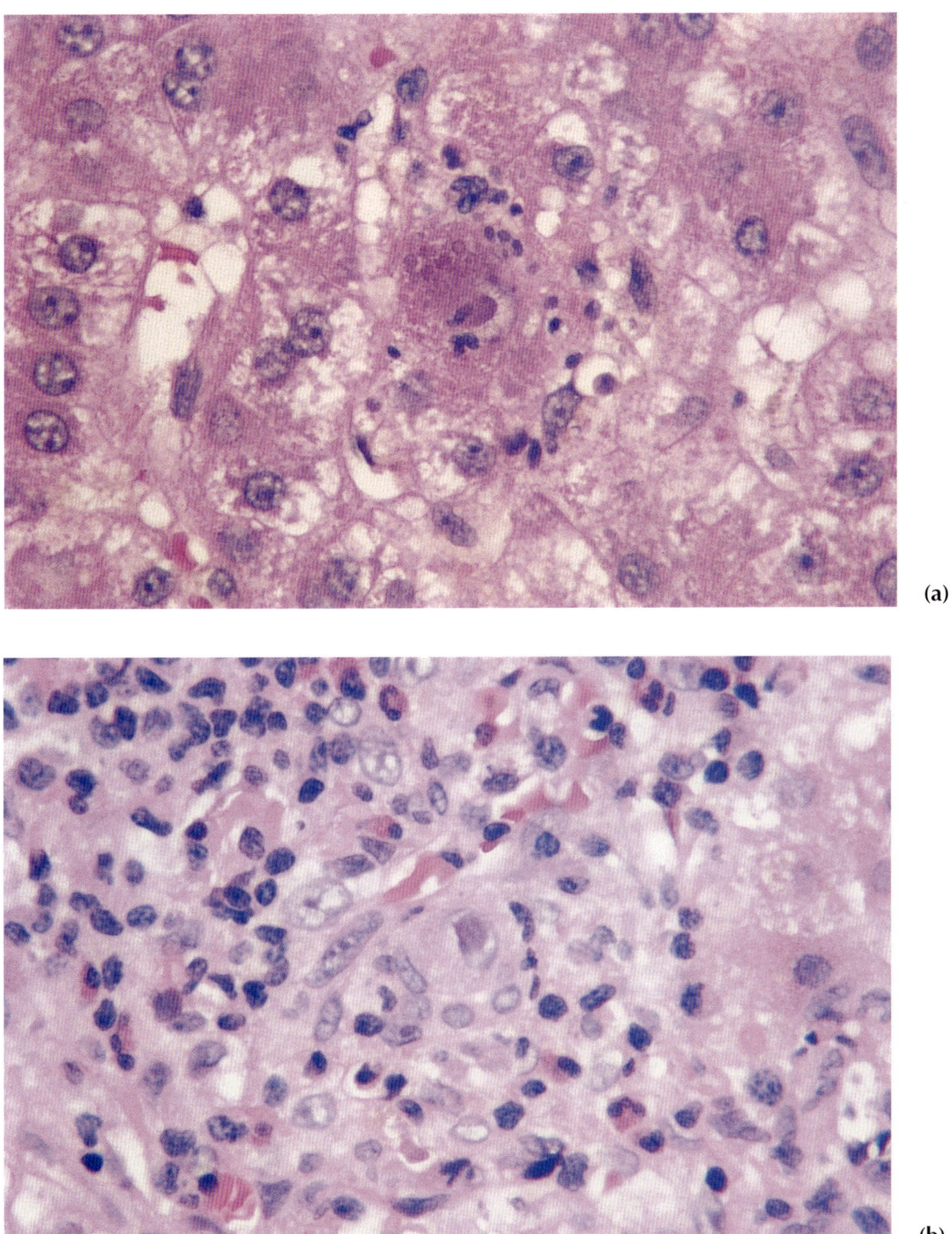

Fig 6.2   Photomicrograph of liver showing features of cytomegalovirus infection: (a) Infection of a hepatocyte (H&E, ×100). (b) Infection of bile duct epithelial cell (×100).

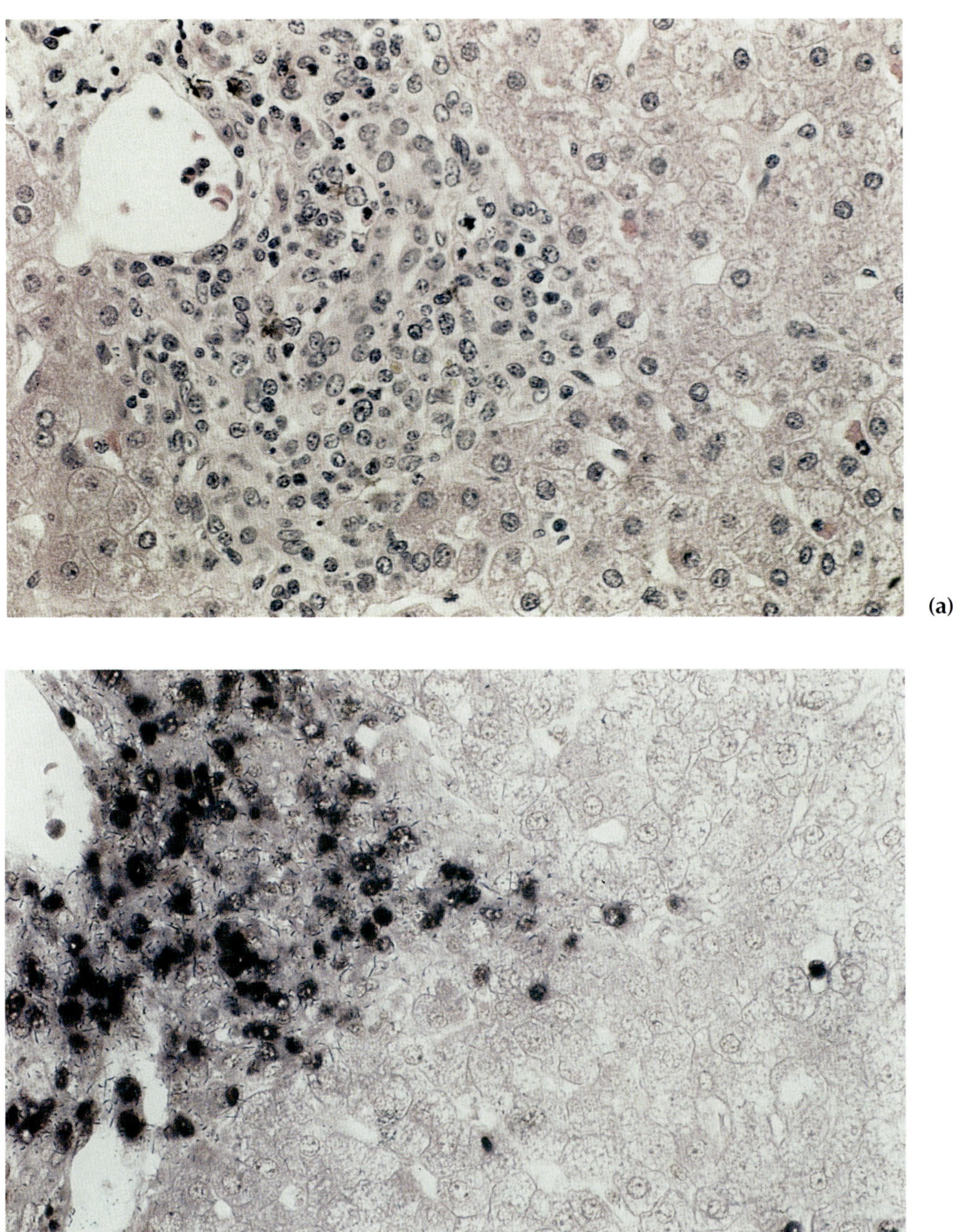

Fig 6.3 Photomicrograph of liver showing features of Epstein–Barr virus infection. (a) H&E, ×100. (b) In situ hybridisation using EBER-1 probe, ×100.

Clinically, overt infections are characterised by fever, sore throat, splenomegaly, lymphadenopathy and, in approximately 5% of patients, jaundice. Serum immunotransferases are elevated in up to 15% of the patients when evaluated.

The immunosuppressed population, including those undergoing bone marrow and solid organ transplantation and those patients with AIDS, have a particularly prominent reaction to the primary EBV infection or EBV reactivation (Markin *et al*, 1990b, 1991; Randhawa *et al*, 1990; Langnas *et al*, 1991; Renard *et al*, 1991). Primary EBV infection in this patient population may present with the clinical symptoms usually found in immunocompetent patients. This infection may develop into a lymphoproliferative disorder or possibly a malignant lymphoma (Langnas *et al*, 1991). Those patients with lymphoproliferative disorders may regress with the decrease in immunosuppressive therapy. Patients with malignant lymphoma, however, fail to regress with modification of immunosuppressive therapy.

The hepatic histological features associated with systemic EBV infection include a prominent inflammatory infiltrate in the portal areas consisting of atypical lymphocytes and plasma cells (Fig. 6.3) (Shaw and Evans, 1988; Markin *et al*, 1990b). There may also be an increase in sinusoidal inflammation in either infectious mononucleosis or lymphoproliferative disorder. In cases where a prominent inflammatory infiltrate is present within the portal areas and consists primarily of atypical lymphocytes, there is a significant danger of misdiagnosing lymphoma. The use of immunoperoxidase staining for immunoglobulins may help to identify the characteristics usually associated with lymphoma, i.e. monoclonal staining patterns. In addition to a portal inflammatory infiltrate, steatosis, cholestasis and individual hepatocyte necrosis may be present. Fulminant hepatic failure has been associated with fatal infectious mononucleosis, X-linked lymphoproliferative disorder (Duncan's disease), and post-transplant lymphoproliferative disorders (Purtilo, 1981).

Adenovirus

Adenoviruses are responsible for a wide variety of infections in humans, including those involving the respiratory tract and the eye. Sporadic outbreaks of hepatitis have been linked to adenoviruses; however, these small outbreaks are not common.

Adenovirus infection rarely occurs in the immunocompetent host. Disseminated infections, however, frequently occur in immunocompromised patients and may result in massive hepatocellular necrosis (Levy *et al*, 1990; Abzug and Levin, 1991; Cames *et al*, 1992; Hierholzer, 1992; Michaels *et al*, 1992). Adenovirus infections are characterised histologically by a prominent 'smokey' or 'blueberry muffin' intranuclear inclusion present within the infected hepatocytes (Fig. 6.4). Prominent collections or necrosis with some granulomatoid inflammation is present, scattered throughout the hepatic parenchyma.

Culturing a liver biopsy for adenovirus in suspected cases may yield cultures that may be used to identify the virus (Cames *et al*, 1992). Reports from Jaffe *et al* at the University of Pittsburgh have shown that adenovirus subtype II and IV are responsible for liver infections (Koneru *et al*, 1987). Other subtypes have not been associated with direct infection in the liver.

Immunoperoxidase staining for adenovirus in paraffin-fixed tissue is variable. Immunoperoxidase staining of frozen tissue, however, may yield positive results. The current standard for identification of adenovirus infection in liver is viral culture.

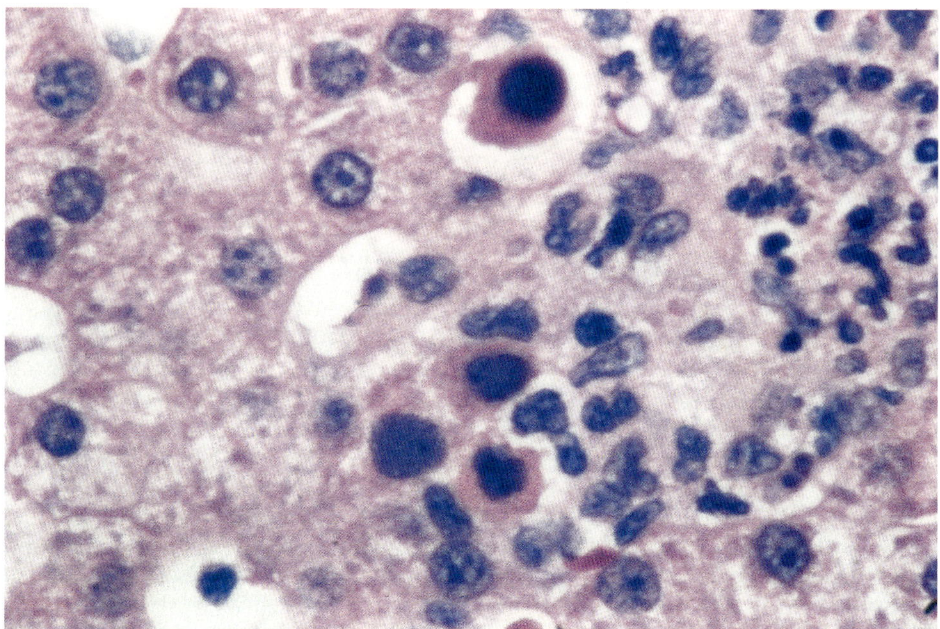

Fig 6.4 Photomicrograph of liver showing features of adenovirus infection (H&E, ×100).

Enteroviruses

The enteroviruses that give rise to hepatic manifestations during systemic infections are limited to Coxsackie B and Echovirus.

The Coxsackie viruses are responsible for a wide variety of clinical illnesses, including myocarditis, myocytis and aseptic meningitis. Serious illness in humans is usually a result of Coxsackie B virus infection (Sun and Smith, 1966; Hosier and Newton, 1985; Read *et al*, 1985). The Coxsackie B virus may be responsible for hepatitis in neonates (Kaplan *et al*, 1983), children and adults. Haemorrhagic necrosis with prominent inflammatory infiltrate has been described in the liver biopsies from infants with culture-proven Coxsackie B virus infections (Iavoroskaia *et al*, 1985).

In adults, bile stasis and small focal collections of lymphocytes are present around the terminal hepatic venule and, in some cases, within the portal tracts. These changes have been identified primarily in patients who have evidence of Coxsackie B virus-induced myocarditis.

The Echoviruses are primarily responsible for respiratory illnesses and aseptic meningitis (Haynes *et al*, 1972). The most common clinical feature associated with Echovirus infection is a prominent fever associated with signs of either respiratory disease or meningitis (Philip and Larson, 1973). Although rarely associated with hepatitis in adults, Echovirus infections in neonates may be overwhelming. Neonates infected with Echovirus may sustain prominent haemorrhagic necrosis of their livers (Krous *et al*, 1973; Drew, 1974). These changes are usually massive enough to be fatal, but an occasional recovery has been recorded.

Paramyxovirus

MEASLES

Measles (rubeola) is a well-known infection resulting in hepatitis. Several studies have shown that the liver disease associated with measles is mild and transitory, resolving in all cases (Ohta *et al*, 1988; Muraoka *et al*, 1991).

The histological changes that have been reported include mild non-specific findings (hepatocellular unrest), nuclear vacuolisation and a mild increase in lymphocytes within the sinusoids. The presence of giant cells has been reported in clinical cases of measles (Bott and Eizenberg, 1982; Ceresa *et al*, 1983). In addition, the presence of viral particles has not been detected in cases of measles hepatitis.

Sporadic syncytial giant cell hepatitis, however, has been reported to be associated with paramyxovirus. In the 10 cases reported by Phillips *et al* (1991), paramyxovirus nucleocapsids were present in all livers examined. In addition, prominent syncytial giant cells were present containing up to 30 nuclei. In half of these cases the patients died, and in the other half the patients underwent transplantation. This group of patients needs to be studied further.

Togavirus

RUBELLA

Rubella is not usually associated with liver disease in the general patient population. Rubella virus, however, may be responsible for neonatal hepatitis (Jannuzzi *et al*, 1976). In some clinical cases of rubella, focal hepatocellular necrosis and cholestasis have been associated with a mild chronic portal inflammatory infiltrate (Zeldis *et al*, 1985; Onji *et al*, 1988). Several cases of massive hepatic necrosis have been reported. Rubella virus has been one of several viruses implicated in the development of extrahepatic and intrahepatic biliary atresia. In a few cases, biliary tract infection with virus has been documented (Haukenes *et al*, 1990).

Arboviruses

The arboviruses are responsible for what is commonly termed 'viral haemorrhagic fever'. 'Viral haemorrhagic fever' is used to refer to diseases associated with disseminated intravascular coagulation and haemorrhage. These clinical features may also be found in systemic herpes virus infections; however, the term 'viral haemorrhagic fever' is usually reserved for use with the arboviruses (Dennis *et al*, 1969).

Viral haemorrhagic fevers with associated hepatic involvement due to arborviruses include yellow fever, Crimean–Congo fever, Rift Valley fever, Dengue fever, Kyasaur Forest disease and Korean haemorrhagic fever. The hepatic lesions associated with these disease are characterised by focal coagulative necrosis that varies in extent and distribution. A prominent inflammatory infiltrate is not usually present in these diseases. Prominent necrotic hepatocytes with karyorrhexis and karyolysis are usually present. Endothelial cells may also be involved in the necrotic process. Reticulin- and Masson-stained sections usually reveal an intact fibrous tissue network in marked contrast to the changes seen in hepatitis due to hepatotropic viruses. In most cases, all cells that contributed to the liver as an organ are involved in the necrotic process. The changes may be suggestive of herpes virus infection; however, a periphery of the lesion is usually well defined as the prominent haemorrhagic ring.

The most common problems associated with these diseases are their contagious nature and high mortality rate. Subclinical-to-mild infections have, however, been identified using serological methods. The presence of serology-positive patients is much higher than was previously thought.

YELLOW FEVER

Yellow fever is an acute infectious disease, usually with a sudden onset and of variable intensity. The arbovirus responsible for yellow fever is transmitted by the mosquito species *Aedes aegypti*. The disease is clinically characterised by fever, jaundice, albuminuria and haemorrhagic tendencies. The usual incubation period for yellow fever virus is 3–6 days (Camain and Lambert, 1966; De *et al*, 1971; Boulos *et al*, 1988).

Yellow fever is endemic in tropical Africa and South America. An acute demise as a result of yellow fever is usually associated with liver failure. Death at a later stage in the disease may be associated with renal failure.

Close examination of the liver reveals a prominent yellow colour, hence the name yellow fever. Histologically, the lesion of yellow fever is classically described as mid-zonal (zone II necrosis with viable cells in zones I and III (Fig. 6.5). Although the classical pattern may be seen, the area of necrosis may extend into zones I and III. Prominent individual hepatocyte necrosis (Councilman bodies) are present (Francis *et al*, 1972; Ricosse *et al*, 1972). Torres bodies (distinct eosinophilic intranuclear inclusions) may also be present (Serie *et al*, 1968; Ricosse *et al*, 1972). Fatty change is prominent and partially responsible for the yellow appearance. Some Kupffer cell hyperplasia may be present. Bile duct proliferation and cholestasis are usually not present.

CRIMEAN–CONGO FEVER

Crimean–Congo fever is a disease caused by the *Bunyavirus* genus of *Arbovirus*. The disease generally occurs in epidemics with the usual clinical features of viral haemorrhagic fever (le Roux, 1984). Its geographical distribution is normally confined to India, Pakistan, the former Soviet Union and Europe. The virus is transmitted to humans by a tick of the *Hyalomma* species.

Clinically, patients present with headache, muscle pain, rigors and vomiting (le Roux, 1984). Haemorrhage usually results in profound systemic shock. Crimean–Congo fever is highly contagious. A significantly mortality (greater than 70%) is the expected outcome (Gear *et al*, 1982; Swanepoel *et al*, 1983).

Histologically, prominent zone III (pericentral) necrosis is present. Massive hepatic necrosis with resultant volume loss and collapse may occasionally be present.

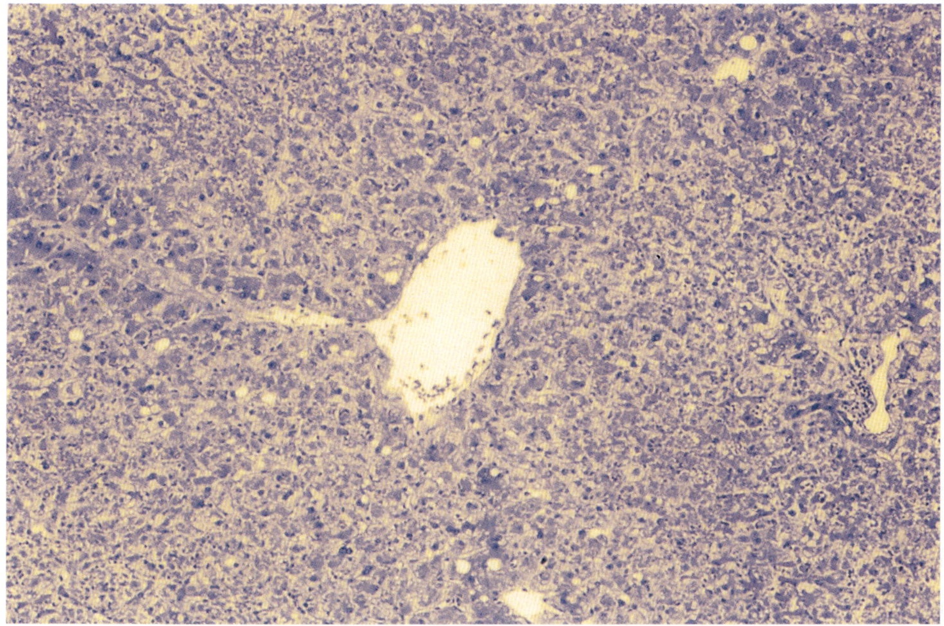

Fig 6.5 Photomicrograph of liver showing features of yellow fever virus infection (H&E, ×100).

DENGUE FEVER

Dengue fever occurs in epidemics and is usually a mild, self-limiting disease. There are four subtypes of the viruses that cause Dengue fever. The mortality rate for Dengue fever is approximately 10%, the usual cause of death being shock (Rosen *et al*, 1989).

Histologically, the liver lesions are similar to those present in Crimean–Congo haemorrhagic fever: zone III necrosis. A characteristic horseshoe-shaped pattern of necrosis may occur around zone III (Fig. 6.6). Mild inflammatory infiltrates composed primarily of neutrophils and lymphocytes may be present (Burke, 1968). Curiously, no prominent haemorrhage is present in the liver in this disease. An occasional necrotic hepatocyte (Councilman-like body) may also be present. Intranuclear inclusions similar to Torres bodies have been described (Teruel, 1991).

RIFT VALLEY FEVER

Rift Valley fever is a viral disease primarily affecting cattle and sheep. Humans may become infected with this disorder as a result of direct contact with animals. Several epidemics of Rift Valley fever have occurred in South America. The incubation period is approximately 3–6 days following exposure. Clinically, patients present with limb pain, muscle pain, backache, vomiting and diarrhoea. Neurological symptoms, including hallucinations, chorea, stupor and coma, may be present. The mortality rate is approximately 30% (McIntosh *et al*, 1980).

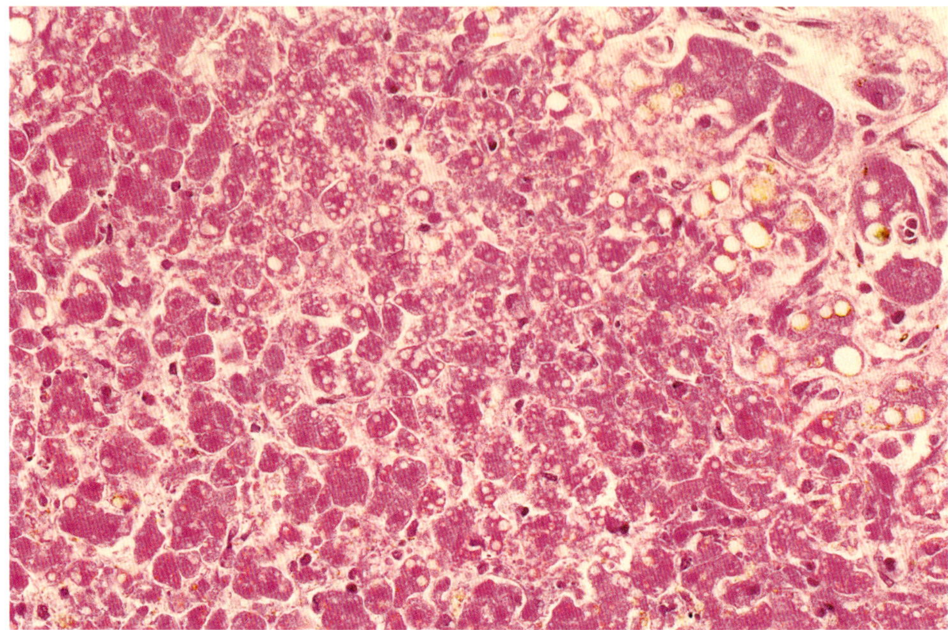

Fig 6.6 Photomicrograph of liver showing features of Dengue fever (H&E, ×100).

The histological findings in Rift Valley fever include focal necrosis in zones II and III with some associated haemorrhage (van Velden *et al*, 1977). Individual hepatocyte necrosis (Councilman-like bodies) may be present. Minimal inflammatory infiltrates may also be present. Electron microscopy shows the presence of the virus, which has a characteristic structure.

KYASAUR FOREST DISEASE

Kyasaur Forest disease is an infectious disorder similar to Rift Valley fever. The clinical and histological features are very similar (Iyer *et al*, 1959), the only histological distinction being the presence of erythrophagocytosis by Kupffer cells.

KOREAN HAEMORRHAGIC FEVER

Korean haemorrhagic fever was first identified after an outbreak of disease in the United Nations troops in Korea (Lee *et al*, 1978). The virus responsible for this disease, hantavirus, is widely found in Siberia and in the Chinese continent. The natural reservoir is the field mouse *Apodemus agrarius* (Lee *et al*, 1981), transmission being via the animal's bite. The clinical syndrome is similar to that of most other haemorrhagic fevers. Renal insufficiency, however, is prominent, presenting as one of the muroid virus nephropathies. A recent outburst of hantavirus infection in North Western New Mexico in the USA resulted in the death of 14 people (*MMWR*, 1993).

The histological pattern is similar to that of the other arboviruses, with focal coagulative necrosis surrounded by a ring of haemorrhage.

Arenaviruses

The arenaviruses are responsible for three diseases: Lassa fever, Argentinian haemorrhagic fever and Bolivian haemorrhagic fever.

LASSA FEVER

Lassa fever is a disease primarily found in Central and Western Africa (*British Medical Journal* Editorial, 1975). The natural reservoir for the Lassa fever virus is the rodent *Mastomys natalensis*. Patients present with fever, pharyngitis, diarrhoea and, in some cases, a haemorrhagic tendency. Renal failure may develop, with albuminuria and casts. Hepatic pain and right upper quadrant tenderness are frequent findings; however, jaundice occurs only rarely. Prominent increases in serum transaminases may be present. The mortality rate is as high as 30% in some areas (Knobloch *et al*, 1980).

Histologically, prominent individual hepatocyte necrosis (Councilman-like bodies) are present (Fig. 6.7). Focal coagulative necrosis is present and may result in bridging. Kupffer cell hyperplasia is prominent, as is lipofuscin deposition. Small focal haemorrhages may occur in a pattern similar to that found in Yellow fever (Edington and White, 1972). Viral particles are easily detected using electron microscopy.

ARGENTINIAN/BOLIVIAN HAEMORRHAGIC FEVER

Argentinian haemorrhagic fever and Bolivian haemorrhagic fever are very similar, patients presenting with clinical features similar to those of Lassa fever (Rugiero *et al*, 1968).

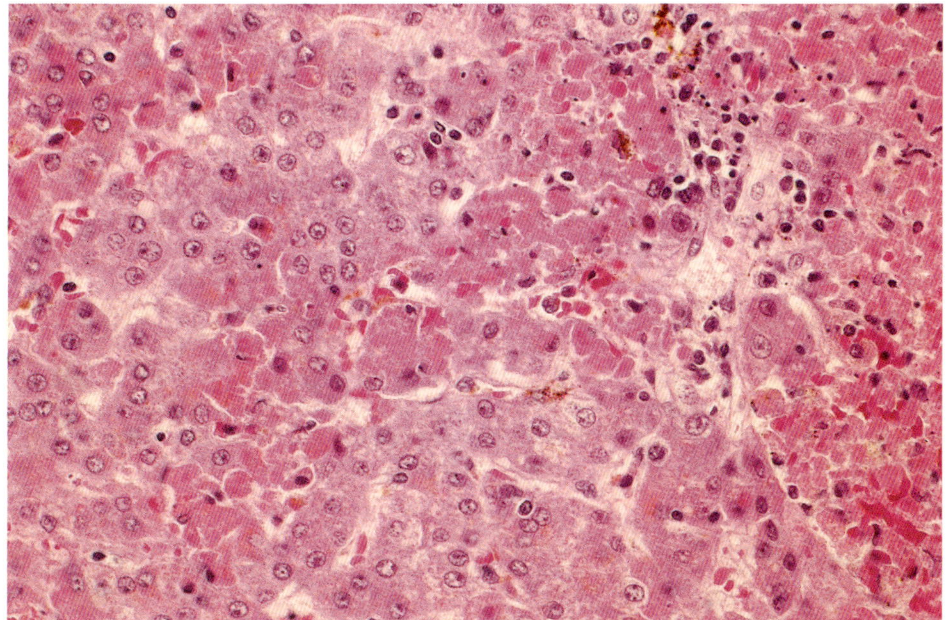

Fig 6.7   Photomicrograph of liver showing features of Lassa fever virus infection (H&E, ×100).

Histologically, focal coagulative necrosis with individual hepatocyte necrosis (Councilman-like bodies) and some briding necrosis may be present (Child *et al*, 1967). Kupffer cell hyperplasia and erythrophagocytosis may also be present. Treatment with immune globulin has been shown to improve the clinical outcome; however, antibodies to Junin virus must be present.

Filoviruses

The filoviruses, more commonly known as the Marburg virus group, are a unique group of viruses. Their structure is highly unusual, characterised by long filamentous structures (Fig. 6.8) (Ellis *et al*, 1978; Baskerville *et al*, 1985).

MARBURG VIRUS

Marburg virus disease is a highly infectious, severe febrile infection first recognised in Marburg, West Germany, in infected laboratory personnel (Gedigk *et al*, 1968) who had been in direct contact with body fluids and tissues from the African Vervet monkey (Siegert, 1970). These monkeys were imported from Uganda, but the original source of the infection has not been determined. Several subsequent epidemics have occurred in Johannesburg, South Africa and Kenya, also without an identified source.

Clinically, patients present with the sudden onset of fever, rigors, headache, myalgia, vomiting and diarrhoea. A prominent macropapular skin rash, lymphadenopathy, conjunctivitis and pharyngitis are seen. A haemorrhagic diathesis and jaundice may also be present. Serum transaminases are usually elevated. The mortality rate is approximately 25% (Martini, 1971).

Histologically, prominent steatosis with focal necrosis and individual hepatocyte necrosis (Councilman-like bodies) are present. The necrotic pattern is ill defined and crosses all three acinar zones. Bridging fibrosis may be present. Prominent basophilic inclusions have, however, been described in necrotic cells. A mild inflammatory infiltrate may be present, consisting primarily of lymphocytes. When patients recover, regeneration of the liver is complete with no resultant fibrosis or cirrhosis (Rippey *et al*, 1984). The electron microscopic appearance of the virus is characteristic. The sexual transmission of Marburg virus has been documented.

EBOLA FEVER

Ebola fever, caused by the Ebola virus, is clinically and histologically similar to Marburg virus disease. Epidemics have occurred in the Sudan and near Zaire, with a mortality rate approaching 50%. Person-to-person transmission can be demonstrated. The histological features are the same as those described for Marburg virus disease (Webb *et al*, 1978).

Parvovirus

The parvovirus family includes the Norwalk agent and several other subtypes including B19. The association of parvovirus B19 infection and hepatocellular damage is usually

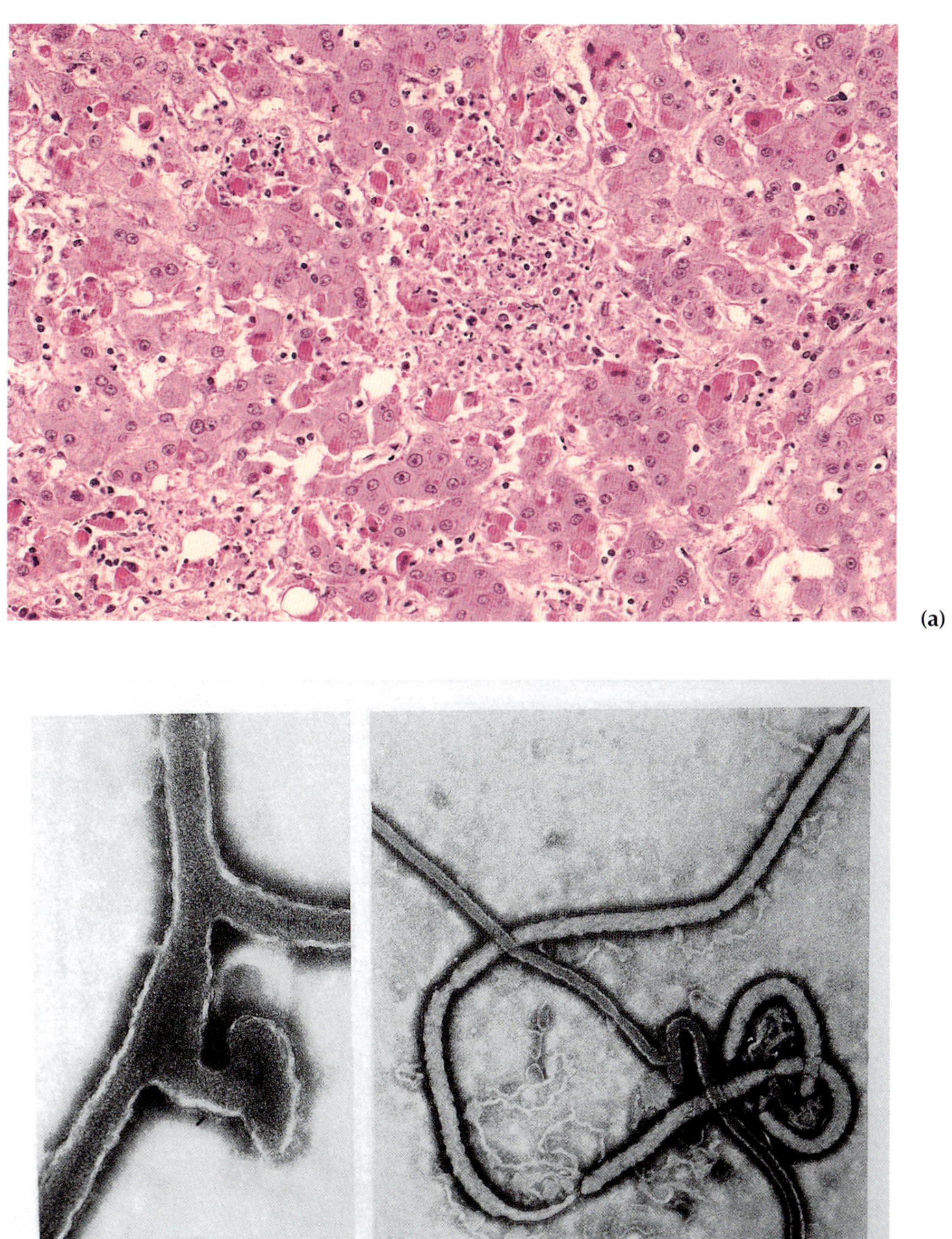

(a)

(b)

Fig 6.8   (a) Photomicrograph of liver infected with Ebola virus (×100). (b) Electromicrograph of liver showing features of Ebola fever virus (×5200). (From F.A. Murphy, 'Marburg and Ebola viruses', Chapter 47 in B.N. Fields (ed.) *Virology*. Reproduced with permission.)

associated with non-hepatic symptoms, including arteritis (Naides *et al*, 1990), and anaemia. Several cases of massive hepatic necrosis (Weiner and Naides, 1992) and fulminant failure associated with aplastic anaemia have been reported (Cattral *et al*, 1994; Langnas *et al*, 1995). Although the pathogenesis is undefined, the association is implausible. Histologically, cases of submassive-to-massive necrosis are histologically similar to those seen in herpes simplex infection. Viral inclusions are not present. Parvovirus B19 DNA may be demonstrated by the polymerase chain reaction in liver tissue. Serum auto-B19 IgM antibodies are also present. Biopsies of parvovirus-infected livers are rare.

Hantavirus

Although no causal relationship has been demonstrated, a high prevalence of hantavirus infection has been demonstrated in a group of Chinese patients in whom no other cause of acute hepatitis could be demonstrated (Meng *et al*, 1997).

References

Abzug, M.J., Levin, M.J. 1991: Neonatal adenovirus infection: four patients and review of the literature. *Pediatrics* **87**(6), 890–6.

Arnold, J.C., Portmann, B.C., O'Grady, J.G., Naoumov, N.V., Alexander, G.J., Williams, R. 1992: Cytomegalovirus infection persists in the liver graft in the vanishing bile duct syndrome. *Hepatology* **16**(2), 285–92.

Aschan, J., Ringden, O., Ljungman, P., Lonnqvist, B., Ohlman, S. 1992: Foscarnet for treatment of cytomegalovirus infections in bone marrow transplant recipients. *Scandinavian Journal of Infectious Diseases* **24**(2), 143–50.

Baskerville, A., Fisher, H.S.P., Neild, G.H., Dowsett, A.B. 1985: Ultrastructural pathology of experimental Ebola haemorrhagic fever virus infection. *Journal of Pathology* **147**(3), 199–209.

Bott, L.M., Eizenberg, D.H. 1982: Congenital rubella after successful vaccination. *Medical Journal of Australia* **i**(12), 514–15.

Boulos, M., Segurado, A.A., Shiroma, M. 1988: Severe yellow fever with 23-day survival. *Tropical and Geographical Medicine* **40**(4), 356–8.

Breinig, M.K., Zitelli, B., Starzl, T.E., Ho, M. 1987: Epstein–Barr virus, cytomegalovirus, and other viral infections in children after liver transplantation. *Journal of Infectious Diseases* **156**(2), 273–9.

British Medical Journal Editorial 1975: Lassa fever. *British Medical Journal* **1**, 173–4.

Burke, T. 1968: Dengue haemorrhagic fever. *Transactions of the Royal Society of Tropical Medicine and Hygiene* **62**, 682–92.

Camain, R., Lambert, D. 1966: Histopathology of the yellow fever livers obtained post-mortem and by hepatic puncture-biopsy during the epidemic in Diourbel (Senegal), November–December 1965. *Bulletin de la Societé Médicale d'Afrique Noire de Langue Francaise* **11**(3), 522–40.

Cames, B., Rahier, J., Burtomboy, G. *et al*. 1992: Acute adenovirus hepatitis in liver transplant recipients. *Journal of Pediatrics* **120**(1), 33–7.

Cattral, M., Langnas, A., Markin, R.S. *et al*. 1994: Aplastic anemia after liver transplantation for fulminant hepatic failure. *Hepatology* **20**(4), 813–18.

Ceresa, S., Rossel, M., Las, H.J., Toro, L., Curotto, D. 1983: Neonatal hepatitis due to rubella virus. *Revista Chilena de Pediatria* **54**(6), 424–7.

Chang, M.H., Huang, H.H., Huang, E.S., Kao, C.L., Hsu, H.Y., Lee, C.Y. 1992: Polymerase chain reaction to detect human cytomegalovirus in livers of infants with neonatal hepatitis. *Gastroenterology* **103**(3), 1022–5.

Child, P.L., MacKenzie, R.B., Valverde, L.R., Johnson, K.M. 1967: Bolivian haemorrhagic fever. A pathological description. *Archives of Pathology* **83**, 434–55.

Climent, C., Velez, R., Capriles, J.A. 1992: Cytomegalovirus infection. *Boletin Asociacion Medica de Puerto Rica* **84**(1), 31–3.

De, H.R.A., Oostburg, B.E., Sitalsing, A.D., Bellot, S.M. 1971: Isolation of yellow fever virus from a human liver obtained by autopsy in Surinam. *Tropical and Geographical Medicine* **23**(1), 59–63.

Dennis, L.H., Reisberg, B.E., Crosbie, J., Crozier, D., Conrad, M.E. 1969: The original haemorrhagic fever: yellow fever. *British Journal of Haematology* **17**(5), 455–62.

Drew, J.H. 1974: Echo II virus infection. A cause of acquired neonatal hepatitis. *Australian Paediatric Journal* **10**, 177–9.

Edington, G.M., White, H.A. 1972: The pathology of Lassa fever. *Transactions of the Royal Society of Tropical Medicine and Hygiene* **66**(3), 381–9.

Ellis, D.S., Simpson, I.H., Francis, D.P., Knobloch Bowen, E.T., Lolik, P., Deng, I.M. 1978: Ultrastructure of Ebola virus particles in human liver. *Journal of Clinical Pathology* **31**(3), 201–8.

Enck, R.E., Betts, R.E., Brown, M.R., Miller, G. 1979: Viral serology (hepatitis B virus, cytomegalovirus, Epstein–Barr virus) and abnormal liver function tests in transfused patients with hereditary hemorrhagic diseases. *Transfusion* **19**(1), 32–8.

Fakan, F. 1977: Generalized varicella and herpes. *Ceskoslovenska Patologie* **13**(3), 95–100.

Francis, T.I., Moore, D.L., Edington, G.M., Smith, J.A. 1972: A clinicopathological study of human yellow fever. *Bulletin of the World Health Organisation* **46**(5), 659–67.

Frank, T.S., Cook, S.M., Del, B.E.A., Wilson, M.D. 1992: A simplified method for detecting cytomegalovirus by polymerase chain reaction from histologic sections of small biopsies. *Modern Pathology* **5**(4), 449–54.

Gear, J.H.S., Thomson, P.D., Hopp, M. *et al.* 1982: Congo–Crimean haemorrhagic fever in South Africa. Report of a fatal case in the Transvaal. *South African Journal* **62**, 576–80.

Gedigk, P., Korb, G., Bechtelsheimer, H. 1968: The pathological anatomy of the Marburg virus disease. *Verhandlungen der Deutschen Gesellschaft für Pathologie* **52**, 317–22.

Haagsma, E.B.I., Klompmaker, I.J., Grond, J.J. *et al.* 1987: Herpes virus infections after orthotopic liver transplantation. *Transplantation Proceedings* **19**(5), 4054–6.

Hart, M.H., Kaufmann, S.S., Vanderhoof, J.A. *et al.* 1991: Neonatal hepatitis and extrahepatic biliary atresia associated with cytomegalovirus infection in twins. *American Journal of Diseases of Children* **145**(3), 302–5.

Haukenes, G., Matre, R., Tonder, O., Myrmel, H., Schrumpf, E. 1990: Measles and rubella antibodies in patients with chronic liver disease. *Journal of Hepatology* **11**(3), 389.

Haynes, R.E., Cramblett, H.G., Hilty, M.D., Azimi, P.H., Crews, J. 1972: Echo virus type 3 infections in children: clinical and laboratory studies. *Journal of Pediatrics* **80**(4), 589–95.

Hierholzer, J.C. 1992: Adenoviruses in the immunocompromised host. *Clinical Microbiology Review* **5**(3), 262–74.

Hondo, R., Kurata, T., Sato, S., Oda, A., Aoyama, Y. 1982: Enzymatic treatment of formalin-fixed and paraffin-embedded specimens for detection of antigens of herpes simplex, varicella-zoster and human cytomegaloviruses. *Japan Journal of Experimental Medicine* **52**(1), 17–25.

Hosier, D.M., Newton, W.A. 1985: Serious Coxsackie infection in infants and children: myocarditis, meningoencephalitis and hepatitis. *American Journal of Diseases of Children* **96**, 251–67.

Iavoroskaia, V.E., Blagerman, S.K., Gicheva, T.A. 1985: Congenital infections due to Coxsackie viruses. *Akusherstvo I Ginekologiia (Mosk)* (4), 20–2.

Iyer, C.G.S., Laxmana Rao, R., Work, T.H., Narashimha Murthy, D.P. 1959: Kyasanur Forest Disease. VI: Pathological findings in three fatal human cases of Kyasanur Forest Disease. *Indian Journal of Medical Science* **13**, 1011–22.

Jannuzzi, C., Campelli, A., Fabbri, A. 1976: Behavior of hemagglutination-inhibiting antibodies against measles and rubella in a group of children with chronic hepatitis. *Bollettino dell Istituto Sieroterapico Milanese* **55**(6), 519–23.

Kaplan, M.H., Klein, S.W., McPhee, J., Harper, R.G. 1983: Group B Coxsackie virus infections in infants younger than three months of age: a serious childhood illness. *Review of Infectious Diseases* **5**(6), 1019–32.

Knobloch, J., McCormick, J.B., Webb, P.A., Dietrich, M., Schumacher, H.H., Dennis, E. 1980: Clinical observations in 42 patients with Lassa fever. *Tropenmedizin und Parasitologie* **31**(4), 389–98.

Koneru, B., Jaffe, R., Esquivel, C.O. *et al.* 1987: Adenovirus infections in pediatric liver transplant recipients. *Journal of the American Medical Association* **258**, 489–92.

Kosai, K., Kage, M., Kojiro, M. 1991: Clinicopathological study of liver involvement in cytomegalovirus infection in infant autopsy cases. *Journal of Gastroenterology and Hepatology* **6**(6), 603–8.

Krous, H.F., Dietzman, D., Ray, C.G. 1973: Fatal infections with Echo virus types 6 and 11 in early infancy. *American Journal of Diseases of Children* **126**, 842–6.

Lancet Editorial 1973a: Oral excretion of E.B. virus. *Lancet* **i**, 811–12.

Lancet Editorial 1973b: Immunopathology of infectious mononucleosis. *Lancet* **ii**, 712–14.

Langnas, A.N., Castaldo, P., Markin, R.S., Stratta, R.J., Wood, R.P., Shaw, B.W. Jr 1991: The spectrum of Epstein–Barr virus infection with hepatitis following liver transplantation. *Transplantation Proceedings* **23**(1), 1513–14.

Langnas, A.N., Markin, R.S., Cattral, M.S., Naides, S.J. 1995: Parvovirus B19 as a possible causative agent of fulminant liver failure and associated aplastic anemia. *Hepatology* **22**, 1661–5.

Lee, H.W., Lee, P.W., Baek, L.J., Song, C.K., Seong, I.W. 1981: Intraspecific transmission of Hantaan virus, etiologic agent of Korean hemorrhagic fever, in the rodent *Apodemus agrarius*. *American Journal of Tropical Medicine and Hygiene* **30**(5), 1106–12.

Lee, H.W., Lee, P.W., Johnson, K.M. 1978: Isolation of the etiologic agent of Korean hemorrhagic fever. *Journal of Infectious Diseases* **137**(3), 298–308.

le Roux, N.J. 1984: Congo–Crimean haemorrhagic fever. *South African Medical Journal* **66**, 514.

Levy, J., Wodell, R.A., August, C.S., Bayever, E. 1990: Adenovirus-related hemophagocytic syndrome after bone marrow transplantation. *Bone Marrow Transplantation* **6**(5), 349–52.

Lopez, T.J.C., Allende, H., Esteban, R., Villegas, G., Esteban, J.I., Guardia, J. 1990: Diagnosis of acute hepatitis caused by herpes simplex virus using in situ hybridization. *Medical Clinics (Barcelona)* **94**(9), 342–3.

McIntosh, B.M., Russell, D., dos Santos, S.I., Gear, J.H. 1980: Rift Valley fever in humans in South Africa. *South African Medical Journal* **58**(20), 803–6.

Makkonen, M., Huttunen, M., Martikainen, A., Saarikoski, S. 1992: Cytomegalovirus hepatitis in late pregnancy. *International Journal of Gynaecology and Obstetrics* **37**(3), 199–201.

Markin, R.S., Stratta, R.J., Woods, G.L. 1990a: Infection after liver transplantation. *American Journal of Surgical Pathology* **14**(supplement), 64–78.

Markin, R.S., Wood, R.P., Shaw, B.W. Jr, Brichacek, B., Purtilo, D.T. 1990b: Immunohistologic identification of Epstein–Barr virus-induced hepatitis reactivation after OKT-3 therapy following orthotopic liver transplant. *American Journal of Gastroenterology* **85**(8), 1014–18.

Markin, R.S., Langnas, A.N., Donovan, J.P., Zetterman, R.K., Stratta, R.J. 1991: Opportunistic viral hepatitis in liver transplant recipients. *Transplantation Proceedings* **23**(1 part 2), 1515–16.

Martini, G.A. 1971: Marburg virus disease, clinical syndrome. In Martini, G.A., Siegart, R. (eds) *Marburg virus disease* Berlin: Springer Verlag, 1–9.

Matveev, V.A., Kazinets, N.M., Sonkina, A.A., Stakhanova, V.M. 1992: Clinical picture of congenital cytomegalovirus infection in infants in their first year of life. *Pediatriia* (1), 44–7.

Meng, G., Lan, Y., Nakagawa, M. *et al.* 1997: High prevalence of hantavirus infection in a group of Chinese patients with acute hepatitis of unknown aetiology. *Journal of Viral Hepatitis* **4**, 231–4.

Michaels, M.G., Green, M., Wald, E.R., Starzl, T.E. 1992: Adenovirus infection in pediatric liver transplant recipients. *Journal of Infectious Disease* **165**(1), 170–4.

MMWR Update 1993: Hanta virus disease United States. *MMWR* **42**(29), 1–12.

Muraoka, H., Sata, M., Hino, T. *et al.* 1991: A study on hepatic dysfunction associated with rubella infection. *Kansenshogaku Zasshi* **65**(5), 597–603.

Naides, S.J., Scharosch, L.L., Foto, F., Howard, E.J. 1990: Rheumatological manifestations of human parvovirus B19 infection in adults. Initial two-year clinical experience. *Arthritis and Rheumatology* **33**, 1297–309.

Ohta, Y., Hashimoto, N., Umeda, N. *et al.* 1988: An adult case of acute hepatitis associated with rubella. *Nippon Shokakibyo Gakkai Zasshi* **85**(5), 1110–13.

Onji, M., Kumon, I., Kanaoka, M., Miyaoka, H., Ohta, Y. 1988: Intrahepatic lymphocyte subpopulations in acute hepatitis in an adult with rubella. *American Journal of Gastroenterology* **83**(3), 320–2.

Pan, S.H., Rosenthal, P., Howard, T.K., Podesta, L.G., Sher, L., Makowka, L. 1992: Evaluation of three cytomegalovirus infection prophylactic regimens in liver transplant recipients. *Transplantation Proceedings* **24**(4), 1466–7.

Philip, A.G.S., Larson, E.J. 1973: Overwhelming neonatal infection with Echo 19 virus. *Journal of Pediatrics* **82**, 391–7.

Phillips, M.J., Blendis, L.M., Poucell, S. *et al.* 1991: Syncytial giant-cell hepatitis. Sporadic hepatitis with distinctive pathological features, a severe clinical course, and paramyxoviral features. *New England Journal of Medicine* **324**(7), 455–60.

Purtilo, D.T. 1981: Fulminant hepatic failure in childhood. *British Medical Journal* **282**(6257), 69 (letter).

Randhawa, P.S., Markin, R.S., Starzl, T.E., Demetris, A.J. 1990: Epstein–Barr virus-associated syndromes in immunosuppressed liver transplant recipients. Clinical profile and recognition on routine allograft biopsy. *American Journal of Surgical Pathology* **14**(6), 538–47.

Read, R.B., Ede, R.J., Morgan, C.P., Moscoso, G., Potmann, B., Williams, R. 1985: Myocarditis and fulminant hepatic failure from Coxsackie virus B infection. *Postgraduate Medical Journal* **61**(718), 749–52.

Renard, T.H., Andrews, W.S., Foster, M.E. 1991: Relationship between OKT3 administration, EBV seroconversion, and the lymphoproliferative syndrome in pediatric liver transplant recipients. *Transplantation Proceedings* **23**(1), 1473–6.

Ricosse, J.H., Loubiere, R., Albert, J.P., Ette, M., Roux, F. 1972: Anatomopathological diagnosis of yellow fever (apropos of the epidemic in Upper Volta in 1969). *Annales d'Anatomie Pathologique (Paris)* **17**(1), 21–38.

Rippey, J.J., Schepers, N.J., Gear, J.H. 1984: The pathology of Marburg virus disease. *South African Medical Journal* **66**(2), 50–4.

Rosen, L., Khin, M.M., Khin, T.U. 1989: Recovery of virus from the liver of children with fatal dengue: reflections on the pathogenesis of the disease and its possible analogy with that of yellow fever. *Research in Virology* **140**(4), 351–60.

Rugiero, H.R., Ruggiero, H.A., Astarloa, L. *et al.* 1968: Argentinian hemorrhagic fever. *Prensa Medica Argentina* **55**(36), 1750–2.

Sano, N., Izumi, K. 1991: Hepatic cytomegalovirus involvement in autopsy cases. *Acta Pathologica Japonica* **41**(9), 668–72.

Serie, C., Lindrec, A., Poirier, A., Andral, L., Neri, P. 1968: Studies on yellow fever in Ethiopia. I: Introduction – clinical symptoms of yellow fever. *Bulletin of the World Health Organisation* **38**(6), 835–41.

Shaw, N.J., Evans, J.H. 1988: Liver failure and Epstein–Barr virus infection. *Archives of Disease in Childhood* **63**(4), 432–3.

Siegert, R. 1970: The Marburg virus (Vervet monkey agent). *Modern Trends in Medical Virology* **2**, 204–40.

Singh, N., Dummer, J.S., Kusne, S. *et al.* 1988: Infections with cytomegalovirus and other herpesviruses in 121 liver transplant recipients: transmission by donated organ and the effect of OKT3 antibodies. *Journal of Infectious Diseases* **158**(1), 124–31.

Stratta, R.J., Shaeffer, M.S., Markin, R.S. *et al.* 1992: Cytomegalovirus infection and disease after liver transplantation. An overview. *Digestive Diseases and Sciences* **37**(5), 673–88.

Sun, N.C., Smith, V.C. 1966: Hepatitis associated with myocarditis: unusual manifestations of infection with Coxsackie Group B, type 3. *New England Journal of Medicine* **274**, 190–3.

Swanepoel, R., Struthers, J.K., Shepherd, A.J., McGillivray, G.M., Nel, M.J., Jupp, P.G. 1983: Crimean–Congo hemorrhagic fever in South Africa. *American Journal of Tropical Medicine and Hygiene* **32**, 1407–15.

Teruel, L.E. 1991: Dengue. A review. *Investigacion Clinica* **32**(4), 201–17.

Tsuda, H. 1993: Liver dysfunction caused by parvovirus B19. *American Journal of Gastroenterology* **88**, 1463.

van Velden, V.D.J., Meyer, J.D., Olivier, J., Gear, J.H., McIntosh, B. 1977: Rift Valley fever affecting humans in South Africa: a clinicopathological study. *South African Medical Journal* **51**(24), 867–71.

Watanabe, K., Tanaka, J., Hatano, M. *et al.* 1984: Generalized neonatal herpes virus infection (cytomegalovirus or herpes virus type 1). *Acta Pathologica Japonica* **34**(4), 847–58.

Webb, P.A., Johnson, K.M., Wulff, H., Lange, J.V. 1978: Some observations on the properties of Ebola virus. In Pattyn, S.R. (ed.) *Ebola virus hemorrhagic fever*. Amsterdam: Elsevier North-Holland/Biochemical Press, 91–4.

Weiner, C., Naides, S.J. 1992: Fetal survival of human parvovirus B19 infection. Spectrum of intrauterine response in twin pregnancy. *American Journal of Perinatology* **9**, 66–8.

Wright, T.L. 1992: Cytomegalovirus infection and vanishing bile duct syndrome: culprit or innocent bystander? *Hepatology* **16**(2), 494–6.

Zeldis, J.B., Miller, J.G., Dienstag, J.L. 1985: Hepatitis in an adult with rubella. *American Journal of Medicine* **79**(4), 515–16.

CHAPTER 7

Pathogenesis of liver cell damage in viral hepatitis

A ALBERTI AND L CHEMELLO

Viruses are thought to cause damage to the cells they infect by one of two general mechanisms, which are not necessarily mutually exclusive (Table 7.1). The first is a direct cytopathic action caused by the intracellular presence and replicative activity of the virus itself. This effect can be reproduced in vitro when appropriate target cells are used to culture the virus. The cell damage is caused by rapidly replicating virus particles or by the accumulation of toxic viral products that interfere with important aspects of cell metabolism. The histopathological reaction is a direct consequence of such interference and reflects the type of metabolic derangement provoked by the virus. Cytopathic viruses more frequently cause acute rather than chronic disease as they are either rapidly suppressed and eliminated by the immune response or produce massive damage from which the host may not survive (Motkins, 1984).

The second mechanism of cell damage occurring in viral infection is that involving antigen non-specific and specific immunological responses against the virus and infected

Table 7.1 Mechanisms of virus-induced cell damage

Direct cytopathic action

Interference with cell metabolism by toxic components
Alteration of protein synthesis by action at the level of the host DNA or RNA
Alteration of cellular cytoskeleton by disruption of filaments and microtubules
Formation of syncytion of multinucleate giant cells by cell-to-cell fusion
Formation of inclusion bodies containing virions or viral proteins

Immune-mediated types

Antigen non-specific
  NK cell cytotoxicity
  Toxic cytokines (e.g. interferons, tumour necrosis factor and interleukins)

Antigen specific
  Antibody and complement-mediated reactions
  Antibody-dependent cellular cytotoxicity reactions
  Cytotoxic T-lymphocytes reactions
  Autoimmune reactions

NK, natural killer

cells (Table 7.1). This mechanism is typical of non-cytopathic viruses that cause acute and chronic disease. The non-specific reaction involves mainly natural killer (NK) cells, while the specific immunological responses are mediated by antibodies, immune complexes and cytotoxic cells. One of the most important effector mechanisms in viral immunopathology involves the activation of cytotoxic T-lymphocytes (CTLs), usually CD8+ CTLs, that recognise short peptides derived from endogenously processed viral proteins and expressed on the surface of infected cells in association with HLA class I molecules (Zinkernagel, 1988). Cytotoxic reactions may also be mediated, in a less conventional pathway, by CD4+ T-lymphocytes that recognise exogenous viral antigens taken up by cells, processed in lysosomes and presented to T-cells in association with HLA class II molecules. Damage to infected cells may also derive from the action of several cytokines that are released at high concentrations at the site of inflammatory reactions, mainly as a consequence of T-cell activation. These cytokines act directly on infected cells (and possibly also on uninfected bystander cells) and represent an important mechanism of amplification of the process of tissue damage in viral diseases. Finally, viruses may initiate autoimmune reactions, which become another potential cause of tissue damage and disease.

In this chapter, we will discuss which of these mechanisms of cell damage are thought to be operative in viral hepatitis.

Viruses and liver disease

The list of viruses able to cause liver damage includes a first group of agents responsible for acute or chronic disease that exclusively or primarily involves the liver – called *hepatotropic viruses* (*see* Chapter 1) – and a second group of viruses which may or may not cause clinically significant liver damage as part of a systemic disease (*systemic viruses*) (*see* Chapter 6).

The hepatotropic viruses causing liver damage are quite different from one another in nature, structure and biology (*see* Chapter 1). Nevertheless, the liver damage they cause and the consequent biochemical changes are similar, sometimes indistinguishable, as a result of the limited repertoire of liver responses to different noxious agents (*see* Chapters 2 and 3).

Both mechanisms of viral cytopathology described above are thought to be operative in viral hepatitis. Direct cytotoxic effects may exist for some or even all hepatitis viruses and consist mainly of histological lesions such as fat and acidophilic degeneration and the swelling and ballooning of hepatocytes. The exact role that direct virus cytotoxicity plays in vivo has been difficult to establish for those hepatitis agents that cannot be successfully cultured in vitro. On the other hand, immune-mediated pathways of cell damage are certainly operative in most forms of viral hepatitis and frequently represent major determinants of liver disease. This conclusion is supported by the observation that liver histology in viral hepatitis is typically characterised by the infiltration of inflammatory cells, mainly macrophages and lymphocytes, which are often found in intimate contact with dying hepatocytes. Furthermore, antibody- as well as T-cell-mediated immune reactions against a variety of viral antigens can be detected in patients infected with any type of hepatitis virus. Autoimmune reactions are also often observed and may have pathogenetic significance.

Our knowledge of the mechanisms of liver damage in viral hepatitis has changed rapidly in the past two decades as a consequence of the extraordinary number of new discoveries in the field, and it is still uncompleted. The main elements on which the interpretation of virus-induced liver damage can be based are the following:

- the pattern of virus replication and expression in infected hepatocytes and its relationship to liver damage;
- the histopathological changes seen in the infected liver;
- the type, kinetics and intensity of the immune response against the virus and virus-infected hepatocytes and their relationship to the type and severity of the liver disease;
- the pattern of virus activity and of liver damage during immunomanipulation and antiviral therapy.

Understanding the pathogenesis of liver damage during infection with hepatotropic viruses is an essential prerequisite for a rational approach to treatment. This will be discussed with particular reference to the mechanism of action of the interferons, which currently represent the only available therapy for chronic viral hepatitis.

Liver damage in hepatitis A

Several genotypes of HAV have been propagated in tissue culture, using hepatoma cells or other types of human and animal cell culture. Unlike picornaviruses, it has been found that HAV propagation in tissue cultures often establishes persistent infection, with active replication that does not interfere with host cell biosynthetic processes and does not usually result in a cytopathic effect (Frosner *et al*, 1979; Provost and Hilleman, 1979). Indeed, most HAV isolates have been found not to be cytopathic in cell cultures, and even the most cytopathic variants of HAV do not usually affect in a significant way host cell protein and RNA synthetic functions (Siegl *et al*, 1991). It should be noted that, while in vitro the infection becomes persistent, chronicity does not occur in vivo.

Although early studies suggested that HAV could be directly cytopathic, the above findings and other recent data indicate that the immune response may be more important than the virus itself in causing hepatocyte death in hepatitis A (Koff, 1998). Indeed, the onset of liver damage in acute hepatitis A does not correlate with the peak of virus replication and shedding in the faeces, which occurs several weeks before the rise in transaminase levels, but instead coincides with the appearance of the immune response to HAV, heralded by the rise in IgM anti-HAV (Fig. 7.1). The histopathological appearance of the liver during typical acute HAV infection also favours the hypothesis that immune-mediated rather than cytopathic events predominate. Indeed, although microvesicular fatty change, focal necrosis and the degeneration of hepatocytes indicate some direct cytopathic effects, a central feature of acute hepatitis pathology is the infiltration of portal tracts and of the lobules by lymphocytes and plasma cells (*see* Chapter 2). In the early phase of disease, these contain NK cells, which are later replaced by CD8+ T-lymphocytes able specifically to kill HAV-infected target cells in a HLA class I-restricted manner.

Recently, the involvement of specific CTLs in the pathogenesis of liver disease caused by HAV has been confirmed in experimentally infected tamarin monkeys (Karayiannis *et al*, 1994). By using autologous cytotoxicity experiments with skin fibroblasts infected with either HAV or recombinant vaccinia virus expressing HAV structural polypeptides, specific cytotoxic T-cell killing in tamarins suffering from acute HAV infection could be demonstrated. Interestingly, HAV-specific cytotoxicity by peripheral blood lymphocytes was at its maximum at the time of peak ALT levels and correlated with liver damage more closely than HAV replication in serum and shedding in faeces. These findings in the

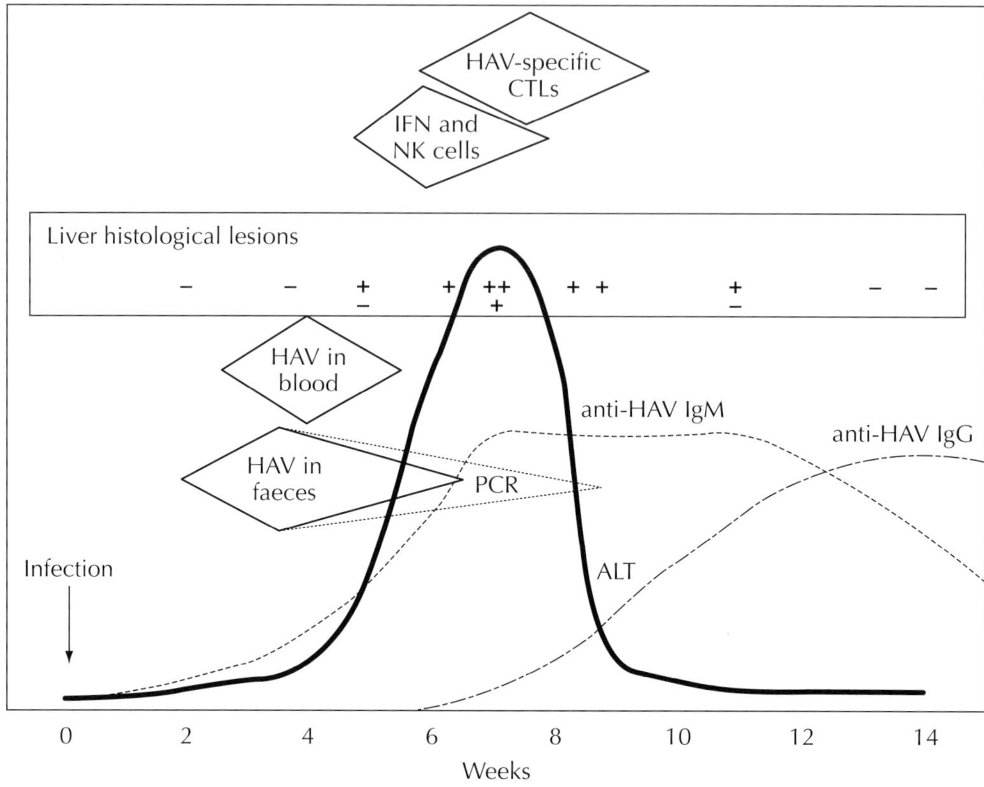

Fig 7.1   Sequence of immune responses and virological events during acute hepatitis A and their relationship to the biochemical and histological activity of liver damage. HAV, hepatitis A virus; CTLs, cytotoxic T-lymphocytes; IFN, interferon; NK, natural killer; PCR, polymerase chain reaction; ALT, alanine amino transference.

experimental animal model appear in full agreement with earlier results demonstrating HAV-specific killing in human beings tested during acute hepatitis A (Vallbracht *et al*, 1986, 1989). Thus CTL-mediated cytotoxicity seems to be the leading cause of tissue damage in hepatitis A.

However, if hepatocyte necrosis directly reflects mainly the cell-mediated immune attack on infected hepatocytes, the extent of HAV replication and the genotype of the infecting virus may also determine, in a more indirect way, the degree of hepatocellular damage by affecting the spread of virus in the liver. When this is particularly extensive, severe and even fulminant hepatitis may supervene, as seen in 1–5% of adult patients with hepatitis A. The observation that acute infection by HAV is usually asymptomatic and mild in children and becomes more aggressive and severe in adults is intriguing and would suggest that certain more cytopathic strains of HAV may become more aggressive in the adult liver or that the antiviral immune response, which is certainly more vigorous in adult life, may be disastrously efficient in individual, perhaps genetically predisposed, cases, particularly in the presence of more active virus replication and extensive spread in the liver. The pathogenesis of fulminant liver failure during hepatitis A remains uncertain and will be discussed, together with other aetiological forms, in a separate section of this chapter.

Liver damage in hepatitis B

The pathogenesis of liver cell damage caused by HBV has been a matter of debate and investigation for more than 20 years, and our understanding of it is still incomplete (Lee, 1998). The concept that HBV is not directly cytopathic was initially based on indirect evidence, derived mainly from clinical observation of an HBV carrier state that may last for many decades without any sign of liver damage. Other clinical observations indicate the fact that, during the acute phase of hepatitis B, peak virus activity occurs much earlier than liver damage (Alberti *et al*, 1979). The transaminase elevation correlates more closely with the appearance of an immune response to HBV, particularly of a T-cell response to surface antigens (Vento *et al*, 1987).

The absence of an important direct cytopathic effect of HBV is further supported by the observation of an inverse relationship between virus and disease activity in chronic infection (Alberti *et al*, 1983) and by data indicating that immunosuppressive therapy dramatically increases HBV replication, while it reduces the severity of liver damage that is instead triggered again at the time of treatment withdrawal (*see* Chapter 5). More recently, a large body of evidence has been provided in the scientific literature unanimously pointing to the conclusion that immune reactions play a major role in the pathogenesis of HBV-related liver damage.

The current interpretation of HBV immunopathology was anticipated more than 10 years ago by early studies that identified HBV antigens (both envelope and nucleocapsid related) on the surface of infected hepatocytes (Alberti *et al*, 1975; Alberti, 1984) as potential targets of the host cytolytic immune reactions and by in vitro cytotoxicity experiments showing that liver cells derived from the liver of patients with chronic hepatitis B were specifically lysed by autologous T-lymphocytes recognising nucleocapsid or surface antigens on target cells (Mondelli *et al*, 1982, 1987). Other studies showed the predominant presence of CD4+ and CD8+ lymphocytes in liver biopsies of patients with chronic hepatitis B, and these cells were often proven to recognise specifically the core antigen of HBV (Penna *et al*, 1991), which has since then been considered to be one of the major targets of the host immune response causing the lysis of infected hepatocytes and, consequently, the liver damage characterising hepatitis B. Definitive evidence has recently been provided indicating that CTLs able specifically to recognise HBcAg in association with a HLA class I molecule are present in the peripheral blood of patients with acute hepatitis B who later recover completely from the infection (Ferrari *et al*, 1991). Using synthetic peptides and recombinant vectors to produce specific systems to test CTL-mediated cytotoxicity, it has been shown that core antigen-specific CTLs are present in acute resolving hepatitis B, being much weaker in patients progressing to chronic infection, independently of the activity of liver disease.

Studies with overlapping synthetic epitopes have identified an HLA-A2 epitope restricted to amino acid residues 18–27 of HBcAg and HLA-B1 and HLA AW68 epitopes restricted to amino acid residues 141–151 (Missale *et al*, 1993). Thus core-specific T-lymphocytes are certainly involved in causing liver damage and the lysis of infected cells in acute hepatitis, while their role in chronic hepatitis is less obvious. Studies conducted during phases of acute exacerbation of chronic hepatitis B have identified the activation of HBcAg/HBeAg-specific T-cells, with an elevation of HBcAg/HBeAg-specific precursor T-cell frequencies (Tsai *et al*, 1992; Jung *et al*, 1995), suggesting that these immune reactions also play an important role during chronic infection and may indeed be a prerequisite for HBeAg seroconversion. Recently, a naturally processed hepatitis B core-derived peptide that is recognised by CD8+ CTLs has been identified in the liver of patients with chronic hepatitis B, further supporting the role of these cells in the pathogenesis of liver disease. The finding that tumour necrosis factor receptors are over-expressed in hepatocytes in patients with more active diseases (Marinos *et al*, 1995) may indicate enhanced CTL activity.

In patients with active chronic hepatitis, cytotoxic T-cells recognising pre-S2 envelope antigens in association with HLA class I and II molecules have also been described, suggesting that CD8+ as well as CD4+ lymphocytes sensitised against the envelope proteins of HBV may act as effector cells in chronic hepatitis B (Barnaba and Balsano, 1992; Nayersina *et al*, 1993). The involvement of these antigens as targets of the T-cell cytotoxic activity has also been confirmed in the transgenic mice model (Ando *et al*, 1993).

Host genetic factors have been shown to be important in determining disease progression (Thursz, 1997). MHC genes have been shown to play a role in influencing the clearance of HBV infection. For example, a case control study in the Gambia revealed an association of the allele DRB1*1302 with clearance of HBV infection (Thursz *et al*, 1995). Other genetic factors that may play a role in clearing HBV include mutations in the mannose-binding protein gene (Thomas *et al*, 1996). This opsonising protein could bind a mannose-terminated carbohydrate chain on HBsAg and facilitate its removal from peripheral blood. TNF polymorphisms may also be important (Thursz, 1997).

Other mechanisms of cell damage that may operate in hepatitis B, particularly in chronic hepatitis with prominent necro-inflammatory activity include (Table 7.2):

- Antibody- and complement-dependent cytotoxicity or antibody-dependent cell-mediated cytotoxicity (ADCC) against hepatocyte membrane-expressed HBeAg.
- Autoimmune reactions mediated mainly by autoantibodies to liver-specific membrane lipoproteins and to the asialoglycoprotein receptors, which have, since the early studies on liver immunopathology, been claimed to be the major cause of piecemeal necrosis (interface hepatitis). These reactions certainly do not have the same importance as in the typical forms of autoimmune hepatitis and most probably play only a marginal role in most cases of hepatitis B. Their significance has been studied in the woodchuck model (Diao and Michalak, 1997).
- Cytotoxic reactions mediated by soluble lymphokines such as gamma-IFN and TNF that are released following the immunological recognition of HBV and act in an unspecific way on infected and possibly also uninfected hepatocytes. This mechanism

Table 7.2 Mechanisms of liver damage in hepatitis B

Type of cell damage	*Pathway*
Immune mediated	
Antibody/complement-mediated cytotoxicity	Anti-HBe reacting with membrane-associated HBeAg
Antibody-dependent cellular cytotoxicity	Autoimmune reaction against liver membrane lipoproteins and asialoglycoprotein receptors
T-cell cytotoxicity	CD8+ and CD4+ T-lymphocytes reacting with nucleocapsid or surface antigens
Cytotoxicity by soluble cytokines	Mediates by interferons, interleukins and tumour necrosis factor
Direct virus cytopathic effects	Overproduction of virions; intracellular accumulation of S/pre-S

of amplification of liver damage in HBV infection has been demonstrated to occur in transgenic mice expressing surface HBV antigens in the hepatocytes.

Although most data strongly indicate that HBV causes liver damage through immune-mediated specific and non-specific mechanisms, other cytotoxic effects may be operative in atypical forms of the disease. A high-level accumulation of HBsAg and of pre-S1 proteins in the cytoplasm of hepatocytes is associated with liver cell degeneration and necrosis in transgenic mice (Chisari *et al*, 1987; Gilles *et al*, 1992), and overexpression of HBcAg in the hepatoblastoma line induces cytopathic changes (Roingeard *et al*, 1990). In patients who develop a recurrence of HBV infection after liver transplantation and during heavy immunosuppression, a novel histological pattern, fibrosing cholestatic hepatitis, and a fulminant clinical course have been described, the suggestion being that HBV may be directly cytopathic in these cases (Lau *et al*, 1992) (*see* Chapter 5).

Liver damage in patients infected by HBV pre-core mutants

In the past decade, great interest has been generated by the discovery that some patients chronically infected with HBV have mainly circulating virus particles that are unable to produce the hepatitis B e antigen because of the presence of point mutations in the pre-core gene (Brunetto *et al*, 1990; Carman, 1989). These mutations have been found to be particularly common in chronic hepatitis B cases seen in Italy, Greece, Israel and Japan, and to associate with a more severe form of liver involvement such as fulminant hepatitis or a severe type of chronic hepatitis. Other studies, however, have not confirmed the role of HBV pre-core mutants in fulminant hepatitis and have shown that these variants of HBV may be found also in patients with mild or minimal liver damage, indicating that their presence is not *per se* linked to severe liver disease. The findings of a prevalence of pre-core mutants among circulating HBV particles is most probably an expression of immune selection. Hepatocytes infected by pre-core mutants do not express HBeAg that may be an important target of the immune response and can therefore survive immune lysis more efficiently than can hepatocytes infected by wild-type HBV. In the phase of a strong immuno-elimination reaction, there would be a drastic reduction of wild-type HBV with the emergence of mutant HBV. This may be the major reason why the HBeAg-negative, anti-HBe-positive profile of hepatitis B, with a predominant population of pre-core mutant HBV in the serum, has been associated with more severe liver damage. The presence of a large proportion of pre-core mutant would therefore be a consequence rather than a cause of the more active destruction of infected hepatocytes. This interpretation is in agreement with clinical and in vitro data indicating that the pre-core mutant HBV is not inherently more cytopathic and is detected mainly in conditions of active HBV immuno-elimination such as acute hepatitis, fulminant hepatitis and the HBeAg/anti-HBe seroconversion phase of chronic HBV infection.

Liver damage in hepatitis D

Liver damage in patients with HDV (and HBV) infection is the result of the concurrent pathogenicity of the two agents, with most probably a synergistic effect. It may be difficult, and often impossible, to discriminate in the individual case the relative contribution of HBV and of HDV in causing liver damage that is, in general, more severe than that seen in hepatitis B alone. Compared with infection by HBV alone, hepatitis D is indeed associated with a higher rate of fulminant hepatitis and with a more severe and progressive course of acute and chronic liver disease (Rizzetto *et al*, 1992). The mechanisms of HDV-related liver damage are poorly understood and may involve both direct cytopathic effects and immune-mediated reactions. There is a general consensus that the former pathway most probably predominates in most patients with hepatitis D. Concomitant immune-mediated liver damage may be an expression of HBV rather than HDV immunopathology. The following observations support the idea that HDV is directly cytopathic:

- In acute hepatitis D, liver damage may occur early in the course of infection, coincident with the first evidence of HDV replication, still in the absence of an antiviral immune response and even before the initiation of HBV replication.
- A relationship has been described between levels of HDV replication, or expression of HDV antigens in the liver, and the severity of liver damage.
- HDV-related liver disease may become particularly severe in immunocompromised and immunosuppressed hosts.
- Hepatitis D often has a relapsing course, phases of severe liver damage alternating with phases of remission, and this behaviour is parallel to HDV replication activity.
- Liver histology in severe forms of hepatitis D is often characterised by prominent signs of hepatocyte degeneration and necrosis, with less striking inflammatory changes (Popper *et al*, 1983; Verme *et al*, 1986).

However, the clinical expression of HDV infection and the severity and histopathological pattern of liver disease show a wide variation world wide, suggesting that host or virus genetic factors are important determinants in the pathogenesis of hepatitis D. One of the most interesting observations in this respect is the report of the existence of different HDV genotypes that might associate with different pathogenicity (Casey *et al*, 1993). At least three distinct HDV genotypes have been identified, and others may exist. The cloning and sequencing of HDV isolates obtained during outbreaks of severe hepatitis D in the Amazon basin in Peru have led to the identification of genotype III of HDV, which appeared responsible for a particularly severe form of hepatitis. The disease was associated with a characteristic histological lesion termed the 'morula cell', with microvesicular steatosis and granular eosinophilic degeneration, typical of direct virus cytotoxicity (*see* Chapter 3). Structural and functional differences between HDV genotypes have been identified that may explain the different pathogenicity. The most striking variation is in the C-terminus part of the D antigen p27 that promotes the packaging of HDV RNA with HBsAg and inhibits the further replication of HDV RNA. This may indeed lead to variations in virus expression, replication and interaction with the host immune system.

Thus, in conclusion, HDV may cause liver damage mainly by direct cytopathic effects, which may differ between different HDV genotypes, thus explaining the wide range in the severity of liver disease. Immune-mediated mechanisms may also be involved, being driven mainly by the associated HBV infection. Various autoantibodies to liver and kidney microsomal antigens have been described in HDV-infected patients, but their contribution to the liver injury is probably minor.

Liver damage in hepatitis C

Hepatitis in patients infected with yellow fever virus, a virus of the *Flaviviridae* family, which includes HCV, is characterised by prominent histological signs of direct hepatocellular damage without a significant inflammatory infiltrate (*see* Chapter 3). The histological hallmarks of direct virus cytotoxicity include cell rounding, shrinkage, nuclear pyknosis, acidophilic degeneration of the hepatocytes and spotty necrosis. At the ultramicroscopic level, damage to the mitochondria and endoplasmic reticulum can be observed. Similar changes have also been reported to occur in the liver of patients with hepatitis C, and early studies of liver biopsies obtained during parenterally acquired non-A, non-B hepatitis, later recognised as classical forms of hepatitis C, led to the conclusion that histological and ultrastructural features were most consistent with direct viral cytotoxicity. Following the discovery of HCV in 1989 (Choo *et al*, 1989), a large body of clinical, histological, biochemical, serological and immunological data has accumulated through the study of natural infection in humans and experimental infection in chimpanzees, but the overall picture of results has been fragmentary and sometimes conflicting, making our current understanding of HCV pathogenicity still largely incomplete.

Available data suggest that both direct virus cytopathogenicity and immune-mediated injury may be operative in hepatitis C. Several observations seem to indicate that HCV replication may directly alter hepatocytes, perhaps without being always cytolytic. This is supported by the finding of steatosis and liver cell degeneration, in the absence of inflammatory infiltrate, in liver biopsies taken from asymptomatic HCV carriers with completely normal transaminase levels. Other patients have spotty necrosis and acidophilic bodies with a minimal lymphocyte infiltrate. Recent data in experimentally infected chimpanzees have shown that the detection of replicating HCV RNA molecules by in situ hybridisation parallels ALT elevation and may occur in hepatocytes in the absence of morphological changes or inflammatory infiltrate, suggesting the HCV may functionally damage hepatocytes without killing them (Negro *et al*, 1992). A few studies in humans have also found, although not consistently, some correlation between serum or hepatic HCV RNA levels and the severity of hepatocyte damage, further supporting the idea that HCV may exert a direct cytopathic effect. In the absence of in vitro cell culture systems to properly assess the HCV direct cytotoxicity, the exact role of this mechanism of liver damage remains undefined in hepatitis C.

The possibility that HCV may exert direct cytopathic effects in the liver should also be considered in the light of the existence of distinct virus genotypes. At least six main genotypes of HCV, and a greater number of subtypes, have been identified (Simmonds *et al*, 1993; Simmonds, 1997). Some of these genotypes, particularly HCV-1b, have been found to associate with more severe disease, particularly after liver transplantation (Nousbaum *et al*, 1995) and with poor response to IFN therapy (Chemello *et al*, 1994) (*see* Chapter 1). Whether these features are dependent on a more aggressive cytopathogenicity compared with other HCV genotypes remains to be defined.

Evidence has recently accumulated suggesting that HCV causes liver disease also through the induction of cytotoxic immune responses. The high rate of chronicity of hepatitis C and the wide spectrum of severity of the associated liver disease activity both favour the hypothesis that the immune response may have a central role in determining the expression of liver damage in hepatitis C. Early in vitro cytotoxicity studies provided evidence that T-lymphocytes derived from peripheral blood mononuclear cells were cytotoxic to autologous hepatocytes in patients with chronic hepatitis C. Taking this line, using peripheral lymphocytes from a patient with chronic hepatitis C, Imawari *et al* (1989) were able to establish a human T-cell clone capable of lysing autologous and allogeneic hepatocytes. This cytotoxic cell clone was not HLA class I restricted and expressed the phenotype of NK cells. Several studies have shown that CD4+ T-lymphocytes reacting with several structural and non-structural HCV-specific proteins, especially those encoded by the core and by the non-structural NS3, NS4 and NS5 regions, are present in the peripheral blood of patients with chronic HCV infection (Ferrari *et al*, 1994). Interestingly, a positive correlation between the CD4+ T-cell response to core proteins and the absence of significant signs of liver damage in the presence of ongoing HCV replication has been observed, suggesting that these cells may play an important role in controlling and limiting HCV pathogenicity (Botarelli *et al*, 1993). These 'healthy' carriers of HCV usually have some degree of hepatocyte degeneration and mild infiltration of lymphocytes on histological examination of the liver (Alberti *et al*, 1992). Levels of virus replication are usually low, suggesting that the immune response is indeed keeping the HCV under control. The virus may, however, escape this immune surveillance, with progression to more overt liver disease.

Together with CD4+ T-lymphocytes, cytotoxic CD8+ cells with specificity for several epitopes encoded by the core, as well as by the E1, E2/NS1 and NS2 regions, have also been clearly demonstrated by direct cloning of lymphocytes from liver biopsy specimens of infected individuals (Koziel *et al*, 1993; Cerny *et al*, 1994), and CD8+ T-cells have been observed in close contact with HCV-infected hepatocytes and apoptotic bodies (Ballardini *et al*, 1995). However, the exact relationship between HLA class I-restricted T-cell-mediated cytotoxicity with specificity for viral epitopes and disease activity and progression is yet to be understood. Increased hepatocyte expression of B7/BB-1, a co-stimulatory molecule for T-cell activation, has been shown to be increased in HCV infection (Mochizuki *et al*, 1997). The result of this will be to increase cytotoxic T-cell generation.

One most important feature of HCV immunopathogenesis is doubtless related to the high rate of virus mutation that occurs mainly within the envelope glycoprotein region (Weiner *et al*, 1992; Yamaguchi *et al*, 1994). The presence of such a hypervariable region may be important for chronicity and for the fluctuating course of liver disease, as a result of the cyclic emergence of escape mutant virus under the pressure of the host immune response. The relevance of sequence variability within the E2 hypervariable region (HVR1) in the evolution of natural HCV infection is supported by the observation of an antibody-driven selection of HVR1 variants. The HVR1 domain has structural characteristics typical of rapidly evolving linear epitopes, such as the V3 loop of the gp120 protein of human immunodeficiency virus (HIV). It has been shown that antibodies against a single HVR1 epitope reach maximum levels several months after the demonstration in serum of the specific hypervariable sequence, and HCV species with different HVR1 sequences become dominant in the follow-up. Recent data (Kumar *et al*, 1994) have provided further support to the role of humoral immunity in promoting rapid HCV mutation and the emergence of escape virus variants. Agammaglobulinaemic patients with HCV infection were found to have a particularly aggressive and severe course of HCV infection in the absence of significant mutation within the envelope proteins. These findings suggest that the mechanism of liver damage and of that causing the emergence of escape HCV mutants and chronicity are distinct. T-cell cytotoxicity against as yet undefined epitopes of HCV may play a central role in liver cell damage, while the humoral immune response may be more relevant in exercising the selective pressure that causes virus mutation, as a consequence of neutralising anti-HCV activity.

Further information on the role of the immune response in determining liver disease in chronic HCV infection derives from clinical observations in patients with chronic hepatitis C treated with immunosuppressive drugs (*see* Chapter 5). In these patients, a reduction in ALT level can be observed while hepatitis C viraemia increases. This behaviour would suggest that liver damage is dependent more on immune reactions than on virus replication. However, partially to contradict this conclusion, there are other retrospective studies indicating that the progression of liver disease towards more severe lesions is more common in patients who have been treated with immunosuppression compared with untreated cases. One possible explanation is that both a minor direct cytopathic effect of HCV and a major immune-mediated mechanism of liver damage co-exist in the natural course of HCV infection. Immunosuppression may then change the ratio between these two pathways by enhancing the former but reducing the latter.

Finally, there is increasing evidence that HCV, as much as and perhaps even more than other hepatotropic viruses, is able to elicit several types of autoimmune reaction, and it is possible that some of them may become implicated in determining liver damage. Patients with HCV are often positive in serum for anti-GOR, an autoantibody directed against a self-antigen that seems to cross-react with HCV-encoded peptides (Mishiro *et al*, 1991). The role of anti-GOR in causing liver damage is, however, largely speculative. Furthermore, around 2–3% of patients with chronic hepatitis C are positive in their serum for liver kidney microsomal autoantibodies (LKM-1). In these patients, immunosuppressive therapy is sometimes effective, while interferons may instead enhance liver damage, suggesting that autoimmunity in chronic hepatitis C may occasionally be not just an epiphenomenon of no pathogenetic significance.

Much interest has recently been generated by the observation that HCV may be found not only in hepatocytes but also in extrahepatic tissues and cells, including lymphocytes. Definitive evidence of active virus replication in lymphocytes is still lacking, but it has been suggested that this may occur, having a central role in the pathogenesis of hepatitis C. The infection of cells involved in the immune response may alter their function and reduce the antiviral response, favouring chronicity. The interaction of HCV with the immune system may also be relevant for the pathogenesis of the extrahepatic manifestations that are characteristic of a subgroup of infected individuals.

The direct infection of lymphocytes or, more probably, chronic stimulation by viral antigens of B-lymphocytes may induce polyclonal or monoclonal expansion with the production of type III or type II cryoglobulins (as seen in patients with HCV-related mixed cryoglobulinaemia). This may eventually lead to the development of low-grade HCV and HGV in B-cell non-Hodgkin's lymphoma (Ellenrieder *et al*, 1998).

Increasing attention is being paid to host genetic factors in determining disease progression and outcome in HCV (Thursz, 1997). MHC type II factors have been shown to be important in influencing the clearance of infection and the severity of liver disease.

Liver damage in hepatitis E

HEV causes a self-limiting disease, and no progression to chronicity has so far been documented. The acute disease may be asymptomatic and mild, or symptomatic with a severe, potentially fatal clinical course. Massive liver necrosis, liver failure and death occur in around 7% of cases. This rises to 32% in women developing acute hepatitis E during the third trimester of pregnancy (Khuroo *et al*, 1981; Mast *et al*, 1994). The mechanisms by which HEV causes liver damage and the determinants of the clinical course and severity of liver disease are still poorly understood (Tsega *et al*, 1991). The severe course seen in pregnant women suggests that immune mechanisms may be important.

The pathogenesis of hepatitis E has been difficult to characterise largely because of limited methods for identifying the agent in serum and liver and for following the events of infection and disease development. Animal models of experimental infection have been established. Hepatitis E has been produced in a variety of non-human primates, including cynomolgus macaques (*Macaca fasciculons*), tamarins, African green monkeys, chimpanzees, rhesus monkeys and owl monkeys (Bradley, 1995). Cynomolgus macaques are the most reliably infected and develop the most marked hepatitis.

The understanding of hepatitis E pathogenesis has been further improved more recently following the development of new techniques to identify HEV, to measure its replication activity and to evaluate the host antiviral immune response. These techniques include immunofluorescence for hepatitis E virus antigens in liver tissue, the polymerase chain reaction to detect HEV levels in serum, bile and faeces, in situ hybridisation and enzyme immunoassays that measure anti-HEV levels in serum. Studies of the pathogenesis of liver damage in hepatitis E have been conducted in animals and humans, and have been based mainly on the sequential and comparative analysis of virus replication activity, liver disease activity and the antiviral immune response.

Interpretation of the results obtained in different studies has been conflicting. Longer *et al* (1993) have monitored the course of experimental HEV infection in cynomolgus macaques by assessing serum levels of ALT, the biliary shedding of HEV, the presence of HEVAg, pathological changes in liver tissue and the serum levels of the anti-HEV response. Several macaques were inoculated with infected bile or faeces, and serial serum, bile and liver specimens were taken to be examined by immune electron microscopy (IEM) for HEV particles, by the polymerase chain reaction for HEV genome, by immunofluorescence for HEVAg and by enzyme immunoassay for anti-HEV.

When liver biopsies were studied by light microscopy, the accumulation of mononuclear cells in lobules and the ballooning and degeneration of hepatocytes, with little necrosis, were seen as soon as 12–15 days after inoculation, still in the absence of a humoral immune response against HEV. In this phase, HEVAg could be detected by immunofluorescence in the liver, and in some animals, this was not accompanied by evident pathological changes. More prominent pathological changes were seen between 18 and 25 days after inoculation, with marked and diffuse swelling of the hepatocytes, accompanied by inflammatory lobular and portal infiltrates of mononuclear cells. These changes were usually seen in the presence of HEVAg and HEV particles and of HEV RNA in bile and faeces, but before the appearance of anti-HEV in serum. Later biopsies, taken more than 30 days after inoculation, showed the most marked degree of necrosis, ballooning and microvesicular steatosis of hepatocytes, at the time of high anti-HEV titre and peak ALT activity. In some animals studied with sequential liver biopsies, the early detection of HEVAg in the liver with HEV RNA shedding in the bile and faeces were not associated with pathological changes and coincided with rather insignificant ALT elevation, while the later appearances of significant histological changes and ALT abnormalities coincided with development of anti-HEV.

This sequence of events is similar to that described by other authors (Fig. 7.2) and suggests that hepatitis E has an initial early phase of HEV replication in the liver that causes a mild direct cytotoxic effect, coinciding with the onset of hepatitis, and a later phase in which more marked liver damage is caused by immune responses, which in turn clear the virus from the liver and determine recovery from the infection. Similar sequential events during acute hepatitis E have also been observed in humans. In a case report of one volunteer study of HEV transmission (Balayan *et al*, 1983), the detection of HEV in stool and of HEV RNA in serum by the polymerase chain reaction correlated with onset of disease, while anti-HEV appeared at peak ALT levels, more than 1 month after disease onset.

All these data, taken together, indicate that HEV pathology is mainly, but not exclusively, immune mediated. It may involve antibody-dependent immune reactions or T-cell effector mechanisms. It has been shown that cytotoxic CD8 cells are the most prominent type of infiltrating lymphocytes in HEV-infected livers, suggesting cell-mediated CTL

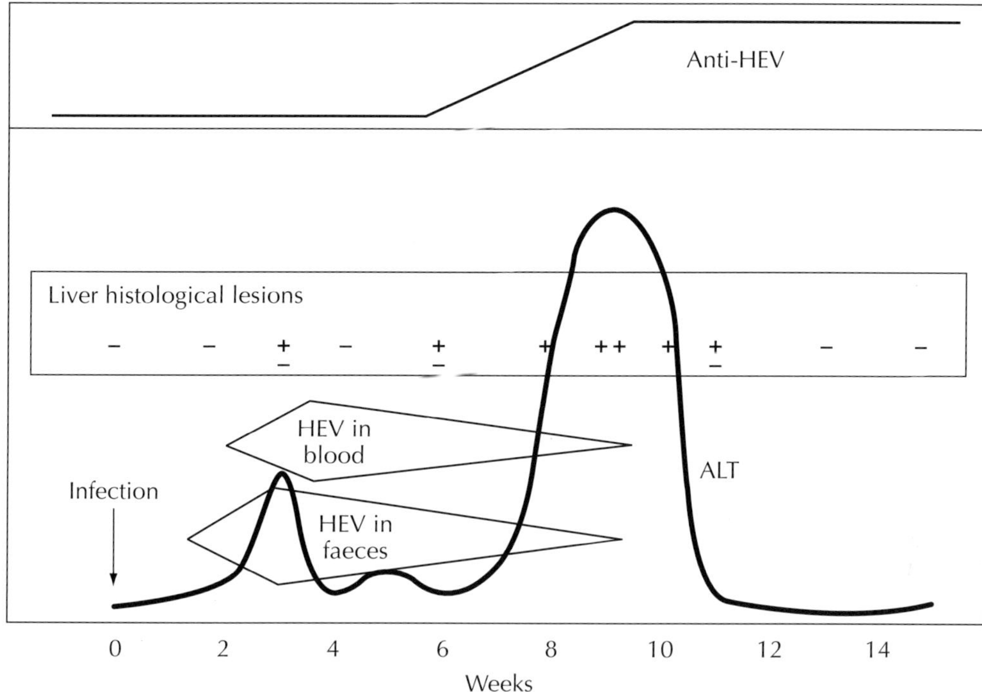

Fig 7.2   Sequence of immune responses and virological events during acute hepatitis E and their relationship to biochemical and histological signs of liver damage. HEV, hepatitis E virus; ALT, alanine amino transference.

necrosis as an important mechanism of liver cell damage. Other studies have suggested that virus replication itself causes liver damage in hepatitis E, and experimentally infected animals with the highest levels of viraemia were also those with the most prominent histopathological changes. It should, however, be noted here that immunosuppression with steroids or cyclosporine did not modify the severity of experimental hepatitis E in macaques studied by Balayan *et al* (1983), although it increased virus excretion. Until more definitive data are obtained, it seems reasonable to conclude that HEV may induce liver damage both by direct cytopathic effects, which are more evident during the early phase of disease, and immune-mediated mechanisms, developing later in the course of hepatitis.

Liver damage in systemic viral infections

A number of viruses cause liver damage as part of a systemic disease (*see* Chapter 6). Some of these agents, like cytomegalovirus and Epstein–Barr virus (EBV), are capable of producing hepatitis as the main clinical picture, while others cause hepatitis occasionally and usually without overt signs and symptoms of liver disease, apart from when they infect neonates or severely immunocompromised hosts. These agents include herpes viruses, measles and rubella viruses, some enteroviruses (such as Coxsackie and Echo viruses) and adenoviruses. Hepatitis is also seen during infection with exotic viruses, including yellow fever and Lassa fever viruses and the agents of Rift Valley and Crimean–Congo haemorrhagic fever. Most of these viruses cause liver damage mainly through direct cytopathic effects, which become particularly severe and may provoke massive hepatic necrosis in immature or immunocompromised hosts, in the absence of an efficient immune response to control the activity and spread of the virus.

Cytomegalovirus hepatitis is usually mild and completely asymptomatic during primary infection as well as during reactivation in the immunocompetent host. The disease is more severe in neonates, in patients receiving chemotherapy, in those with AIDS or in those who have received an allograft (*see* Chapter 5). In these cases, there are a large number of inclusion bodies in the hepatocytes, as well as vascular endothelium and bile epithelium, together with extensive liver damage and necrosis, accompanied by scarce inflammatory infiltrates, indicating that cytomegalovirus is directly cytolytic in the liver and that a normal immune response is required to limit the severity of the infection.

EBV hepatitis during infectious mononucleosis is characterised by portal and sinusoidal mononuclear cell infiltration with little hepatic necrosis, being immunopathologically mediated by activation in the liver, as elsewhere, of reactive T-lymphocytes.

Hepatitis due to herpes simplex and varicella–zoster viruses occurs usually during generalised infection and is more common and severe in neonates and in immunocompromised children and adults. The liver damage may become massive and the course occasionally fatal. Liver histology shows focal or confluent hepatocellular necrosis with scanty inflammatory infiltrates, confirming that the main mechanism of liver damage is a direct cytopathic effect of the virus itself, with nuclear inclusion bodies and large multinuclear hepatocytes appearing in the liver.

A similar mechanism of cell damage is also involved in causing liver injury during measles, rubella, enterovirus and adenovirus infections, again affecting particularly neonates and immunocompromised hosts. Direct virus cytopathogenicity with moderate or insignificant inflammatory cell infiltrates also characterises hepatitis during yellow fever, and Lassa fever (*see* above). However, in other forms of viral haemorrhagic fever, direct cell damage by the virus may co-exist with immunologically mediated cell injury.

Pathogenesis of fulminant hepatitis of viral aetiology

The reasons why viral hepatitis may develop into a fulminant disease with massive liver cell destruction are still largely unknown. All hepatotropic viruses may cause fulminant liver failure, but with significantly different frequency. HAV and HBV are more often involved, while HCV is an extremely rare cause of severe acute hepatitis. Several hypotheses have been proposed to explain massive hepatic necrosis during viral hepatitis:

- a direct cytopathic effect of a particularly aggressive virus strain, such as in some forms of hepatitis D or in hepatitis B due to HBV mutants (Carman *et al*, 1991);
- an exaggerated immune response by the host against virus-infected hepatocytes or with a massive deposition of immune complexes in the liver, a mechanism proposed mainly for hepatitis B;
- a major role of host factors, such as genetic predisposition, to the enhancement of liver damage, favoured by pre-existing liver disease with reduced liver cell mass or hepatocyte degeneration, steatosis, membrane instability, reduced blood flow and oxygen supply, and an accumulation of oxygen free radicals;

- overproduction of 'toxic' virus products such as pre-S, core or pre-core proteins of HBV;
- a massive release of cytotoxic cytokines such as interleukin-2 (IL-2) and TNF by inflammatory cells infiltrating the liver; FAS-mediated pathways of cell death by apoptosis may play a relevant role as the CD95 receptor (APO-1/FAS) and its mRNA expression have been increased during fulminant hepatitis (Galle *et al*, 1995);
- the synergistic effect of more than one virus, as typically seen in patients with HBV/HDV co-infection or superinfection.

The possibility that fulminant hepatitis may be caused by this last mechanism appears quite convincing. Recent evidence indicates that, while HCV alone is only exceptionally associated with fulminant disease (Wright *et al*, 1992), many patients with acute liver failure are found to have concurrent HBV and HCV infection (Feray *et al*, 1993). A recent report highlights the role of hepatitis A superinfection precipitating fulminant hepatitis in patients with chronic hepatitis C (Vento *et al*, 1998). The hypothesis that multiple infection by hepatotropic viruses may play a major role in fulminant hepatitis is consistent with many of the pathogenetic mechanisms previously described. In fact, superinfection by a hepatotropic virus in a liver already infected by another agent has the highest probability of occurring in an already damaged liver with a larger number of infiltrating inflammatory cells, which may be recruited to release large amount of cytokines. Certainly, in the case of HDV and HBV, superinfection by HDV produces more severe disease than does co-infection. Furthermore, virus expression may be modified by the interaction between the two agents (Pontisso *et al*, 1992), with an enhanced production of defective particles and side-products of disturbed replication that are not exported and accumulate in the cells. It should, however, be underlined that most of these mechanisms proposed to explain massive hepatic necrosis are, and will most probably remain, speculative, such as a consequence of factors that are intrinsic to fulminant hepatitis, a rare disease, often impossible to predict and characterised by a rapid clinical course. All these features usually do not allow the setting-up of adequate pathogenetic studies in these patients.

Pathogenetic rationale and mechanism of action of interferon therapy in chronic viral hepatitis

In this section, we will briefly discuss the rationale of the administration of exogenous IFN to treat chronic viral hepatitis and the different mechanisms of action of such treatment in chronic hepatitis B and C.

About 30–40% of patients with chronic hepatitis B clear HBeAg and HBV DNA permanently when treated with IFN-α, and this effect seems to derive from a combination of antiviral and immunomodulatory mechanisms. On the other hand, 20–30% of patients with chronic hepatitis C also develop a sustained response associated with decrease of the virus after IFN therapy. The rationale for treating patients with chronic hepatitis B with IFN-α lies in the observation that they have a reduced capacity to produce endogenous IFN.

The first effect seen in chronic hepatitis B after the administration of IFN-α is an immediate fall in serum HBV DNA levels, most probably as a consequence of direct antiviral effects. The suppression of HBV replication may remain the only effect of IFN, and such cases usually show only a transient response, virus replication recurring soon after the cessation of IFN administration. In other patients, typically in those who will become permanent responders with a definitive loss of HBV replication, a sharp rise in serum transaminase levels may be observed after the initial suppression of HBV activity (Fig. 7.3). This hepatitis 'flare' most probably reflects enhancement of the immune-mediated lysis of infected (and possibly also uninfected) liver cells. The appearance of the ALT peak is usually delayed after 5–8 weeks into treatment, suggesting the recruitment of specific CTLs (rather than NK cells). It may reflect the need to reach, by the early direct antiviral effect, a significant reduction in the levels of circulating virions and viral antigens that would otherwise 'paralyse' cytotoxic T-cells. IFN-α most probably promotes the ALT flare by optimising the presentation of viral antigens at the hepatocyte surface to the CTLs. This effect may be mediated by the enhancement of HLA class I expression in the presence of already activated, antigen-specific cytotoxic T-cells. On the other hand, IFN-α is most probably ineffective in the absence of activated T-cells and would not favour the activation of resting T-cells. This explains why the patients who respond to IFN therapy are those who, pre-treatment, had more active disease and who are also most likely to undergo spontaneous anti-HBe seroconversion and loss of HBV replication if left untreated.

Although it has been reported that a higher degree of HLA class I display on hepatocytes correlates with a successful response to IFN, some authors have suggested that HLA class II display may also have a role. However, IFN-α is not as good as IFN-γ in inducing HLA class II antigens, and recent data correlating ALT levels, HLA class I antigen display on the hepatocytes, serum beta-2-microglobulin levels and intrahepatic CD8+ cells seem to support the hypothesis that IFN potentiates HLA-restricted CD8+ cell cytotoxicity. Thus, IFN therapy seems to act in hepatitis B by the combination of direct antiviral effects and enhancement of the host immune response against infected

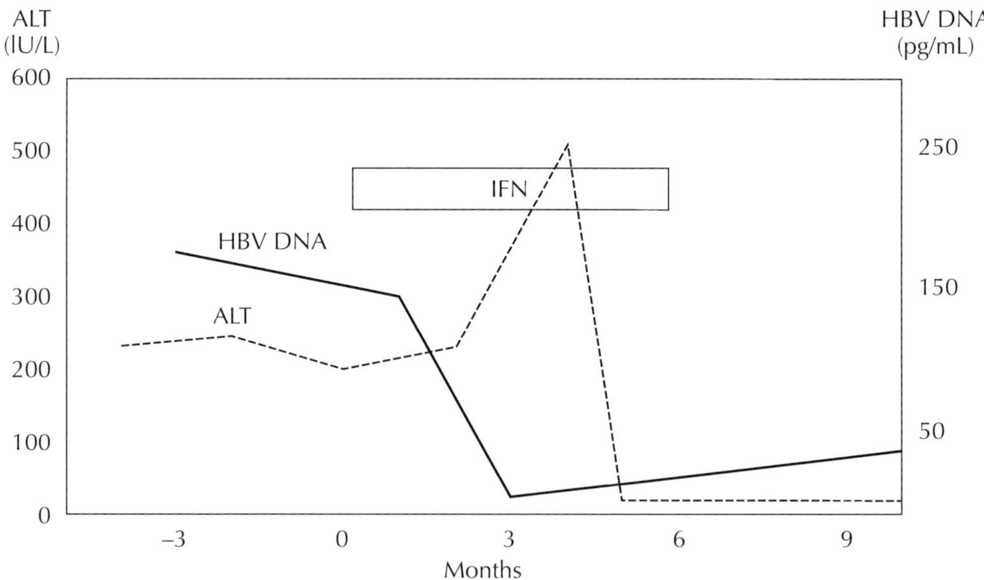

Fig 7.3 Changes in alanine amino transference (ALT) and serum hepatitis B virus (HBV) DNA during interferon therapy (IFN) in a HBeAg-2 positive patient with chronic hepatitis B, showing a sustained response.

hepatocytes. Full expression of the latter mechanism seems essential to achieve a permanent cure. The kinetics of serum HBV DNA and of ALT levels during IFN therapy are characterised by a behaviour opposite to that of the two parameters (Fig. 7.3), thus confirming that liver damage in hepatitis B, including that occurring during IFN therapy, is not related to the activity of HBV itself but to the immune response that clears infected cells, thus reducing the number of released virions.

IFN therapy is also used widely in chronic hepatitis C, based on the results of several randomised trials that have confirmed its efficacy in about 15–30% of patients. The profile of the ALT response to IFN and its relation to the virus replicative activity is quite different from the behaviour in hepatitis B, suggesting that therapy is here acting through different mechanisms. As shown in Figure 7.4, in patients with hepatitis C, there is indeed an almost absolute parallelism between ALT and HCV RNA levels, both during and after therapy, indicating that IFN is here acting mainly as an antiviral agent able to establish the suppression of virus activity which, in turn, induces the suppression of disease activity. Interestingly, even in patients who do not have a virological response to treatment with IFN, necro-inflammatory activity in the liver may decrease; the mechanism for this is unknown. The parallelism between serum HCV RNA and ALT levels indicates that, in chronic hepatitis C, virus cytotoxicity plays a more direct role in the mechanism of liver damage compared with the case in hepatitis B.

Most recently, the pathogenetic mechanisms involved in the response to IFN treatment in patients with chronic hepatitis C have been analysed in detail by studying the relationship of HCV genotype and tissue expression, the hepatocellular expression of HLA-A, B and C and ICAM-1 molecules, and the response to treatment (Ballardini *et al*, 1995). Patients not responding to therapy were usually infected by HCV-1b and displayed higher scores of HCV-positive hepatocytes, HLA-A, B and C and ICAM-1

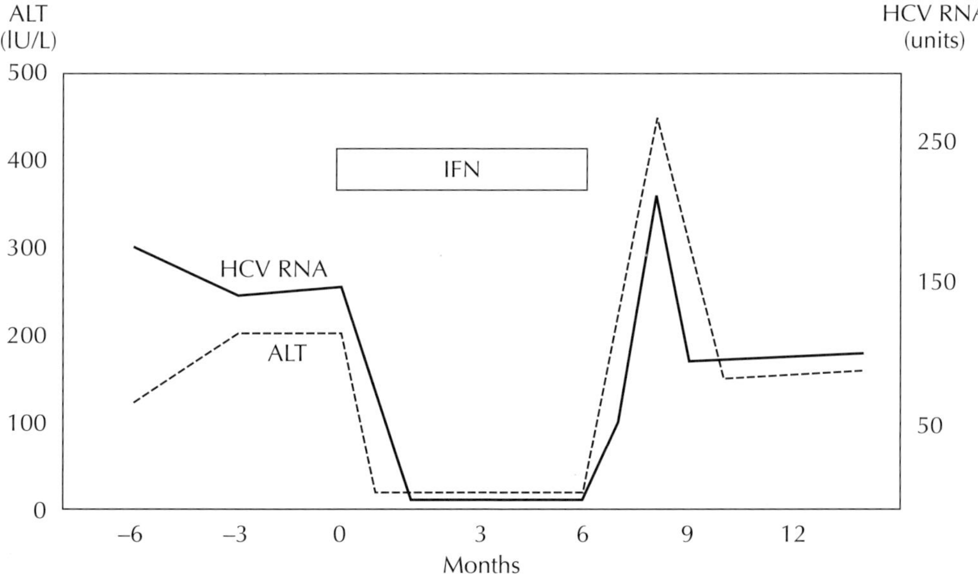

Fig 7.4 Changes in alanine amino transference (ALT) and hepatitis C virus (HCV) RNA during interferon therapy (IFN) in a patient with chronic hepatitis C, showing a transient response followed by relapse after treatment withdrawal.

molecules. In these patients, CD8+ T-cells were often observed in close contact with infected hepatocytes and cells undergoing acidophilic degeneration, and their numbers in the lobules correlated with the severity of the biochemical activity of liver damage. These observations suggest that T-cell-mediated cytotoxicity could play an important role in liver damage in these patients and that their poor response to exogenous IFN could reflect the presence of a strong activation of the endogenous IFN system, possibly induced by HCV replication itself and leading to IFN resistance. Indeed, a prompt and complete response to exogenous IFN was observed in patients who had no signs of pre-treatment activation of the endogenous IFN system, usually infected by HCV genotypes other than 1b. Further analysis of these issues would eventually allow the definition of more effective strategies for the treatment of patients infected with different strains of HCV.

References

Alberti, A. 1984: The role of hepatitis B virus replication and hepatocytes membrane expression in the pathogenesis of HBV-related hepatic damage. In Chisari, F. (ed.) *Advances in hepatitis research*. Masson Publishing, 134–43.

Alberti, A., Realdi, G., Tremolada, F. *et al.* 1975: HBsAg on liver cell surface in viral hepatitis. *Lancet* **i**, 346.

Alberti, A., Diana, S., Eddleston, A.L.W.F., Williams, R. *et al.* 1979: Change in hepatitis B virus DNA polymerase in relation to the outcome hepatitis type B. *Gut* **20**, 190–5.

Alberti, A., Tremolada, F., Fattovich, G. *et al.* 1983: Virus replication and liver disease in chronic hepatitis B virus infection. *Digestive Diseases and Sciences* **28**, 962–6.

Alberti, A., Gerlich, W.H., Herrmann, K.H., Pontisso, P. 1990: Nature and display of hepatitis B virus envelope proteins and the humoral immune response. *Seminars in Immunopathology* **12**, 5–23.

Alberti, A., Morsica, G., Chemello, L. *et al.* 1992: Hepatitis C viremia and liver disease in symptom-free individuals with anti-HCV. *Lancet* **340**, 697–8.

Ando, K., Moriyama, T., Wirth, S. *et al.* 1993: Mechanisms of class I restricted immunopathology: a transgenic mouse model of fulminant hepatitis. *Journal of Experimental Medicine* **178**, 1541–4.

Balayan, M.S., Andjaparize, A.G., Cook, E.H. *et al.* 1983: Evidence for a virus in non-A, non-B hepatitis transmitted via the fecal oral route. *Intervirology* **20**, 23–31.

Ballardini, G., Groff, P., Pontisso, P. *et al.* 1995: Hepatitis C virus (HCV) genotype, tissue HCV antigens, hepatocellular expression of HLA-A, B, C and intercellular adhesion-1 molecules. *Journal of Clinical Investigation* **95**, 2067–75.

Barnaba, V., Balsano, F. 1992: Immunologic and molecular basis of viral persistence. The hepatitis B virus model. *Journal of Hepatology* **114**, 391–400.

Botarelli, P., Brunetto, M.R., Minutello, M.A. *et al.* 1993: T-lymphocyte response to hepatitis C virus in different clinical courses of infection. *Gastroenterology* **104**, 580–7.

Bradley, D.W. 1995: Hepatitis E virus: a brief review of the biology, molecular virology and immunology of a novel virus. *Journal of Hepatology* **22**, 140–5.

Brunetto, M., Stemler, M., Bonino, F. *et al.* 1990: A new hepatitis B virus strain in patients with severe anti-HBe positive chronic hepatitis B. *Journal of Hepatology* **10**, 258–61.

Carman, W.F., Jacina, M.R., Hadziyannis, S. *et al.* 1989: Mutation preventing formation of 'hepatitis B e antigen' in patients with chronic hepatitis B infection. *Lancet* **ii**, 588–90.

Carman, W.F., Fagan, E.A., Hadziyannis, S. *et al.* 1991: Association of precore genomic variant of hepatitis B virus with fulminant hepatitis. *Hepatology* **14**, 219–22.

Casey, J.L., Brown, T.L., Colan, E.J. *et al.* 1993: A genotype of hepatitis D virus that occurs in northern South America. *Proceedings of the National Academy of Sciences of the USA* **90**, 9016–20.

Cerny, A., McHutchinson, J., Pasquinelli, C. *et al.*1994: Hepatitis C virus-specific cytotoxic T lymphocytes restricted by HLA-A2 are present in the peripheral blood of patients with chronic hepatitis C. In Nishiokata, K., Suzuki, H., Mishiro, S., Oda, T. (eds) *Viral hepatitis and liver disease*. Tokyo: Springer-Verlag, 190–4.

Chemello, L., Alberti, A., Rose, K., Simmonds, P. 1994: Hepatitis C serotype and response to interferon therapy. *New England Journal of Medicine* **330**, 143.

Chisari, F.V., Filippi, P., Buras, J. *et al.* 1987: Structural and pathological effects of synthesis of hepatitis B virus large envelope polypeptide in transgenic mice. *Proceedings of the National Academy of Sciences of the USA* **84**, 6909–13.

Choo, Q.-L., Kuo, G., Weiner, A.J. *et al.* 1989: Isolation of a cDNA clone derived from a blood-borne non-A, non-B viral hcpatitis genome. *Science* **244**, 359–62.

Diao, J., Michalak, T.I. 1997: Virus-induced anti-asialoglycoprotein receptor autoimmunity in experimental hepadnaviral hepatitis. *Hepatology* **25**, 689–96.

Durazzo, M., Michel, G., Philip, T. *et al.* 1992: Anti-GOR in hepatitis D; specific association with hepatitis C virus. Superinfection. *Hepatology* **16**, 76A.

Ellenrieder, V., Weidenbach, H., Frickhofen, N. *et al*, 1998: HCV and HGV in B-cell non-Hodgkin's lymphoma. *Journal of Hepatology* **28**, 34–9.

Feray, C., Gigou, M., Samuel, D. *et al.* 1993: Hepatitis C virus RNA and hepatitis B virus DNA in serum and liver of patients with fulminant hepatitis. *Gastroenterology* **104**, 549–55.

Ferrari, C., Bertoletti, A., Penna, A. *et al.* 1991: Identification of immunodominant T cell epitopes of the hepatitis B virus nucleocapsid antigen. *Journal of Clinical Investigation* **88**, 214–22.

Ferrari, C., Valli, A., Galati, L. *et al.* 1994: T-cell response to structural and nonstructural hepatitis C virus antigens in persistent and self-limited hepatitis C virus infections. *Hepatology* **19**, 286–95.

Frosner, G.G., Deinhardt, F., Scheid, R. *et al.* 1979: Propagation of human hepatitis A virus in a hepatoma cell line. *Infection* **7**, 303–6.

Galle, P.R., Hofmann, W.J., Walczak, H. *et al.* 1995: Involvement of the CD95 (APO-1/Fas) receptor and ligand in liver damage. *Journal of Experimental Medicine* **182**, 1223–30.

Ganem, D., Varmus, H.E. 1987: The molecular biology of the hepatitis B viruses. *Annual Review of Biochemistry* **56**, 651–93.

Gilles, P.N., Guerrette, D.L., Ulevitch, R.J. *et al.* 1992: HBsAg retention sensitises the hepatocyte to injury by physiological concentrations of interferon-gamma. *Hepatology* **16**, 655–63.

Houghton, M., Weiner, A., Han J. *et al.* 1991: Molecular biology of the hepatitis C viruses: implications for diagnosis, development and control of viral diseases. *Hepatology* **14**, 381–8.

Imawari, M., Nomura, M., Kaieda, T. *et al.* 1989: Establishment of a human T cell clone for both autologous and allogenic hepatocytes from chronic hepatitis patients with non-A, non-B hepatitis. *Proceedings of the National Academy of Sciences of the USA* **86**, 2883–7.

Jung, M.C., Diepòlder, H.M., Spengler, U. *et al.* 1995: Activation of a heterogeneous hepatitis B (HB) core and e antigen-specific CD4+ T-cell population during seroconversion to anti-HBe and anti-HBs in hepatitis B virus infection. *Journal of Virology* **69**, 3358–68.

Karayiannis, P., O'Rourke, S., Waters, J. *et al.* 1994: Studies of cytotoxic T lymphocytes activity in tamarins with acute hepatitis A virus infection. In Nishiokata, K., Suzuki, H., Mishiro, S., Oda, T. (eds) *Viral hepatitis and liver disease*. Tokyo: Springer-Verlag, 155–7.

Khuroo, M.S., Teli, M.R., Skidmore, S. *et al.* 1981: Incidence and severity of viral hepatitis in pregnancy. *American Journal of Medicine* **70**, 252–5.

Koziel, M., Dudley, D., Afdhal, N. *et al.* 1993: Hepatitis C virus (HCV): specific cytotoxic T lymphocytes recognize epitopes in the core and envelope proteins of HCV. *Journal of Virology* **67**, 7522–32.

Kumar, U., Monjardino, J., Thomas, H.C. *et al.* 1994: Hypervariable region of hepatitis C virus envelope glycoprotein (E2/NS1) in an agammaglobulinemic patient. *Gastroenterology* **106**, 1072–5.

Lau, J.Y.N., Davies, S.E., Bain, V.S. *et al.* 1992: High level expression of hepatitis B viral antigens in fibrosing cholestatic hepatitis. *Gastroenterology* **102**, 956–62.

Lee, W, 1998: Hepatitis B virus infection. *New England Journal of Medicine* **337**, 1733–46.

Lemon, S.M., Ping, L.-H., Day, S. *et al.* 1990: Immunobiology of hepatitis A virus. In Hollinger, B., Lemon, S., Margolis, H. (eds) *Viral hepatitis and liver disease*. Williams & Wilkins, 20–4.

Lemon, S.M., Robertson, B.H. 1994: Taxonomic classification of hepatitis A virus. In Nishioka, K., Suzuki, H., Mishiro, S., Oda, T. (eds) *Viral hepatitis and liver disease*. Springer-Verlag, 50–3.

Longer, C.F., Denny, S.L., Caudill, J.D. *et al*. 1993: Experimental hepatitis E: pathogenesis in cynomolgus macaques (*Macaca fascicularis*). *Journal of Infectious Disease* **168**, 602–9.

Marinos, G., Naoumov, N.V., Rossol, S. *et al*. 1995: Tumor necrosis factor receptors in patients with chronic hepatitis B virus infection. *Gastroenterology* **108**, 1453–63.

Mast, E., Polish, L. Favorov, M. *et al*. 1994: Hepatitis E among refugees in Kenya: minimal apparent person-to-person transmission, evidence for age-dependent disease expression and new serologic assays. In Nishioka, K., Suzuki, H., Mishiro, S., Oda, T. (eds) *Viral hepatitis and liver disease*. Tokyo: Springer-Verlag, 375–8.

Mishiro, S., Takeda, K., Hoshi, Y. *et al*. 1991: An autoantibody cross-reactive to hepatitis C virus core and a host nuclear antigen. *Autoimmunity* **10**, 269–73.

Missale, G., Redeker, A., Person, J. *et al*. 1993: HLA-A31 and HLA-Aw68 restricted cytotoxic T cell responses to a single hepatitis B virus nucleocapsid epitope during acute viral hepatitis. *Journal of Experimental Medicine* **117**, 751–62.

Mochizuki, K., Hayashi, N., Katayama, K. *et al*. 1997: B7/BB-1 expression and hepatitis activity in liver tissues of patients with chronic hepatitis C. *Hepatology* **25**, 713–18.

Mondelli, M., Vergani, G.M., Alberti, A. *et al*. 1982: Specificity of T cell cytotoxicity to autologous hepatocytes in chronic hepatitis B virus infection: evidence that T cells are directed against HBV core antigen expressed on hepatocytes. *Journal of Immunology* **129**, 2773–9.

Mondelli, M., Bortolotti, F., Pontisso, P. *et al*. 1987: Definition of hepatitis B virus (HBV) specific target antigens recognized by cytotoxic T cells in acute HBV infection. *Clinical and Experimental Immunology* **68**, 242–50.

Motkins, A.L., Oldstone, M.B.A. 1984: *Concepts in viral pathogens*. New York: Springer-Verlag.

Nayersina, R., Fowler, P., Guilhot, S. *et al*. 1993: HLA-A2 restricted cytotoxic T lymphocyte response to multiple hepatitis B surface antigen epitopes during hepatitis B virus infection. *Journal of Immunology* **150**, 4659–71.

Negro, F., Pacchioni, D., Shimizu, Y. *et al*. 1992: Detection of intrahepatic replication of hepatitis C virus RNA by in situ hybridization and comparison with histopathology. *Proceedings of the National Academy of Sciences of the USA* **89**, 2247–51.

Nousbaum, J.B., Pol, S., Nalpas, B. *et al*. 1995: Hepatitis C virus type 1b (II) infection in France and Italy. *Annals of Internal Medicine* **122**, 161–8.

Penna, A., Chisari, F.V., Bertoletti, A. *et al*. 1991: Cytotoxic T lymphocytes recognize an HLA-A2 restricted epitope within the hepatitis B virus nucleocapsid antigen. *Journal of Experimental Medicine* **174**, 1565–70.

Pontisso, P., Ruvoletto, M.G., Fattovich, G. *et al*. 1993: Clinical and virological profiles in patients with multiple hepatitis virus infections. *Gastroenterology* **105**, 1529–33.

Popper, H., Thung, S.N., Gerber, M.A. *et al*. 1983: Histologic studies of severe delta agent infection in Venezuelan indians. *Hepatology* **3**, 906–12.

Provost, P.J., Hilleman, M.R. 1979: Propagation of human hepatitis A virus in cell culture in vitro. *Proceedings of the Society of Experimental Biology and Medicine* **160**, 213–21.

Rizzetto, M., Hadziyannis, S., Hansson, B.G. *et al*. 1992: Hepatitis delta virus infection in the world; epidemiological patterns and clinical expression. *Gastroenterology International* **5**, 18–32.

Roingeard, P., Romet-Lemonne, J.I., Leturcq, D. *et al*. 1990: Hepatitis B virus core antigen (HBcAg) accumulation in an HBV nonproducer clone of HepG2-transfected cells is associated with cytopathic effect. *Virology* **179**, 113–20.

Schlicht, H., Von Brunn, A., Theilmann, L. *et al*. 1991: Antibodies in anti-HBe positive patient sera bind to an Hbc protein expressed on the cell surface of human hepatoma cells: implications for virus clearance. *Hepatology* **13**, 57–61.

Siegl, G., Nuesch, J., Weitz, M. 1991: Replication and protein processing of hepatitis A virus. In Hollinger, B., Lemon, S. (eds) *Viral hepatitis and liver disease*. Baltimore: Williams & Wilkins, 25–30.

Simmonds, P. 1997: Clinical relevance of hepatitis C virus genotypes. *Gut* **40**, 291–3.

Simmonds, P., Holmes, E.C., Cha, T.-A. *et al.* 1993: Classification of hepatitis C virus into six major genotypes and a series of subtypes by phylogenetic analysis of the NS5 region. *Journal of General Virology* **74**, 2391–9.

Thomas, H.C., Foster, G.R., Semiya, H., McIntosh, D., Turner, M.W., Sepperfield, J.A. 1996: Mutations of gene of mannose-binding protein associated with chronic hepatitis B viral infection. *Lancet* **348**, 1417–19.

Thursz, M.R. 1997: Host genetic factors influencing the outcome of hepatitis. *Journal of Viral Hepatitis* **4**, 215–20.

Thursz, M.R., Kwiatkowski, D., Allsopp, C.E.M., Greenwood, B.M., Thomas, H.C., Hill, A.V.S. 1995: Association between an MHC class II allele and clearance of hepatitis B virus in The Gambia. *New England Journal of Medicine* **332**, 1065–9.

Tsai, S.L., Chen, P.J., Lai, M.Y. *et al.* 1992: Acute exacerbations of chronic type B hepatitis are accompanied by increased T cell responses to hepatitis B core and e antigens: implications for hepatitis B e antigen seroconversion. *Journal of Clinical Investigation* **89**, 87–96.

Tsega, E., Krawczynski, K., Hansson, B.G. *et al.* 1991: Outbreak of acute hepatitis E virus infection among military personnel in northern Ethiopia. *Journal of Medical Virology* **34**, 232–6.

Vallbracht, A., Gabriel, P., Maier, K. *et al.* 1986: Cell-mediated cytotoxicity in hepatitis A virus infection. *Hepatology* **6**, 1308–14.

Vallbracht, A., Maier, K., Stierhof, D. *et al.* 1989: Liver derived cytotoxic-T cells in hepatitis A virus infection. *Journal of Infectious Diseases* **160**, 209–17.

Vento, S., Rondanelli, E.G., Ranieri, S. *et al.* 1987: Prospective study of cellular immunity of hepatitis B virus antigens from the early incubation phase of acute hepatitis B. *Lancet* **ii**, 119–22.

Vento, S., Garafano, T., Renzini, C. *et al.* 1998: Fulminant hepatitis associated with hepatitis A virus superinfection in patients with chronic hepatitis C. *New England Journal of Medicine* **338**, 286–90.

Verme, G., Amoroso, P., Lettieri, G. *et al.* 1986: A histologic study of hepatitis delta virus liver disease. *Hepatology* **6**, 1303–7.

Weiner, A.J., Geysen, H.M., Christopherson, C. *et al.* 1992: Evidence for immune selection of hepatitis C virus (HCV) putative envelope glycoprotein variants: potential role in chronic HCV infections. *Proceedings of the National Academy of Sciences of the USA* **89**, 3468–72.

Wright, T.L., Mamish, D., Combs, C. *et al.* 1992: Hepatitis C virus not found in fulminant non-A, non-B hepatitis. *Lancet* **115**, 111.

Yamaguchi, K., Tanaka, E., Higashi, K. *et al.* 1994: Adaptation of hepatitis C virus for persistent infection in patients with acute hepatitis. *Gastroenterology* **106**, 1344–8.

Zinkernagel, R.M. 1988: Virus-triggered AIDS: a T-cell-mediated immunopathology? *Immunology Today* **9**, 370–2.

CHAPTER 8

Viral hepatitis and liver cancer

E TABOR

Hepatocellular carcinoma (HCC), one of the most important and fascinating human cancers, was one of the first human cancers to be shown to be associated with virus infections. Its close association with HBV and the development of safe and effective vaccines for the prevention of HBV infection have led to the prospect of a viral vaccine that may function as an anti-cancer vaccine. In recent decades, a rising incidence of HCC associated with chronic HCV infection has been noted. The association of HCC with these two very different viruses (HBV, the partially double-stranded DNA virus that replicates through an RNA intermediate with a reverse transcriptase; HCV, the positive-sense, single-stranded RNA virus) has provided two important models for the pathogenesis of HCC and for viral oncogenesis in general.

HCC is one of the most common cancers in males in certain areas of the world. Patients with HCC succumb early, except for those few patients in highly technological societies where early detection and excision of the tumour can be accomplished. Even in countries where such early detection is possible, the reported mortality from HCC is high, for example 18 per 100 000 of the male population per year in Japan (Bosch and Muñoz, 1991). This is not significantly different from the HCC mortality rates in males in countries without such early diagnosis, such as Greece (16 per 100 000) and Singapore (24 per 100 000). In females, mortality from HCC is lower than among males (5–7 per 100 000 in these countries). In some geographical areas, the incidence of HCC (the mortality rate is not available but is certainly identical to incidence) is even higher (China: males 34, females 11; Mali: males 48, females 15).

Historical aspects

Before the availability of tests to detect infection with the human hepatitis viruses, researchers had noticed clinical and pathological evidence of an association between HCC and what we now know as chronic HBV infection. For example, in 1963, Higginson reported that HCC was found in sub-Saharan Africa and South East Asia in young adult males whose livers often had the pathological findings of 'post-hepatitic' or 'post-necrotic' cirrhosis, a finding also noted following hepatitis of presumed viral aetiology. On the basis of these observations, Higginson formulated the hypothesis that damage to the liver in childhood by a virus predisposed to the development of HCC following some other hepatotoxic event later in life (Higginson, 1963). This hypothesis is still the basis of much of the thinking today about how HCC develops.

A geographical association between HCC and presumed or known viral hepatitis has also been recognised for decades. Higginson (1963) noted that there were high prevalences of HCC, cirrhosis, viral hepatitis and malnutrition in Africa and Asia, including the tribal areas of South Africa, compared with a low prevalence of all of these factors in the USA, UK, Guatemala and urban portions of South Africa. The geographical association was confirmed when serological tests for HBV became available. For example, Szmuness (1978) observed that, in northern Europe and the USA (low-prevalence areas for HBV), HCC was found at autopsy in 0.2–1.6% of deaths from all causes, compared with 2.4–6.8% in Africa and Asia (high-prevalence areas for HBV). The highest rates of HCC were noted in those areas with a prevalence of HBsAg greater than 5% (Szmuness, 1978).

The first serological test for HBV was developed in 1964, and by 1970 Sherlock *et al* (1970) published the first report of an association between HBsAg in serum and HCC. This association was subsequently confirmed in countries throughout the world, a higher prevalence of HBsAg being detected as the assays became more sensitive. The application of sensitive assays for HBsAg and tests for anti-HBc permitted the detection of active HBV infection in more than 68% of HCC patients in Africa, compared with 12% in the general population (Tabor *et al*, 1977). Similar associations were found among Caucasian patients from the USA (Tabor *et al*, 1977) and Greece (Trichopoulos *et al*, 1978). Active HBV infection was detected in up to 47% of HCC patients in the USA, compared with few (Tabor *et al*, 1977; Yarrish *et al*, 1980) or none (Yarrish *et al*, 1980) among controls.

The development of HCC in prospectively followed populations and in families

New cases of HCC have been documented among prospectively followed asymptomatic HBsAg-positive individuals and in those with HBsAg-positive cirrhosis. In a classic study, Beasley *et al* (1981) prospectively followed 22 707 Chinese men in Taiwan for an average of 3.3 years each; the incidence of new cases of HCC was 1158 per 100 000 HBsAg-positive men, compared with an incidence of 5 per 100 000 HBsAg-negative men, a relative risk for the development of HCC among HBsAg carriers of 223. Testing of stored serial sera from three Eskimo and other Alaskan native HCC patients showed that HCC was diagnosed from 6 to 12 years after they became HBsAg-positive (Heyward *et al*, 1982; Lanier *et al*, 1987). In other studies, HCC developed up to 3 years (Nomura *et al*, 1982), up to 6 years (Kubo *et al*, 1978) and up to 14 years (Lanier *et al*, 1987) after the first HBsAg-positive samples in 34 patients in whom the time of onset of HBV infection was not documented.

Members of the same family who are infected with HBV may develop HCC. Although one cannot rule out other factors or co factors in such family clusters, the common factor among them is usually the presence of chronic HBV infection; all cases were HBsAg-positive when testing was done in several studies (Denison *et al*, 1971; Ohbayashi *et al*, 1972; Tepfer, 1972; Johnson *et al*, 1976; Sung and Chen, 1978; Gilmore *et al*, 1981; Lanier *et al*, 1987; Lok and Lai, 1988). Additional factors could be other viruses, non-infectious chemical carcinogens and genetic factors. However, if genetic factors are important, it appears that histocompatibility antigens do not play a role (Kew *et al*, 1979; Gilmore *et al*, 1981). In most reported cases, the family members were male; this is similar to the gender distribution of HCC in general. A familial inability to respond immunologically to HBV antigens may be a factor in the development of HCC and has been documented among HCC patients or their families in Africa and Asia (Larouzé *et al*, 1976; Sung and Chen, 1980; Ryder *et al*, 1985). However, the nature of the impairment and any role it has in carcinogenesis have not been identified.

The role of HBV infection in early life in the aetiology of HCC

The risk of developing HCC after HBV infection exists mainly for those whose HBV infection is acquired in early life. Cases of HCC in those whose chronic HBV infection begins in adulthood have only rarely been observed (Heyward *et al*, 1982; Norman *et al*, 1993). In areas of a high prevalence of HBV and HCC, much of the population becomes infected with HBV at birth or in early childhood. As many as 90% of HBV infections in the newborn period and early childhood have been shown to result in chronic infections, compared with about 10% for HBV infections acquired in adulthood. (Most chronic HBV infections continue for the duration of the patient's lifetime, the annual clearance rate being about 1%.) Consistent with these observations are the long intervals that elapse before the onset of HCC after the acquisition of chronic HBV infection, as discussed above. The long time period between the acquisition of HBV and the detection of HCC makes it difficult to identify precisely what other factors could contribute to the carcinogenesis, although long-term hepatic inflammation and/or cirrhosis remain important possible factors.

The presence of HBV DNA in HCC cells

HBV DNA has been identified by hybridisation techniques to be integrated in the HCC tumour DNA in all (Summers *et al*, 1978; Bréchot *et al*, 1981; Shafritz *et al*, 1981) or most (Koshy *et al*, 1981; Horiike *et al*, 1989) HCC patients with HBsAg in their serum, as well as in some HCC patients with only anti-HBc or anti-HBs in their serum (Bréchot *et al*, 1981, 1982; Shafritz *et al*, 1981). Two well-studied HCC cell lines producing HBsAg, PLC/PRF/5 and Hep3B, contain integrated HBV sequences. HBV DNA is also often detectable in the non-tumourous liver tissue from patients with HCC, with either the same or a different hybridisation pattern from that of the tumour cells (Bréchot *et al*, 1981; Shafritz *et al*, 1981) and may be integrated and/or extrachromosomal (Shafritz *et al*, 1981). The integration of HBV DNA into HCC and non-tumorous liver and its potential to interfere with the molecular processes of the hepatocyte provide a possible mechanism by which HBV could participate in hepatocarcinogenesis.

HCC patients with no HBV serum markers can be found to have HBV DNA integrated in the HCC tumour DNA (in 0–75% of cases) using hybridisation techniques (Bréchot *et al*, 1981, 1982, 1985; Hino *et al*, 1984; Cobden *et al*, 1986; Imazeki *et al*, 1986; Pontisso *et al*, 1987; Dunk *et al*, 1987; Walter *et al*, 1988; Horiike *et al*, 1989) and the polymerase chain reaction method (Paterlini *et al*, 1990). Those with no HBV serological markers who can be shown to have integrated HBV DNA in the DNA of their HCC must have had atypical HBV infections or an atypical immune response to the infection, because the absence of HBV serological markers would usually be sufficient to rule out a role for HBV.

Mechanisms of HBV-associated hepatocarcinogenesis

CIRRHOSIS

Cirrhosis is found in 80% or more of patients with HBV-associated HCC in many studies (Akagi *et al*, 1982; Tiribelli *et al*, 1989; Okuda *et al*, 1989), and its role in the aetiology of the HCC has been controversial. It is not known whether HBV causes HCC directly or whether HCC develops as a sequel to HBV-induced inflammation that also leads to cirrhosis. HCC developing in transgenic mice created with an HBV gene fragment (Dunsford *et al*, 1990) may provide a model for the latter process; it has been suggested that inflammation and regenerative hyperplasia in these mice in response to the HBV large envelope protein led to HCC. In a study of 180 HBsAg-positive patients with cirrhosis followed prospectively for up to 17 years, Ikeda *et al* (1993) reported that HCC developed in 7% of patients at 3 years, 14% at 5 years, 27% at 10 years and 27% at 15 years (but no increase occurring in HBsAg-positive cirrhosis after 8.5 years). In some studies, the average age at diagnosis of HCC is higher in patients with extensive cirrhosis than in those with moderate or no cirrhosis, suggesting a longer pre-clinical phase (Obata *et al*, 1980; Okuda *et al*, 1982); however, cirrhosis can be found even in children with HCC; for example, 95% of children under the age of 9 years with HCC in Taiwan were reported to have cirrhosis (all being HBsAg-positive) (Hsu *et al*, 1987).

MOLECULAR CHANGES AND THE 'MULTIPLE-HIT THEORY'

Multiple genetic changes occurring successively to a previously normal cell may be associated with the stages of 'initiation', 'promotion' and 'progression' of cancer. Within this theory, it is possible that HBV could provide 'initiation' of carcinogenesis because, in most cases of HBV-associated HCC, the HBV infection began either in utero, at birth or in early childhood (Tabor, 1991). Alternatively, the ongoing HBV infection could function as a regenerative stimulus to the liver (promotion) and/or a potential source of interference with normal host gene function (progression) over a period of many years. Within this 'multiple-hit' theory of carcinogenesis, it is possible that HBV could function as an initiator in some cases, a promoter in some cases and an agent of progression in others. It also has been suggested that HBV could function as both an initiator and a promoter in the same patient (Trichopoulos *et al*, 1987).

These genetic changes could occur in a variety of cellular genes that control growth, including oncogenes, growth factor genes and tumour suppressor genes. The changes probably occur in sequence, a conclusion based on the infrequency of genetic changes in general and the apparently long time between the HBV infection in early life and the appearance of HCC. It may be that the cumulative effect of the genetic changes is more important that the order in which they occur.

No common integration site of HBV within the HCC genome has been found (Zhou *et al*, 1987; Harrison *et al*, 1990), even though HBV integration in HCC can occur with up to 10 integrated copies of the HBV genome per HCC cell (at 10 different sites) (Tokino *et al*, 1987). In the absence of a consistent integration site, HBV could affect growth-controlling genes at distant sites by transactivation. HBV has at least two transactivating proteins that have been identified. The protein product of a truncated sequence of the pre-S2/S region of HBV has been shown to be capable of transactivating the c-myc promoter in vitro (Kekulé *et al*, 1990). The HBV X protein, which has been shown to be able to transactivate retroviral long terminal repeats, has been shown to be capable of increasing the rate of transcription of the oncogenes c-*fos* and c-*myc* by transactivation in vitro (Balsano *et al*, 1991). HBV X protein activates the transcription factor AP-1, which is a common pathway by which some growth factors and oncogenes function (Kekulé *et al*, 1992), so it is possible that this is a mechanism (or one of several mechanisms) by which HBV X protein could lead to carcinogenesis. The possible role of *X* gene transactivation in hepatocarcinogenesis is supported by reports that mice transgenic for the HBV *X* gene develop HCC in 90% of males (Kim *et al*, 1991) (although *X* gene transgenic mice in some other laboratories did not develop HCCs).

TUMOUR SUPPRESSOR GENE MUTATIONS

Mutations of the tumour suppressor gene *p53* are commonly found in human cancers, including HCC. The normal or wild-type *p53* gene plays an important role in the regulation of cell growth, as well as in inducing programmed cell death (apoptosis), including cell death after damage to its DNA.

p53 mutations, mostly at codon 249, have been found in 50% of HCCs in patients from some geographical regions in which aflatoxin contamination of the diet occurs at a high level, for example South Africa and parts of China (Bressac *et al*, 1991; Hsu *et al*, 1991) (Fig. 8.1). Mutations in HCCs at this codon have been ascribed to the high levels of aflatoxin contamination of food, since the type of mutation usually seen, G to T transversion, can be produced by experimental aflatoxin exposure in bacteria and rats. *p53* codon 249 mutations have been reported in the human hepatoblastoma cell line Hep G2 after treatment with aflatoxin B_1 (Aguilar *et al*, 1993). However, HCCs resulting from aflatoxin exposure in four non-human primates included only one HCC with a *p53* mutation, and that was a mutation at a site other than codon 249 (Fujimoto *et al*, 1992). *p53* mutations also are found in human HCCs from low-aflatoxin areas of the world (Hsia *et al*, 1992) (Fig. 8.2), but these include no (Murakami *et al*, 1991) or few (Oda *et al*, 1992; Sheu *et al*, 1992) mutations at codon 249. In general, there is a consensus that aflatoxin probably plays a role in codon 249 mutations of *p53* and the associated HCCs, although it is not possible at present to rule out other concomitant factors that could be responsible for the codon 249 mutations in HCC in high-aflatoxin areas.

Mutations of *p53* have been found more frequently in human cancers of advanced stages or grades than in early lesions, indicating that, in at least some cancers, mutations of *p53* are events that occur late in the course of carcinogenesis and may play a role in cancer progression (Tabor, 1994). This is also the pattern in HCC; *p53* mutations have been reported in 50% of poorly differentiated, 36% of moderately differentiated and no well-differentiated HCCs (Murakami *et al*, 1991; similar results reported by Nishida *et al*, 1993; Konishi *et al*, 1993; Teramoto *et al*, 1994). In patients with multifocal HCC, *p53* mutations were usually found in only one of the nodules (Oda *et al*, 1992), and *p53* mutations were not found among 18 HCCs less than 2 cm in diameter (Murakami *et al*, 1991). These observations support the hypothesis that *p53* mutations are a late occurrence.

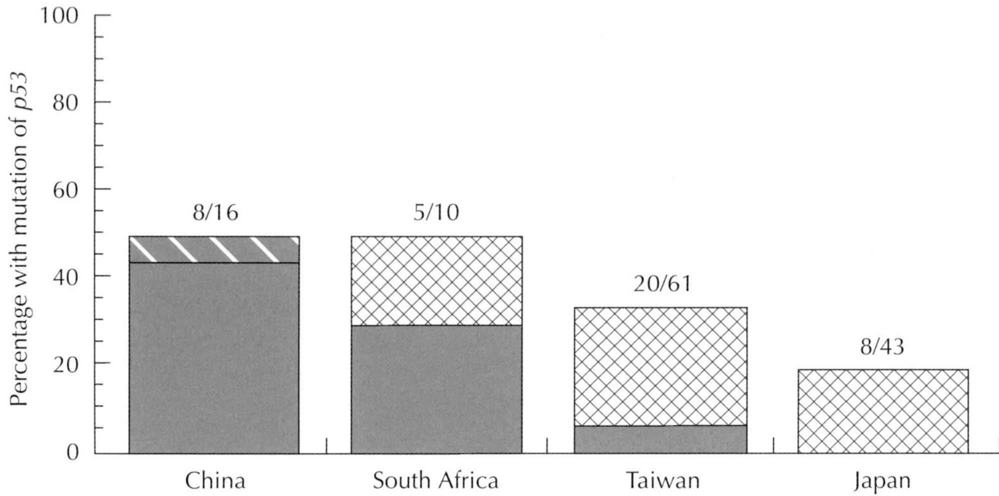

Fig 8.1 Percentage of patients with p53 mutations in hepatocellular carcinoma detected by sequencing or single-strand conformation polymorphism (SSCP). Patients are from four countries: China (Hsu *et al.*, 1991), South Africa (Bressac *et al.*, 1991), Taiwan (Sheu *et al.*, 1992) and Japan (Murakami *et al.*, 1991). ■, mutation at p53 codon 249 (G to T transversion); ▨, mutation at p53 codon 249 (a G to C transition, which results in the same amino acid change as a G to T transversion); ⊠, mutation at a p53 locus other than codon 249.

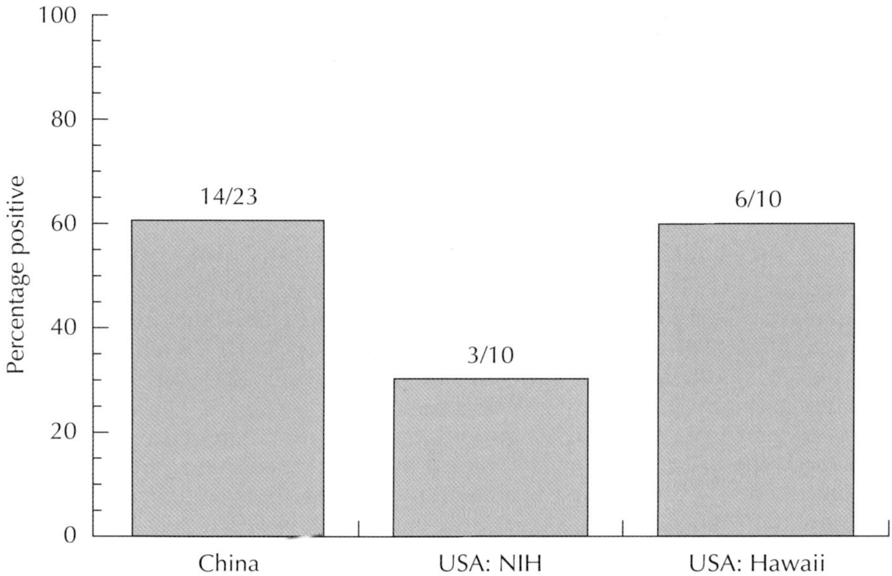

Fig 8.2 Detection of probable mutant p53 in hepatocellular carcinoma tissue by immunohisto-chemistry. Patients are from China and two geographical areas of the USA (Hsia *et al.*, 1992).

Even in the absence of a *p53* mutation, the functions of normal *p53* can be inactivated when p53 protein becomes bound by viral or other cellular proteins. For example, the transforming proteins (oncoproteins) of three DNA tumour viruses (SV40 T antigen, adenovirus E1B antigen and human papilloma virus E6 protein) can form stable complexes with wild-type p53 and either prevent its normal function (T antigen, E1B antigen) or induce its degradation (E6 protein). Similarly, the cellular protein mdm2 can bind to p53 and inactivate it. In certain other human tumours, the amplification of mdm2 and the mutation of *p53* appear to be mutually exclusive mechanisms of tumorigenesis. It is not yet known whether components of HBV can bind to p53 and inactivate it; several reports of such binding by HBV X protein in vitro have been published (Feitelson *et al*, 1993; Wang *et al*, 1994), but additional information will be needed before the significance of these findings can be established. It has been reported that HBV X protein blocks p53-mediated apoptosis, giving a selective advantage to those hepatocytes expressing viral genes (Wang *et al*, 1995).

Mutation or deletion of the *RB* tumour suppressor gene can also be found in some human HCCs. The identification of HCCs that have deletions or mutations of the *RB* gene as well as mutations of the *p53* gene suggests that these together could contribute to carcinogenesis. Loss of heterozygosity at the *RB* gene has been reported in six out of seven (86%) HCCs with a *p53* mutation compared to none out of 17 HCCs without a *p53* mutation (the overall prevalence of changes in both the *RB* and *p53* genes being six out of 24, i.e. 25%) (Murakami *et al*, 1991). All of the seven with abnormalities of *p53* (and of *RB* in six) were poorly or moderately differentiated HCCs. Others have also found a frequent concordance of *p53* and *RB* gene abnormalities in human HCC (Hsia *et al*, 1994) and in human HCC cell lines (Farshid *et al*, 1994). It is possible that *RB* and *p53* mutations occurring together may contribute to hepatocarcinogenesis in some patients.

It has also been demonstrated that reduced p21[WAF1/CIP1], a cyclin-dependent kinase inhibitor, is predominantly regulated by p53 and that reduced expression of this protein may play a role in the development of HCC (Hui *et al*, 1997).

THE ROLE OF TRANSFORMING GROWTH FACTOR ALPHA

Transforming growth factor alpha (TGF-α) is present at elevated levels in human hepatocellular carcinoma as well as in other cancers. TGF-α is an autocrine regulator of cell growth and regeneration. Transgenic mice created with a human or rat TGF-α gene develop HCC in up to 67% of males (Jhappan *et al*, 1990; Sandgren *et al*, 1990). Increased levels of TGF-α have been reported in the urine of HCC patients (Yeh *et al*, 1987).

TGF-α, which is undetectable in the normal human liver by immunohistochemistry, was detected in HCCs from 27 out of 33 (82%) patients from the USA and China, and in adjacent non-tumorous liver from 31 out of 33 patients (94%) (Hsia *et al*, 1992). The detection of TGF-α in those tissues was closely linked to HBV; it was found more frequently in patients with HBsAg in the adjacent non-tumorous liver, and staining of consecutively cut sections of tissue showed that, in the majority of patients, it was overexpressed in the same hepatocytes in which HBsAg was detected. In a related study, TGF-α expression was shown to be significantly upregulated by the presence of integrated HBV DNA in a hepatoblastoma cell line transfected with HBV compared with untransfected cells (Tabor *et al*, 1992).

·Liver regeneration associated with chronic HBV infection could be responsible for increased TGF-α expression. TGF-α expression has been shown to increase dramatically during liver regeneration after partial hepatectomy in rats (Mead and Fausto, 1989) and in association with liver regeneration in humans with chronic hepatitis (Castilla *et al*, 1991). The detection of both TGF-α and HBsAg in HCC patients in the same hepatocytes in non-tumorous liver tissue containing signs of regeneration and dysplasia (Hsia *et al*, 1992), suggests that their interaction in a regenerating liver could contribute to hepato-carcinogenesis. The overexpression of TGF-α (and/or other liver growth factor[s]), accompanied by the HBV-associated inactivation of one or more tumour suppressor gene functions, could provide a mechanism by which this could occur.

HCV and HCC

Despite the close association now known to exist between chronic HCV infection and HCC in some countries, theoretical mechanisms remain difficult to devise. It is possible that HCV infection functions as an 'initiator' of carcinogenesis. However, since HCV is not an integrating virus, the inflammation and cirrhosis caused by HCV may function as a 'promoter' in the development of HCC.

The strongest association between HCV and HCC noted to date has been found in Japan, where the incidence of HCC has doubled in the past 25 years and all of the increase has been due to HCV-associated cases (Nishioka *et al*, 1991; Okuda, 1991). Furthermore, in Japan, over 70% of HBV-negative HCC cases have anti-HCV compared with 1% of the general population in Japan (Tabor and Kobayashi, 1992) (Fig. 8.3). In the USA, 30–52% of HCC patients have anti-HCV in the absence of HBV serological markers (study by Tong, described in Tabor and Kobayashi, 1992; Di Bisceglie *et al*, 1994) (Fig. 8.4).

HCC patients with anti-HCV can usually be shown to have active HCV infections. Between 70% and 94% of HCC patients with anti-HCV have HCV RNA detectable by polymerase chain reaction in their sera (Tabor and Kobayashi, 1992; Park *et al*, 1993; Di Bisceglie *et al*, 1994). In studies of small numbers of HCC patients with anti-HCV, HCV RNA was detected in most cases in both HCC and non-tumorous liver, or only in the non-tumorous liver tissue (Yoneyama *et al*, 1990; Chou *et al*, 1991; Miyamura *et al*, 1991). HCV RNA also has been reported in serum from 66% of HBsAg-negative HCC patients who had no detectable anti-HCV (Park *et al*, 1993); if confirmed in larger studies, these observations indicate a role of HCV in the aetiology of even greater numbers of HCCs.

HCV is a non-integrating virus (Yoneyama *et al*, 1990; Tabor and Kobayashi, 1992), so its role in carcinogenesis must occur via different mechanisms from that of HBV or retroviruses. Seven well-documented cases have been reported in which chronic non-A, non-B hepatitis, which was most probably caused by HCV, had been prospectively followed and had progressed to HCC over periods of 2–18 years (reviewed in Tabor and Kobayashi, 1992). In a few cases, HCC appears to have been associated with HCV despite the apparent elimination of the virus in the long interval before the onset of HCC. Di Bisceglie *et al* (1994) reported the development of HCC in an anti-HCV-positive patient who had been treated with IFN-α, resulting in normal ALT levels for several years before the HCC was detected. In two other prospectively followed patients with chronic HCV infection, cirrhosis developed within 1 year and HCC was detected 5 and 9 years respectively after the onset of HCV infection (Di Bisceglie *et al*, 1994).

It is possible that cirrhosis could be the mechanism by which HCV contributes to HCC. Cirrhosis can usually be found in over 80% of anti-HCV-positive (HBsAg-negative)

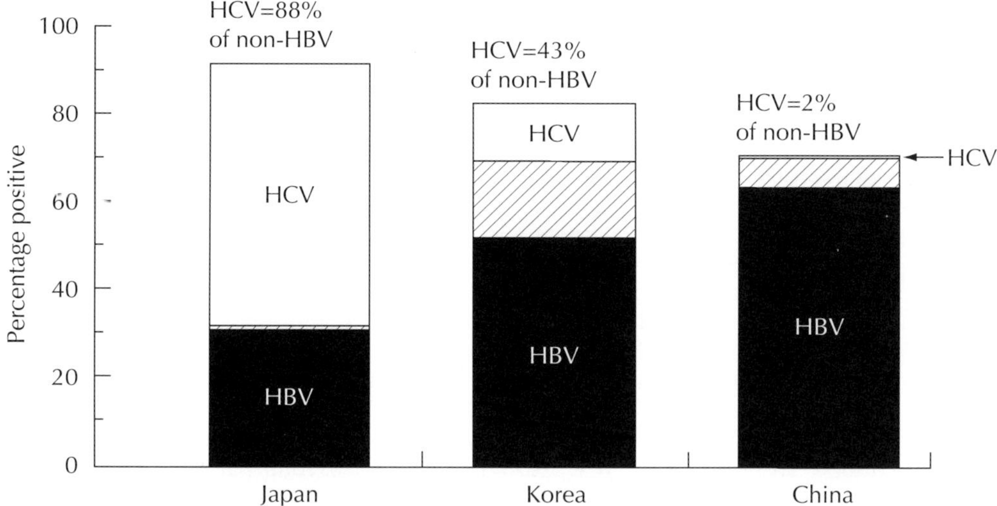

Fig 8.3   Percentage of hepatocellular carcinoma patients with serological evidence of infection with hepatitis B virus (HBV) (■), hepatitis C virus (HCV) (□) or both (▨). Patients are from Japan (Kiyosawa *et al.*, 1984), Korea (Lee *et al.*, 1992), and China (Okuno *et al.*, 1994).

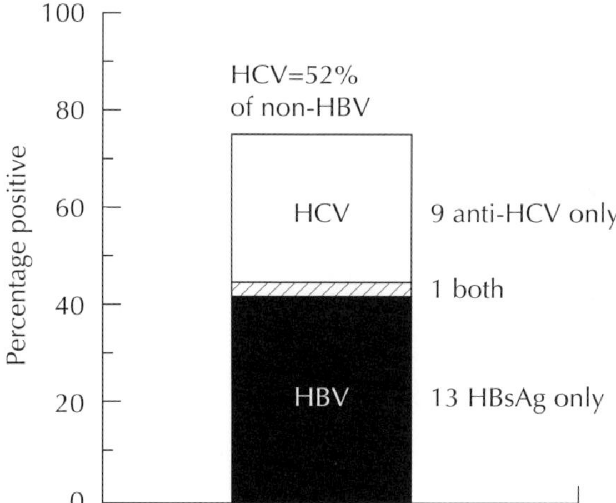

Fig 8.4   A study of 31 hepatocellular carcinoma patients in the USA (Di Bisceglie *et al.*, 1994), showing the percentage of patients with serological evidence of infection with hepatitis B virus (HBV) (■), hepatitis C virus (HCV) (□) or both (▨).

HCC patients, and it has been reported in 100% of such patients from two US populations (Hasan *et al*, 1990; Di Bisceglie *et al*, 1994). In a prospectively followed patient with chronic non-A, non-B hepatitis, presumably due to HCV, the progression to HCC was documented in five biopsies and an autopsy, progressing through a series of histological findings of unresolved viral hepatitis, chronic persistent hepatitis, chronic active hepatitis, to cirrhosis with HCC (Kiyosawa *et al*, 1984). In a study of 349 anti-HCV-positive (HBsAg-negative) cirrhosis patients followed prospectively for up to 17 years, Ikeda *et al* (1993) found that the cumulative HCC prevalence increased throughout the follow-up period. This was in contrast to those with HBsAg-positive cirrhosis, whose prevalence of HCC did not increase after 8.5 years. At 3 years, the prevalence of HCC was 10% among anti-HCV-positive patients with cirrhosis, at 5 years 21%, at 10 years 53% and at 15 years 75% (Ikeda *et al*, 1993).

One of the mysteries of the apparent association of HCV infection and HCC is the far higher incidence of HCV-associated HCC in Japan (greater than 22 per 100 000 male population, by calculation) than in the USA (less than 0.6 per 100 000 white male population, by calculation), whereas the prevalence of HCV is about 1% in the general population in both countries. Heterogeneity of HCV sequences has been suggested as a possible explanation, perhaps with different HCV strains in the two countries having different carcinogenic potential. HCV genotype 1b, which is more common in Japan than in the USA, has been found to be somewhat more common in Japanese patients with HCC (76% of isolates) than among Japanese blood donors infected with HCV (55%) (Ichimura *et al*, 1994), although this difference is not great enough to explain entirely the higher incidence of HCC in Japan. Substantial nucleotide sequence variations have been reported among HCV-infected HCC patients, including four patterns among eight patients (Yuwen *et al*, 1994), two patterns among five patients (Kato *et al*, 1990), five patterns among five patients (Honda *et al*, 1993), and four patterns among four patients (Chou *et al*, 1991). In a few cases, multiple HCV variants have been found within the liver of the same HCC patient (Kato *et al*, 1990).

ONCOGENES, TUMOUR SUPPRESSOR GENES AND HCV-ASSOCIATED HCC

Few studies have been conducted in HCV-associated HCC to analyse the condition of tumour suppressor genes and oncogenes. *p53* mutations were found within exons 5–10 in four out of 15 (27%) Japanese HCC patients with serological evidence of HCV but not HBV infection (recalculated from Konishi *et al*, 1993; the authors state that the prevalence was not significantly different from that of HBV-infected HCC patients in the same study, but it is difficult to evaluate based on the data in the report). In another study, 27 HCC patients with detectable HCV RNA in non-tumorous liver or HCC tissue (21 [78%] of whom had anti-HCV) were analysed for *p53* mutations in exons 4, 5, 7 and 8; either a mutation or loss of heterozygosity at *p53* was present in 12 out of 27 (44%) with HCV infection (two with HBV as well) (Teramoto *et al*, 1994). This was not significantly different from the prevalence they detected in HCC patients with HBV infection alone (five out of 10; 50%) or those with neither HCV nor HBV (one out of eight; 13%, not a significant difference). *p53* mutations are believed to occur late in the process of carcinogenesis in most human tumours, including HCC (Murakami *et al*, 1991). Since the early detection of HCC in Japan is superior to that in most other countries, late mutations in genes such as *p53* may be underrepresented in studies of HCC.

Co-infection with HBV and HCV in some HCC patients

Some geographical areas have high prevalences of chronic infections with both HBV and HCV. In such areas, some HCC patients are infected with both viruses. This has led to speculation that infection with both viruses could contribute to hepatocarcinogenesis.

The suggestion that HBV and HCV could function as additive risk factors for HCC in patients who are infected by both viruses is not a new idea; before the identification of either virus, the possibility of successive infection by two viruses, one in childhood and one later in life, was suggested (Higginson, 1963). In a recent symposium, it was reported that patients with cirrhosis developed HCC approximately twice as frequently (27% during a 3–5-year period) if they had chronic infection with both HBV and HCV compared with those with infection by either virus alone (15% with HBsAg alone and 10% with anti-IICV alone) (Benvegnu *et al*, described in Tabor, 1994). Other investigators have reported a relative risk for HCC of 20.0 for patients with HBsAg and anti-HCV compared with 11.0 for patients with HBsAg alone and 6.3 for those with anti-HCV alone (Kaklamani *et al*, 1991). The presence of both HBsAg and anti-HCV in serum has been reported in 14 HCC patients from Japan (Tabor and Kobayashi, 1992) and several members of two families in the USA (Tong, described in Tabor and Kobayashi, 1992). In a study of HCC patients from Zambia and Uganda, six out of eight with HCV RNA in their serum also had HBsAg in their serum (Yuwen *et al*, 1994), although most HCC patients in those two countries have HBsAg in their serum.

The possible role of alcohol and alcoholic cirrhosis in HCC

The excessive use of alcoholic beverages causing cirrhosis can lead to HCC, with an increased risk found in most studies to be associated with drinking more than 60 g of alcohol (about five drinks) per day (Austin, 1991). In a review of studies of alcohol as a possible cause of HCC, the summary relative risk was 2.1 for HCC, the relative risk ranging up to eight in studies conducted in the USA, Japan, Finland and elsewhere (Austin, 1991). The role of alcohol may vary by country; micronodular (alcoholic) cirrhosis has been reported to be common in patients with HCC studied at autopsy in Japan and Italy (Tiribelli *et al*, 1989). Most investigators feel that some HCCs have an alcoholic aetiology, although the presence of cirrhosis in most cases makes it difficult to rule out cirrhosis as the common denominator of viral and alcoholic cases. It has been estimated that no more than 15% of HCCs in the USA result from the excessive use of alcohol (Austin, 1991). Di Bisceglie *et al* (1994) found a history of excessive alcohol use in only five out of 17 (29%) HBsAg-negative HCC patients in the USA. However, the incidence of liver cancer (cancer registries cite 'liver cancer' rather than separating 'HCC' from other liver cancers) in a country such as France (4–6 per 100 000 male population), where the use of alcohol is proverbially high and begins at an early age, is essentially the same as that in European countries where it is generally thought that less alcohol is consumed, for example Switzerland (4–10 per 100 000 male population) (Bosch and Muñoz, 1991).

There is no evidence based on a review of multiple studies of alcohol and HCC (Austin, 1991), that alcohol or alcoholic cirrhosis and HBV interact leading to HCC. Ikeda *et al* (1993), in a prospective study of 262 HBsAg-positive patients with cirrhosis, found that alcohol consumption resulted in no increased risk of developing HCC.

There have been conflicting studies evaluating whether HCV interacts with alcoholic cirrhosis in the aetiology of HCC. In a study of 202 HCC patients in Japan, there was no significant difference in the prevalence of anti-HCV among those whose alcohol use was 'very high' (62% anti-HCV), 'high' (59%) or 'low or none' (69%) (Miyamura *et al*, 1991). In a prospective study of 364 anti-HCV-positive patients with cirrhosis (349 of whom were HBsAg-negative), excessive alcohol intake was significantly associated with an increased likelihood of developing HCC (Ikeda *et al*, 1993). In a retrospective study of 133 cirrhosis patients in Japan, the risk from alcohol use and anti-HCV in the presence of cirrhosis appeared to be somewhat additive (81% of anti-HCV-positive patients with alcoholic cirrhosis had developed HCC compared with 56% of those without alcoholic cirrhosis) (Yamauchi *et al*, 1993), although anti-HCV was the only significant risk factor for HCC.

Summary

HCC is closely associated with infection by either of two viruses: HBV or HCV. HBV DNA can be shown to be integrated into the HCC genome of most HCC patients with serological evidence of HBV infection. In most such patients, chronic HBV infection began at or shortly after birth; HBV integration occurs at some point in time, and HCC develops many years thereafter. Over 80% of these patients have cirrhosis in the adjacent non-tumourous liver, and this may contribute to hepatocarcinogenesis in many of these patients. Molecular mechanisms of carcinogenesis may explain the role of HBV in these patients. The tumour suppressor gene *p53* has been found to be mutated in up to 60% of HCCs; many of these HCCs also have mutations of the *RB* tumour suppressor gene. These mutations may act in conjunction with mutations or overexpression of oncogenes and overexpression of hepatic growth factors such as TGF-α, ultimately leading to HCC. Several HBV proteins are capable of transactivating oncogenes, a process that could interfere with cellular control of growth. Mechanisms by which HCV leads to HCC are more obscure at present. However, there is a clear association between HCV and HCC; in Japan, HCV-associated cases have been responsible for a doubling of the incidence of HCC in the past 25 years. Cirrhosis is found in 80% of HCV-associated HCC cases, and preliminary reports indicate that up to 44% of cases have *p53* mutations. A relatively small number of HCC cases may result from the combination of alcohol use and HCV (but not HBV) infection or of co-infection with HBV and HCV, although these observations are preliminary.

References

Aguilar, F., Hussain, S.P., Cerutti, P. 1993: Aflatoxin B$_1$ induces the transversion of G-T in codon 249 of the p53 tumor suppressor gene in human hepatocytes. *Proceedings of the National Academy of Sciences of the USA* **90**, 8586–90.

Akagi, G., Furuya, K., Otsuka, H. 1982: Hepatitis B antigen in the liver in hepatocellular carcinoma in Shikoku, Japan. *Cancer* **49**, 678–82.

Austin, H. 1991: The role of tobacco use and alcohol consumption in the etiology of hepatocellular carcinoma. In Tabor, E., Di Bisceglie, A.M., Purcell, R.H. (eds) *Etiology, pathology, and treatment of hepatocellular carcinoma in North America*. The Woodlands, TX: Portfolio, 57–75.

Balsano, C., Avantaggiati, M.L., Natoli, G. *et al*. 1991: Transactivation of c-*fos* and c-*myc* protooncogenes by both full-length and truncated versions of the HBV-X protein. In Hollinger, F.B., Lemon, S.M., Margolis, H. (eds) *Viral hepatitis and liver disease*. Baltimore: Williams & Wilkins, 572–6.

Beasley, R.P., Hwang, L.Y., Lin, C.C., Chien, C.S. 1981: Hepatocellular carcinoma and hepatitis B virus: a prospective study of 22 707 men in Taiwan. *Lancet* **ii**, 1129–33.

Bosch, F.X., Muñoz, N. 1991: Hepatocellular carcinoma in the world: epidemiologic questions. In Tabor, E., Di Bisceglie, A.M., Purcell, R.H. (eds) *Etiology, pathology, and treatment of hepatocellular carcinoma in North America*. The Woodlands, TX: Portfolio, 35–54.

Bréchot, C., Hadchouel, M., Scotto, J. *et al*, 1981: State of hepatitis B virus DNA in hepatocytes of patients with hepatitis B surface antigen-positive and -negative liver diseases. *Proceedings of the National Academy of Sciences of the USA* **78**, 3906–10.

Bréchot, C., Nalpas, B., Couroucé, A. *et al*. 1982: Evidence that hepatitis B virus has a role in liver-cell carcinoma in alcoholic liver disease. *New England Journal of Medicine* **306**, 1384–7.

Bréchot, C., Degos, F., Lugassy, C. *et al*, 1985: Hepatitis B virus DNA in patients with chronic liver disease and negative tests for hepatitis B surface antigen. *New England Journal of Medicine* **312**, 270–6.

Bressac, B., Kew, M., Wands, J., Ozturk, M. 1991: Selective G to T mutations of *p53* gene in hepatocellular carcinoma from southern Africa. *Nature* **350**, 429–31.

Castilla, A., Prieto, J., Fausto, N. 1991: Transforming growth factors β_1 and α in chronic liver disease: effects of interferon alpha therapy. *New England Journal of Medicine* **324**, 933–40.

Chou, W.-H., Yoneyama, T., Takeuchi, K., Harada, H., Saito, I., Miyamura, T. 1991: Discrimination of hepatitis C virus in liver tissues from different patients with hepatocellular carcinomas by direct nucleotide sequencing of amplified cDNA of the viral genome. *Journal of Clinical Microbiology* **29**, 2860–4.

Cobden, I., Bassendine, M.F., James, O.F.W. 1986: Hepatocellular carcinoma in northeast England: importance of hepatitis B infection and ex-tropical military service. *Quarterly Journal of Medicine* **60**, 855–63.

Denison, E.K., Peters, R.L., Reynolds, T.B. 1971: Familial hepatoma with hepatitis-associated antigen. *Annals of Internal Medicine* **74**, 391–4.

Di Bisceglie, A.M., Simpson, L.H., Lotze, M.T., Hoofnagle, J.H. 1994: Development of hepatocellular carcinoma among patients with chronic liver disease due to hepatitis C viral infection. *Journal of Clinical Gastroenterology* **19**, 222–6.

Dunk, A.A., Spiliadis, H., Sherlock, S. *et al*. 1987: Hepatocellular carcinoma and the hepatitis B virus: a study of British patients. *Quarterly Journal of Medicine* **62**, 109–16.

Dunsford, H.A., Sell, S., Chisari, F.V. 1990: Hepatocarcinogenesis due to chronic liver cell injury in hepatitis B virus transgenic mice. *Cancer Research* **50**, 3400–7.

Farshid, M., Hsia, C.C., Tabor, E. 1994: Alterations of the RB tumour suppressor gene in hepatocellular carcinoma and hepatoblastoma cell lines in association with abnormal p53 expression. *Viral Hepatitis* **1**, 45–53.

Feitelson, M.A., Zhu, M., Duan, L.-X, London, W.T. 1993: Hepatitis B x antigen and p53 are associated *in vitro* and in liver tissues from patients with primary hepatocellular carcinoma. *Oncogene* **8**, 1109–17.

Fujimoto, Y., Hampton, L.L., Luo, L., Wirth, P.J., Thorgeirsson, S.S. 1992: Low frequency of *p53* gene mutation in tumors induced by aflatoxin B_1 in nonhuman primates. *Cancer Research* **52**, 1044–6.

Gilmore, I.T., Harrison, J.M., Parkins, R.A. 1981: Clustering of hepatitis B virus infection and hepatocellular carcinoma in a family. *Journal of the Royal Society of Medicine* **74**, 843–5.

Harrison, T.J., Lin, Y., Stamps, A.C., Dusheiko, G.M., Zuckerman, A.J. 1990: Hepatitis B virus-associated hepatocellular carcinoma in African patients. *Cancer Detection and Prevention* **14**, 457–60.

Hasan, F., Jeffers, L.J., De Medina, M. *et al*. 1990: Hepatitis C-associated hepatocellular carcinoma. *Hepatology* **12**, 589–91.

Heyward, W.L., Bender, T.R., Lanier, A.P., Francis, D.P., McMahon, B.J., Maynard, J.E. 1982: Serological markers of hepatitis B virus and alpha-fetoprotein levels preceding primary hepatocellular carcinoma in Alaskan Eskimos. *Lancet* **ii**, 889–91.

Higginson, J. 1963: The geographical pathology of primary liver cancer. *Cancer Research* **23**, 1624–33.

Hino, O., Kitagawa, T., Koike, K. *et al*. 1984: Detection of hepatitis B virus DNA in hepatocellular carcinoma in Japan. *Hepatology* **4**, 90–5.

Honda, M., Kaneko, S., Unoura, M., Kobayashi, K., Murakami, S. 1993: Sequence analysis of putative structural regions of hepatitis C virus isolated from 5 Japanese patients with hepatocellular carcinoma. *Archives of Virology* **128**, 163–9.

Horiike, N., Michitaka, K., Onji, M., Murota, T., Ohta, Y. 1989: HBV-DNA hybridization in hepatocellular carcinoma associated with alcohol in Japan. *Journal of Medical Virology* **28**, 189–92.

Hsia, C.C., Kleiner, D.E., Axiotis, C.A. *et al.* 1992: Detection of *p53* mutations by immunohistochemistry in hepatocellular carcinoma: association with hepatitis B virus in patients from high- and low-aflatoxin regions. *Journal of the National Cancer Institute* **84**, 1638–41.

Hsia, C.C., Di Bisceglie, A.M., Kleiner, D.E., Farshid, M., Tabor, E. 1994: RB tumor suppressor gene expression in hepatocellular carcinomas from patients infected with the hepatitis B virus. *Journal of Medical Virology* **44**, 67–73.

Hsu, H., Wu, M.-Z., Chang, M.-H., Su, I.-J., Chenn, D.-S. 1987: Childhood hepatocellular carcinoma develops exclusively in hepatitis B surface antigen carriers in three decades in Taiwan: report of 51 cases strongly associated with rapid development of liver cirrhosis. *Journal of Hepatology* **5**, 260–7.

Hsu, I.C., Metcalf, R.A.,, Sun, T., Welsh, J.A., Wang, N.J., Harris, C.C. 1991: Mutational hotspot in the *p53* gene in human hepatocellular carcinomas. *Nature* **350**, 427–8.

Hui, A.-M., Kanai, Y., Sakamoto, M., Tsuda, H., Hirohashi, S. 1997: Reduced p21[WAF1/CIP1] expression and p53 mutation in hepatocellular carcinomas. *Hepatology* **25**, 575–9.

Ichimura, H., Tamura, I., Kurimura, O. *et al.* 1994: Hepatitis C virus genotypes, reactivity to recombinant immunoblot assay 2 antigens and liver disease. *Journal of Medical Virology* **43**, 212–15.

Ikeda, K., Saitoh, S., Koida, I. *et al.* 1993: A multivariate analysis of risk factors for hepatocellular carcinogenesis: a prospective observation of 795 patients with viral and alcoholic cirrhosis. *Hepatology* **18**, 47–53.

Imazeki, F., Omata, M., Yokosuka, O., Okuda, K. 1986: Integration of hepatitis B virus DNA in hepatocellular carcinoma. *Cancer* **58**, 1055–60.

Jhappan, C., Stahle, C., Harkins, R.N., Fausto, N., Smith, G.H., Merlino, G.T. 1990: TGFα overexpression in transgenic mice induces liver neoplasia and abnormal development of the mammary gland and pancreas. *Cell* **61**, 1137–46.

Johnson, P., Wansbrough-Jones, M., Eddleston, A.L.W.F., Williams, R., Calne, R.Y., Maycock, W.d'A. 1976: Familial occurrence of HBsAg-positive hepatoma: treatment by orthotopic liver transplantation and specific immunoglobulin. *Digestion* **14**, 524 (abstract).

Kaklamani, E., Trichopoulos, D., Tzonou, A. *et al.* 1991: Hepatitis B and C viruses and their interaction in the origin of hepatocellular carcinoma. *Journal of the American Medical Association* **265**, 1974–6.

Kato, N., Hijikata, M., Ootsuyama, Y., Nakagawa, M., Ohkoshi, S., Shimotohno, K. 1990: Sequence diversity of hepatitis C viral genomes. *Molecular Biology and Medicine* **7**, 495–501.

Kekulé, A.S., Lauer, U., Meyer, M., Caselmann, W.H., Hofschneider, P.H., Koshy, R. 1990: The *preS2/S* region of integrated hepatitis B virus DNA encodes a transcriptional transactivator. *Nature* **343**, 457–61.

Kekulé, A.S., Lauer, U., Weiss, L., Hofschneider, P.H., Koshy, R. 1992: *Trans*-activation by hepatitis B virus X protein is mediated via a tumour promoter pathway. *Archives of Virology* (supplement) **4**, 63–4.

Kew, M.C., Gear, A.J., Baumgarten, I., Dusheiko, G.M., Maier, G. 1979: Histocompatibility antigens in patients with hepatocellular carcinoma and their relationship to chronic hepatitis B virus infection in these patients. *Gastroenterology* **77**, 537–9.

Kim, C., Koike, K., Saito, I., Miyamura, T., Jay, G. 1991: HBx gene of hepatitis B virus induces liver cancer in transgenic mice. *Nature* **351**, 317–20.

Kiyosawa, K., Akahane, Y., Nagata, A., Furuta, S. 1984: Hepatocellular carcinoma after non-A, non-B posttransfusion hepatitis. *American Journal of Gastroenterology* **79**, 777–81.

Konishi, M., Kikuchi-Yanochita, R., Tanaka, K. *et al.* 1993: Genetic changes and histopathological grades in human hepatocellular carcinomas. *Japanese Journal of Cancer Research* **84**, 893–9.

Koshy, R., Maupas, P., Müller, R., Hofschneider, P.H. 1981: Detection of hepatitis B virus-specific DNA in the genomes of human hepatocellular carcinoma and liver cirrhosis tissues. *Journal of General Virology* **57**, 95–102.

Kubo, Y., Okuda, K., Musha, H., Nakashima, T. 1978: Detection of hepatocellular carcinoma during a clinical follow-up of chronic liver disease: observations in 31 patients. *Gastroenterology* **74**, 578–82.

Lanier, A.P., McMahon, B.J., Alberts, S.R., Popper, H., Heyward, W.L. 1987: Primary liver cancer in Alaskan natives 1980–1985. *Cancer* **60**, 1915–20.

Larouzé, B., London, W.T., Saimot, G. *et al.* 1976: Host responses to hepatitis-B infection in patients with primary hepatic carcinoma and their families: a case/control study in Senegal, West Africa. *Lancet* **ii**, 534–8.

Lee, H.-S., Yoon, J.H., Kim, W., Kim, C.Y. 1992: Relative role of hepatitis B virus and hepatitis C virus in HBsAg-negative patients with chronic liver disease in Korea: determination of serum HBV DNA using polymerase chain reaction and of serum anti-HCV using ELISA. *Korean Journal of Internal Medicine* **42**, 8–15.

Lok, A.S.F., Lai, C.-L. 1988: Factors determining the development of hepatocellular carcinoma in hepatitis B surface antigen carriers: a comparison between families with clusters and solitary cases. *Cancer* **61**, 1287–91.

Mead, J.E., Fausto, N. 1989: Transforming growth factor-α may be a physiological regulator of liver regeneration by means of an autocrine mechanism. *Proceedings of the National Academy of Sciences of the USA* **86**, 1558–62.

Miyamura, T., Saito, I., Yoneyama, T. *et al.* 1991: Role of hepatitis C virus in hepatocellular carcinoma. In Hollinger, F.B., Lemon, S.M., Margolis, H. (eds) *Viral hepatitis and liver disease* Baltimore: Williams & Wilkins, 559–62.

Murakami, Y., Hayashi, K., Hirohashi, S., Sekiya, T. 1991: Aberrations of the tumor suppressor *p53* and retinoblastoma genes in human hepatocellular carcinoma. *Cancer Research* **51**, 5520–5.

Nishida, N., Fukuda, Y., Kokuryu, H. *et al.* 1993: Role and mutational heterogeneity of the *p53* gene in hepatocellular carcinoma. *Cancer Research* **53**, 368–72.

Nishioka, K., Watanabe, J., Furuta, S. *et al.* 1991: A high prevalence of antibody to the hepatitis C virus in patients with hepatocellular carcinoma in Japan. *Cancer* **67**, 429–33.

Nomura, A., Stemmermann, G.N., Wasnich, R.D. 1982: Presence of hepatitis B surface antigen before primary hepatocellular carcinoma. *Journal of the American Medical Association* **247**, 2247–9.

Norman, J.E., Beebe, G.W., Hoofnagle, J.H., Seeff, L.B. 1993: Mortality follow-up of the 1942 epidemic of hepatitis B in the U.S. Army. *Hepatology* **18**, 790–7.

Obata, H., Hayashi, N., Motoike, Y. *et al.* 1980: A prospective study on the development of hepatocellular carcinoma from liver cirrhosis with persistent hepatitis B virus infection. *International Journal of Cancer* **25**, 741–7.

Oda, T., Tsuda, H., Scarpa, A., Sakamoto, M., Hirohashi, S. 1992: Mutation pattern of the *p53* gene as a diagnostic marker for multiple hepatocellular carcinoma. *Cancer Research* **52**, 3674–8.

Ohbayashi, A., Okochi, K., Mayumi, M. 1972: Familial clustering of asymptomatic carriers of Australia antigen and patients with chronic liver disease or primary liver cancer. *Gastroenterology* **62**, 618–25.

Okuda, K. 1991: Hepatitis C virus and hepatocellular carcinoma. In Tabor, E., Di Bisceglie, A.M., Purcell, R.H. (eds) *Etiology, pathology, and treatment of hepatocellular carcinoma in North America*. The Woodlands, TX: Portfolio, 119–26.

Okuda, K., Nakashima, T., Sakamoto, K. *et al.* 1982: Hepatocellular carcinoma arising in noncirrhotic and highly cirrhotic livers: a comparative study of histopathology and frequency of hepatitis B markers. *Cancer* **49**, 450–5.

Okuda, K., Nakashima, T., Kojiro, M., Kondo, Y., Wada, K. 1989: Hepatocellular carcinoma without cirrhosis in Japanese patients. *Gastroenterology* **97**, 140–6.

Okuno, H., Xie, Z.-C., Lu, B.-Y. *et al.* 1994: A low prevalence of anti-hepatitis C virus antibody in patients with hepatocellular carcinoma in Guangxi Province, southern China. *Cancer* **73**, 58–62.

Park, Y.M., Yoon, S.K., Chung, K.W., Kim, B.S. 1993: Detection of HCV RNA using reverse transcription and nested polymerase chain reaction in chronic non-A, non-B liver diseases in Korea. *Gastroenterologica Japonica* **28**(supplement 5), 12–16.

Paterlini, P., Gerken, G., Nakajima, E. *et al.* 1990: Polymerase chain reaction to detect hepatitis B virus DNA and RNA sequences in primary liver cancers from patients negative for hepatitis B surface antigen. *New England Journal of Medicine* **323**, 80–5.

Pontisso, P., Stenico, D., Diodati, G. *et al.* 1987: HBV-DNA sequences are rarely detected in the liver of patients with HBsAg-negative chronic active liver disease and with hepatocellular carcinoma in Italy. *Liver* **7**, 211–15.

Ryder, R.W., Whittle, H.C., Ajdukiewicz, A.B., Tulloch, S., Yvonnet, B. 1985: Response of children of patients with primary hepatocellular carcinoma to hepatitis B virus vaccine. *Journal of Infectious Diseases* **151**, 187–91.

Sandgren, E.P., Luetteke, N.C., Palmiter, R.D., Brinster, R.L., Lee, D.C. 1990: Overexpression of TGFα in transgenic mice: induction of epithelial hyperplasia, pancreatic metaplasia, and carcinoma of the breast. *Cell* **61**, 1121–5.

Shafritz, D.A., Shouval, D., Sherman, H.I., Hadziyannis, S.J., Kew, M.C. 1981: Integration of hepatitis B virus DNA into the genome of liver cells in chronic liver disease and hepatocellular carcinoma: studies in percutaneous liver biopsies and post-mortem tissue specimens. *New England Journal of Medicine* **305**, 1067–73.

Sherlock, S., Fox, R.A., Niazi, S.P., Scheuer, P.J. 1970: Chronic liver disease and primary liver-cell cancer with hepatitis-associated (Australia) antigen in serum. *Lancet* **i**, 1243–7.

Sheu, J., Huang, G., Lee, P. *et al.* 1992: Mutation of *p53* gene in hepatocellular carcinoma in Taiwan. *Cancer Research* **52**, 6098–100.

Summers, J., O'Connell, A., Maupas, P., Goudeau, A., Coursaget, P., Drucker, J. 1978: Hepatitis B virus DNA in primary hepatocellular carcinoma tissue. *Journal of Medical Virology* **2**, 207–14.

Sung, J.-L, Chen, D.-S. 1978: Clustering of different subtypes of hepatitis B surface antigen in families of patients with chronic liver diseases. *American Journal of Gastroenterology* **69**, 559–64.

Sung, J., Chen, D. 1980: Maternal transmission of hepatitis B surface antigen in patients with hepatocellular carcinoma in Taiwan. *Scandinavian Journal of Gastroenterology* **15**, 321–4.

Szmuness, W. 1978: Hepatocellular carcinoma and the hepatitis B virus. Evidence for a causal association. *Progress in Medical Virology* **24**, 40–69.

Tabor, E. 1991: Strongly supported features of the association between hepatitis B virus and hepatocellular carcinoma. In Tabor, E., Di Bisceglie, A.M., Purcell, R.H. (eds) *Etiology, pathology, and treatment of hepatocellular carcinoma in North America.* The Woodlands, TX: Portfolio, 107–17.

Tabor, E. 1994: Tumor suppressor genes, growth factor genes, and oncogenes in hepatitis B virus-associated hepatocellular carcinoma. *Journal of Medical Virology* **42**, 357–65.

Tabor, E., Kobayashi, K. 1992: Commentary: Hepatitis C virus, a causative infectious agent of non-A, non-B hepatitis: prevalence and structure. Summary of a conference on hepatitis C virus as a cause of hepatocellular carcinoma. *Journal of the National Cancer Institute* **84**, 86–90.

Tabor, E., Gerety, R.J., Vogel, C.L. *et al.* 1977: Hepatitis B virus infection and primary hepatocellular carcinoma. *Journal of the National Cancer Institute* **58**, 1197–200.

Tabor, E., Farshid, M., Di Bisceglie, A., Hsia, C.C. 1992: Increased expression of transforming growth factor α after transfection of a human hepatoblastoma cell line with the hepatitis B virus *Journal of Medical Virology* **37**, 271–3.

Tepfer, B.D. 1972: Hepatoma and HAA. *Annals of Internal Medicine* **76**, 145–6 (letter).

Teramoto, T., Satonaka, K., Kitazawa, S., Fujimori, T., Hayashi, K., Maeda, S. 1994: *p53* gene abnormalities are closely related to hepatoviral infections and occur at a late stage of hepatocarcinogenesis. *Cancer Research* **54**, 231–5.

Tiribelli, C., Melato, M., Crocé, L.S., Giarelli, L., Okuda, K., Ohnishi, K. 1989: Prevalence of hepatocellular carcinoma and relation to cirrhosis: comparison of two different cities of the world – Trieste, Italy, and Chiba, Japan. *Hepatology* **10**, 998–1002.

Tokino, T., Fukushige, S., Nakamura, T. *et al.* 1987: Chromosomal translocation and inverted duplication associated with integrated hepatitis B virus in hepatocellular carcinoma. *Journal of Virology* **61**, 3848–54.

Trichopoulos, D., Tabor, E., Gerety, R.J. *et al.* 1978: Hepatitis B and primary hepatocellular carcinoma in a European population. *Lancet* **ii**, 1217–19.

Trichopoulos, D., Day, N.E., Kaklamani, E. *et al.* 1987: Hepatitis B virus, tobacco smoking and ethanol consumption in the etiology of hepatocellular carcinoma. *International Journal of Cancer* **39**, 45–9.

Walter, E., Blum, H.E., Meier, P. *et al.* 1988: Hepatocellular carcinoma in alcoholic liver disease: no evidence for a pathogenetic role of hepatitis B virus infection. *Hepatology* **8**, 745–8.

Wang, X.W., Forrester, K., Yeh, H. *et al.* 1994: Interaction with hepatitis B virus X protein inhibits p53 transcriptional activity and p53 association with ERCC3. *Proceedings of the American Association for Cancer Research* **35**, 585 (abstract).

Wang, X.W., Gibson, M.K., Vermeulen, W. *et al.* 1995: Abrogation of p53-induced apoptosis by the hepatitis B virus X gene. *Cancer Research* **55**, 6012–16.

Yamauchi, M., Nakahara, M., Maezawa, Y. *et al.* 1993: Prevalence of hepatocellular carcinoma in patients with alcoholic cirrhosis and prior exposure to hepatitis C. *American Journal of Gastroenterology* **88**, 39–43.

Yarrish, R.L., Werner, B.G., Blumberg, B.S. 1980: Association of hepatitis B virus infection with hepatocellular carcinoma in American patients. *International Journal of Cancer* **26**, 711–15.

Yeh, Y.C., Tsai, J.F., Chuang, L.Y. *et al.* 1987: Elevation of transforming growth factor α and its relationship to the epidermal growth factor and α-fetoprotein levels in patients with hepatocellular carcinoma. *Cancer Research* **47**, 896–901.

Yoneyama, T., Takeuchi, K., Watanabe, Y. *et al.* 1990: Detection of hepatitis C virus cDNA sequence by the polymerase chain reaction in hepatocellular carcinoma tissues. *Japanese Journal of Medical Science and Biology* **43**, 89–94.

Yuwen, H., Bayley, A.C., Cairns, J., Tabor, E. 1994: Hepatocellular carcinoma: lack of association with a unique hepatitis C virus nucleotide sequence. *Journal of Infectious Diseases* **169**, 706–7 (letter).

Zhou, Y., Butel, J.S., Li, P., Finegold, M.J., Melnick, J.L. 1987: Integrated state of subgenomic fragments of hepatitis B virus DNA in hepatocellular carcinoma from mainland China. *Journal of the National Cancer Institute* **79**, 223–31.

Index